SPIRITUAL Effects of Live Food

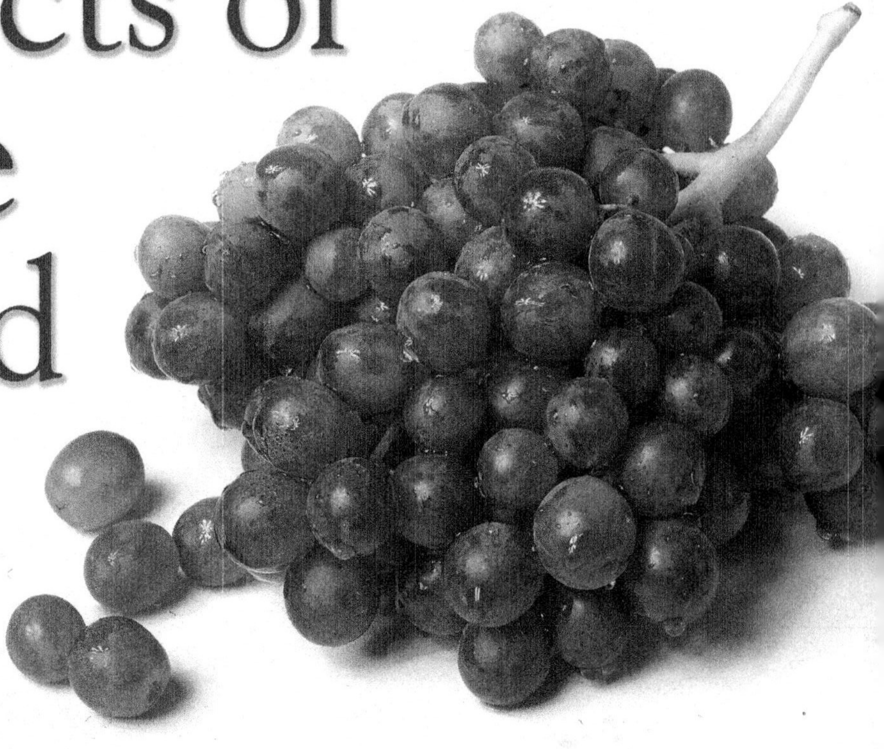

Diet for a New Age

Spiritual Effects of Live Food

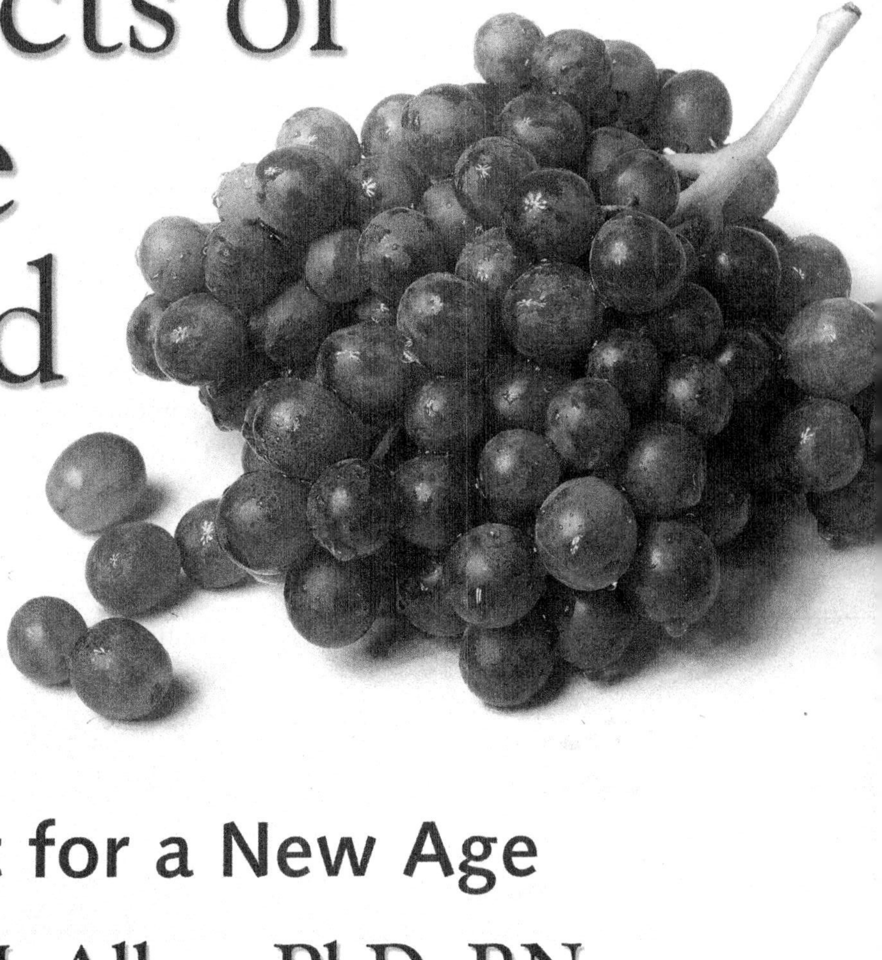

Diet for a New Age

Janet J. Allen, PhD, RN

EWH Press

MICHIGAN, 2014

Published by EWH Press
PO Box 537
Leslie, MI 49251
www.ewhpress.com

ISBN 978-0-9834438-8-9
EWH Press first printing, February 2015

Cover and book design by Terrie MacNicol
Cover photo by Miriam Garcia
Edited by Jeff Stoner

Printed in the United States of America

Dedication

This book is dedicated to promoting a peaceful world
where everyone wins and thrives.

Acknowledgments

Special thanks to Carol Parrish-Harra, Ann Wigmore, Victoria Boutenko, Mark Gillen, Betty Carper, Karen Petersmarck, Creative Health Institute, Sancta Sophia Seminary, Institute for Bioenergy Studies, members of MidMichigan Writers, and the hosts of unseen helpers.

Disclaimer

This material is for information and educational purposes only and is not intended as medical, psychological, or spiritual advice. The author and publisher accept no responsibility for any consequences, adverse or wonderful, resulting from adopting the lifestyle herein described. Anyone who suspects a problem is urged to seek individual professional advice, and then make decisions based upon their own intuition. This is not a peer-reviewed scientific paper; it offers yet another perspective on wellness and the cause of dis-ease. The opinions and beliefs expressed here are those of the author backed with information from other writers so the reader may continue her own search for truth.

How Clarity of Mind is Influenced by Diet

I would not interfere with any creed of yours
Or want to appear that I have all the cures.
There is so much to know…So many things are true…
The way my feet must go may not be best for you…
And so, I give this spark of what is light to me.
To guide you through the dark but not tell you what to see.

— Unknown Author

Found in *Fresh, The Ultimate Live-Food Cookbook* by Sergei Boutenko and Valya Boutenko (Berkely, CA: North Atlantic Books, 2008), 7.

Table of Contents

Chapter 7 | Blocked Energy is Illness 137

Preface

Part philosophy, part theology, and part nutrition, the premise of this book is that adopting an organic, uncooked, living vegan diet, which still contains the life force energy from the Earth and sun, will increase the free flow of vital energy in and around a person's body. This increase of energy flow can have profound effects on physical and mental/emotional health. Surprisingly, it can speed the expansion of spiritual consciousness as well, which is vital in this new age of tumultuous events and increasing intensity of radiant celestial energies.

There are myriad names for the energy core of which all entities are a part and from which life energy flows: river of consciousness, the all, divine intelligence, the universe, universal law, all that is, goddess, god, allah, yahweh, nature, and cosmic fire, to name a few. They are not capitalized any more than you would capitalize 'human' or 'animal.' To show that the name of this intelligence does not matter, a different one is used at every opportunity in this book, illustrating how unnecessary it is to fight over a name. Multiple terms are also used for the vital energy which enervates all living things—prana, chi, manna, and love, for example.

The feminine version of pronouns, instead of the conventional male form, has been predominately used in hopes this will allow the reader to become comfortable with both—toward a goal of equality and peace.

All of us are on a quest for higher consciousness, but not all are aware of that yet. The Law of Attraction and the basic premise of energy healing declare that where attention and intent go, so goes energy; those who are seeking and longing for information will bring it to themselves. Writers share experiences and those who are drawn to it will find a piece of their own truth. This material is hereby blessed and delivered to those who vibrate with it.

This is not a raw food recipe how-to book, but rather more of a why-to book. No attempt is made to instruct the reader on how to transition or to give individual food advice. Instead, she is directed to the 'nutritionist-within' for meal plans. Each person can decide if changes she experiences are physical or emotional detoxification symptoms or signs that action is needed.

I believe in my core that what I have written is true. Where possible, I have given sources and information from others who have similar opinions if you wish to continue your study of an aspect that appeals to you. I am grateful to all my teachers and mentors in person, in word, and in spirit, and I give my blessing to all who take up the dance.

Here are some thoughts to consider:

- ♥ The ideas expressed in this book are largely unconventional and often contradict modern medicine, religion, and other philosophies in current society.
- ♥ There is always a temptation to *resist* new material or information that seems to be contrary to commonly accepted professional practice.
- ♥ Think of them first in the hypothetical sense. If they resonate, improve them and become the teacher yourSELF. Approach with an open heart and mind. What if they are true?

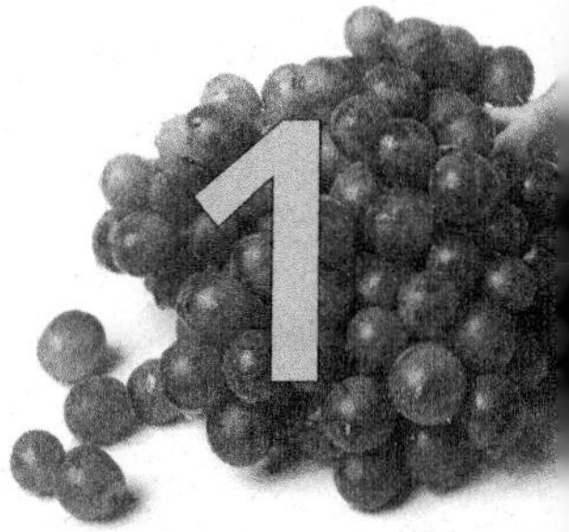

Life on Earth is a Spiritual Journey

What we consume on a daily basis is…there in order to convey its forces to the body, to rouse the body to activity…the important thing is the vitality of the forces in the food.

— Rudolf Steiner

MY SPIRITUAL JOURNEY

My early exposure to holistic spiritual studies was an overwhelming time of great anxiety. I could not inhale the material quickly enough and wanted the information to jump into me without time-consuming reading or meditating. The dogma and rhetoric of religion made my brain fuzzy, and I wanted to sink my teeth into the 'real truth.' I will be forever grateful to an unknown spiritual guide who simply smiled at my eagerness and said, "Just pick a place that appeals to your heart and get started on the path. You can only get on from the place you are standing."

In 1997 I was a nurse practitioner in a private practice—single, with grown children and little grandchildren. I owned a home with six acres, a nice garden and an efficient car. My retirement fund was proceeding according to plan, and by all outward signs I was successful, attractive, and confident. I thought my only issue was that I had been dumped by my lying, cheating boyfriend in the middle of my first energy healing class, which I had been convinced was going to help me understand the universe. It did, but not in the sweet way

I had imagined. Ironically, it was this same boyfriend who led me to ancient teachings, profoundly changing my spiritual life, my physical life, and my beliefs.

My First Dark Night of the Soul

I remember it as if it were an hour ago, my first 'dark night of the soul'—I was reclining on my bed reading a bright red version of Elizabeth Haich's book *Initiations* shortly after the break up with my boyfriend. Suddenly the bed seemed to start vibrating and I jumped off, scared out of my mind. I then realized it was I who was vibrating! It felt like I had just grabbed an electric fence and could not let go. I thought my heart was pounding and my teeth were chattering, but probably they were not. I had no idea what was happening. As I recall, the part I had been reading was Elizabeth's puzzlement as to where her parents were—not the parents in this life, but her parents in a past life. I paced the floor and whenever I stopped walking, I felt more terrified, so I kept pacing. Being a good nurse, I called a doctor friend who came immediately; and since she thought I was having a panic attack, she brought me some Valium. I dutifully took one, grateful that I would soon feel normal again. I didn't—I felt worse and was terribly eager for the pill to wear off. At least I was pretty sure the pill would wear off. I was not so sure about the vibrating.

It felt like I had just grabbed an electric fence and could not let go.

After this initial 'crisis,' the panicky feeling kept escalating at 'illogical' (to me) times. It especially increased near sunset or when I was in a confined space, like when I was with a patient in an examination room. I cried nearly constantly for a year, composing myself to keep working, but continuing the sobbing when I walked out of the clinic each night. Instinctively, I knew this crying was part of a healing process and tried to enhance it by renting all the saddest movies I could find—like *Places in the Heart, Terms of Endearment,* and *Beaches*—and watched them over and over, sobbing for myself. It was one of the only things that made me feel sane. I also felt better when I was in nature—barefoot in the grass, hugging a tree, or listening to Native American flute music. Sometimes, while at work, I would feel an 'attack' coming on and have to go to the bathroom for a quick cry. It worked a lot better than Valium.

I spent every day I had off (and lots of money) visiting psychics, holistic practitioners, and buying oils and flower essences. But I kept taking classes and reading because I could not, *not*. I told one spiritual teacher that I thought I was losing my mind and she said, "Well, go ahead." Others told me bits and pieces of what it all meant, what I could do, and what my future looked like. I learned it had little to do with the boyfriend directly, but that he had come to direct me in a profound way to the spiritual path and that he would then disappear from my life, which came to pass. I was told that I was to build a 'center' of sorts, for there were to be some very scary times ahead. I was to have a place where people of like mind could gather and then reach out energetically to others who are seeking and attract them to the center.

All this time, I thought I was dying! But the odd thing was that I did not think I would feel better dead. In fact, I was pretty sure that I needed to stay in my body and find answers before I could have the 'privilege' of dying. I never thought of killing myself because of this. I set my Aries mind and determined that I would learn the truth, however beautiful it was.

All this time, I thought I was dying! But the odd thing was that I did not think I would feel better dead.

Adopting a Raw Vegan Diet

In spring of 2002, John Robbins's book *Diet for a New Planet* convinced me to become a vegetarian. Then, feeling better, more clear-headed, and having always been one to ask "unanswerable" questions, my mind began probing even deeper into the causes of the illnesses I witnessed every day in my practice. After studying the effects of negative emotions on the body, I noticed the strong element of fear in medical settings, surrounding disease, and at the prospect of aging. Above all I kept asking why we become ill, and why we have to wait to get sick in order to get well.

As often happens when asking for peace of mind, ideas were presented to me. I was invited in March of 2003 to hear a talk by Victoria Boutenko, who came to the United States from Russia with her husband and two children to teach Russian history and within two years they all became severely ill. The enthusiasm of that mother and the delicious taste of the raw supper she served made a huge impression on me. The Boutenkos told how their son reversed insulin dependent diabetes, how their daughter recovered from severe asthma, and how Victoria herself overcame life-threatening heart disease. Her husband proved he was no longer crippled with arthritis by doing hand-springs in the aisle. Knowing that from a medical perspective these conditions are usually considered permanent, I began changing immediately to a raw diet. I gradually learned how to make familiar cooked foods in a raw version and found that avoiding cooked food took a lot of will power.

Above all I kept asking why we become ill, and why we have to wait to get sick in order to get well.

As I began the transition to a live vegetarian diet, the 'panic' attacks subsided. I now believe they were initiations—incoming energies responding to my longing and my request to be more 'spiritual,' not yet knowing exactly what that meant. (One must be careful of what one asks for!) By cleansing the energy 'circuits' of my body, I made it easier for the energies to flow without resistance, fear, and discomfort. I continued the path through physical and emotional detoxification, and now (years later) I have sudden unexplained attacks of intense (almost painful) joy—random, senseless, periods of giddy exhilaration. I still have times of discouragement and of feeling misunderstood, but I have gradually come to understand that each of us treads a different path, in the solitude of our mind and in our own time. At some point, most people will choose to see the beautiful truth within themselves.

Undergoing Physical Changes

Although never diagnosed with anything 'deadly,' I had fought the standard aging battles with constipation, obesity, fatigue, and depression. I had constant aching, swelling, and stiffness in my knees, fingers, back, and right shoulder, as well as low blood sugar, splitting finger tips, and yeast infections. These rapidly reversed after adopting a raw vegan diet.

By cleansing the energy 'circuits' of my body, I made it easier for the energies to flow without resistance, fear, and discomfort.

A skin rash described by my doctor as psoriasis caused my ears and arms to itch intensely and exude fluid profusely for several years before it disappeared. I changed the towel on my pillow daily. My arms and torso would itch and then weep enough to drip. I also suffered TMJ, constant runny nose, and headaches. Diet and exercise never seemed to produce the svelte figure I missed. I had been eating exactly what the latest 'pyramid' told me to consume and got sicker and fatter.

With the living diet, these things rapidly became non-issues. They never returned, even though my age progressed normally. Now I wake up in a new body, transformed from the old one that did not want to get out of bed and needed caffeine to get to work. The morning headache and fog are gone; instead there is a clear link with 'guidance' upon awakening.

My hair, which had been turning quite gray, began to change back to its original reddish brown. In the first year, I dropped forty pounds and my energy kept growing. Pitting edema, abdominal pain, depression, and fatigue all diminished and slowly went away. My bone density stayed stable. My blood pressure and pulse went below 'normal,' my cholesterol in the low normal range, and the tests for B-12 stayed normal.

As a nurse, I had worked at all stages of disease, from office exams to emergency room and intensive care. I saw people suffering and angry about it. I saw them rot away in inches, screaming in pain and anguish. They had been instructed on the basic functions of life—how to prepare food, how to clean their houses, kill bugs and germs, and which brands to choose. Even when they went to church and followed all the rules, they found themselves helpless and at the mercy of the medical system. Going into a 'predicted dark prognosis tunnel,' their diseases progressed as 'planned' for them, and within a specified time they were either in pain, blunted of mind, tied to a sterilized sheet with tubes coming from every natural and several unnatural orifices—or dead. Some tried to keep a cheerful face and not complain and were treated better for their deception. Others rallied back in whatever way they could and were medicated for their rage. To be fair, medical personnel are mostly good people, honestly trying to help. They might suspect the causes of disease but it is rarely discussed with patients, in medical literature, or at conferences. They are strictly taught to avoid 'blaming the patient' for her condition.

It became my personal goal to avoid *becoming* a patient—a 'prisoner' in a hospital bed. There had to be answers to my questions.

It became my personal goal to avoid becoming a patient—a 'prisoner' in a hospital bed.

Spiritual Discoveries

The lying, cheating boyfriend I mentioned earlier had introduced me to metaphysical concepts far different from my Presbyterian roots: ancient teachings, past lives, spiritual readers, and spiritual healing. You can never tell how the path will be revealed because he, in essence, became my first spiritual teacher—although unwittingly, I believe. I then found teachers everywhere and each led to others as rapidly as I could physically keep up. I studied Esoteric Healing, a method of using spiritual energy to benefit another person, with Barbara Briner, a medical doctor who also had become interested in 'complementary medicine.' I met a person in Briner's class who led me to Sancta Sophia Seminary, a modern 'mystery school' in Oklahoma. Books, like *The Power of Positive Thinking,* by Norman Vincent Peale, literally fell off the shelf in my lap. I studied hypnosis, herbal therapy, Emotional Freedom Technique, aromatherapy, magnets, meditation, Feng Shui, crystals, numerology, micronutrient and enzyme therapy, conventional and alternative nutrition, astrology, intuitive development, handwriting analysis, facial reading, reflexology, yoga, ancient philosophy, and read dozens of books on relationships.

Each path was the 'miracle answer of the day' as I dug into it, only to find another 'vein of gold' leading in a different direction. Each 'light bulb' in my 'tunnel of darkness' made me ask, "What am I NOT seeing now?" This always led to the next brilliant discovery. I kept an open mind. No matter how hard I resisted each 'truth' (all were true), I learned enough to know that wisdom lies inside me, if I would only *shut up and listen.*

No matter how hard I resisted each 'truth' (all were true), I learned enough to know that wisdom lies inside me, if I would only shut up and listen.

We are all following on the flagstones laid by those who went before us. They left enough evidence for us to choose which stones will support our next step and which will pull us into the current of fear. I am following wise, benevolent path-builders and will be followed by much greater minds. There are no distinctions between student and teacher.

THE LAW OF ATTRACTION

Along my evolving spiritual journey, I was introduced to the Law of Attraction, which states we have attracted what we experience. I vehemently resisted accepting the concept because it was so much easier and comfortable to blame my parents, the government, germs—anyone or anything outside myself. That way, I did not need to assume responsibility.

But when a tiny step is taken either mentally or physically, a huge decision has been made which ripples out into the body and the environment. That decision brings similar waves back again and again. Changing my diet brought clarity of mind I literally could never have imagined. Yes, I am responsible. I get both the credit and the blame.

But when a tiny step is taken either mentally or physically, a huge decision has been made which ripples out into the body and the environment.

The unbreakable Law of Attraction means also that each person attracts the exact energetic match to their pattern of thought, belief, words, and actions. Financial status, relationships, health, and spiritual life are set up by our past thoughts, but in each moment a new thought can be chosen which can produce a different tomorrow. Words that come from our mouths produce the food that goes into our mouth ("I'll have a cheeseburger"). Conversely, what goes into our mouths profoundly affects the words that come out of it and thereby our entire life circumstance. If we forgive ourselves and begin to take better care of ourselves, others will, too.

I had a passion, an unquenchable thirst to learn about spiritual truth. I read every book I could find about what happens before life begins and after we die. I wanted to know why we are born and how we get born into the families we do. Why does one person get obsessed with spirit and another fascinated with horror? Are ghosts real? Do we need to be afraid? Where are we all going and why? I was obsessed with *why*???????????

WHAT I LEARNED ABOUT THE CONNECTION BETWEEN SPIRITUAL CONSCIOUSNESS AND DIET

Diet profoundly affects all aspects of your life. Others with whom I have shared the experience of living food have found similar benefits, but the life style changes are not easy to sustain. Addictions to the old ways of eating and thinking are so hard-wired, that we fear we may die from the physical detoxification withdrawal symptoms, the mental/emotional healing crises, or the dark nights of the soul. These come when contact is made with the light and our energy (and our bowels) begins to flow naturally. We fearfully cling to dangerous old ways, like horses running back into the burning barn or a drug addict searching for a deadly fix. We struggle and nearly drown the messengers who try to save us, even though something tells us the message is true.

We struggle and nearly drown the messengers who try to save us, even though something tells us the message is true.

A compassionate diet that focuses on plant-based food eliminates the need for animal suffering, leads to becoming aware of the truths inside us, and fosters a better understanding of the role of humanity in the universe. Searing heat denatures and destroys the life-enhancing energy of the food we consume, subsequently draining the energy systems of the body by forcing it to use its own precious chi to energize the dead food. Live food enlivens living bodies.

I came to call my diet CLOVER—Complete (whole food), Local (within 100 miles), Organic (no toxic chemicals), Vegan (plant based), Exquisite (taste, smell, and appearance), and Raw (not ever heated above 118°F). More on this in Chapters 6, 7, 8, and 9.

Live food enlivens living bodies.

Meditation (quieting the mind and feeling connected to the basic oneness of the cosmos) is difficult, even for experienced meditators. It's not easy to find even an hour a day that is uninterrupted and quiet. The idea that diet can help quiet the mind and make 'plugging-in' easier may seem strange at first, but is well worth considering (more on meditation in Chapter 10).

It is the pure and simple diet that the body needs to channel the pure energies now reaching Earth (see Chapter 3). Each human is called to contain and radiate as much light as possible and to ignite the light in others (Chapter 6). With enlightenment comes responsibility as the student becomes an awakened teacher—a way-shower, a flashlight in the darkness. Diet is a choice (at least in this country for most of the population). It is a matter of literally 'putting your money where your mouth is.' Each person chooses a diet that resonates with the vibration of her current consciousness. Conversely, that consciousness can be raised by raising the vibration of the diet. Although medical providers try, no one can be 'ordered' or 'prescribed' any diet changes unless the patient agrees. A person's diet choices are very personal and sensitive. In fact, discussing diet often seems to raise more anger and defensiveness than do discussions of religion or politics. Guilt and shame must be kept out of the teaching. What we eat is our choice—pure and simple.

I can only speak from my own experience that changing to a diet of 'manifested sunlight' is worth the struggle for the rewards, which come gradually and continuously. We learn in our own way to follow that ancient Greek inscription "Know Thyself" by learning to get out of our logical left brain and listen to our intuitive right brain. We can examine our own behavior and thoughts for clues to emotional blocks. The raw vegetarian diet seems to calm and condition the cells to be open and receptive, but we still must ask for enlightenment and do the spiritual work.

A person's diet choices are very personal and sensitive. In fact, discussing diet often seems to raise more anger and defensiveness than do discussions of religion or politics.

What happens on the mental and emotional level becomes physical. Candace Pert, a professor of physiology and biophysics, says, "The body *is* the subconscious mind."[1] The physical vehicle (body) is a direct reflection of the intent (usually unconscious) of the owner. If

---

1 Candace B. Pert, Ph.D., "Your Body is Your Subconscious Mind, New Insights into the Body-Mind Connection" Audio tape from Sounds True, circa 1995.

pure beauty and health are intended, then the purest of food, water, air, and thought will be selected. All disease is reversible if there is enough will and life force energy left to affect the change. The body is a holy temple with complete self-healing capabilities. There is no 'natural aging switch.' Poor habits manifest as gradual accumulation of toxic debris and contorted negative thoughts, making us ill and sad. The very best way to detox the body is not with herbs and therapies but to simply quit 'toxing' it. Live food contains the life-giving energy from the sun and the core of love; it heals pain.

All disease is reversible if there is enough will and life force energy left to affect the change.

THE NEW AGE

A diet of flesh may have matched the vibration of prehistoric humans, but the increase in consciousness since then and the new energies stirring the population call for new ways of living. This New Age of light is a time when humanity will realize that each of us is made of love and that fear, anger, and pain are all self-inflicted obstacles. There is a change in the quality and intensity of the love that has been sustaining life since before the Earth was born. This is making the contrasts between love and fear appear more pronounced. (More on the New Age in Chapter 3.)

The very best way to detox the body is not with herbs and therapies but to simply quit 'toxing' it.

In the age of light, humans will realize they *are* part of the 'divine all' and that physical bodies are just as sacred as the soul. Perfect health and senses are not only possible but are the natural way. Each person will seek health by consulting the divine healer within and become conscious of the implications of even the most mundane habit of daily life. A conscious person craves nature and food as it comes from the tree, the Earth, or the plant—divine gifts that cannot be improved by cooking. A compassionate vegan diet, prepared with love, and eaten in moderation with gratitude brings a peace like nothing else.

A compassionate vegan diet, prepared with love, and eaten in moderation with gratitude brings a peace like nothing else.

Peace attracts peace and it flows to others. Peace, respect and love are contagious! Dark is caused by blocking the light, fear is caused by blocking love, and disease is caused from a block in life force energy. Cure dark by seeking light, cure fear by accepting love, and cure disease by increasing the flow of life force energy.

The Earth and all living beings live in cycles like heartbeats, breaths, ocean waves, days, years, and ages. As each day fades and night begins, what was hidden by the brilliance of the sun becomes astonishingly beautiful—the moon, the stars, and our own inner wisdom. The same is true when one 'age' fades and another one dawns; both personal chronological ages and ages of the Earth. Going within to search for the beauty, the brilliance, and the love is what the New Golden Age is all about. Religion and history look mainly at the past while science and spirituality look to the future. Spirit and science are finally coming to agree—the cosmos is infinite, as is the tiny fractal of it found in each human. As above, so below.

MY RESEARCH STUDY

Being excited about the effects I experienced from the living food diet, when it came time to write my dissertation in holistic wellness at Sancta Sophia Seminary, I conducted a pilot study to gather information on changes perceived by people who experienced the raw vegan diet. A pilot study is not intended to be definitive or prove anything—only to begin to search out questions for further research. Little research had ever been done on the effects of a raw vegan diet and none on the spiritual effects. My small pilot study was done at the Creative Health Institute in Michigan, a residential living food teaching facility.

A pilot study is not intended to be definitive or prove anything—only to begin to search out questions for further research.

The results of the study (it was also called Spiritual Effects of Live Food, or S.E.L.F.), were astonishingly positive. If any marketable service or product could perform anywhere near this well, it would be a 'diamond mine.' The only major 'side effect' of this 'therapy' might be the temporary physical and/or emotional discomforts of detoxification and withdrawal that are often part of the process. (The study is described in Chapter 2 and details are provided in appendices A, B, and C.)

SOME KEY CONCEPTS FOUND IN THIS BOOK

♥ **All that exists in space is energy, Lots Of Vital Energy—LOVE, found in every beating heart.**

Matter (physical material) is composed of love. Love gives birth to matter, and will ultimately save matter. Matter matters very much because it is the physical manifestation of spiritual energy. Various forms of love divide themselves into material elements of iron, oxygen, etc., and also into vibrations, like thoughts, emotions, and higher spiritual rays.

♥ **Good health and, ultimately, peace are caused by the unbounded free flow of vital love energy—the 'juice' of the universe.**

This intelligent love energy connects us with each other and the whole. Every atom, molecule, and cell is plugged into this energy and is part of the Divine organizing plan. Tiny cells arrange themselves into organisms—plants and animals—and then the breath of life is summoned.

♥ **Life is a fine thread linking an organism with the Divine whole.**

Living organisms generate or create love. Living food enhances the vibrations of a living animal and assists it to heal and become conscious.

♥ Life ignites life, similar to the lighting of one candle from another.

Living things produce other living things and lend their love to nourish and sustain life. Animals and plants reproduce but in addition we affect the people and environment around us all the time.

♥ Living matter responds to love and dies without it.

A lack of love gives the illusion that we are somehow separate from the source of love, spawning a deep existential longing, when in fact; we are *part* of it, made of it, breathe it, and eat it every day. Feeling separated from love creates a longing and a search. The more terrible the longing, the more intense is the search. We are searching for ourselves, but we sometimes glimpse that bliss when we fall in love with another, thinking they are that for which we long. Meher Baba, a spiritual teacher from India who taught in the early 20th century, wrote, "To attain union is so impossibly difficult because it is impossible to become what you already are! Union is nothing other than knowledge of oneself…"[2]

♥ Often the longing for love is so great that, not knowing what else to do, we 'self-medicate' with consciousness-dulling substances—alcohol, drugs, and cooked flesh, but this further blocks the 'thread of life.'

Living things are growing and seeking ways to reproduce themselves. They contain the thread from which they were 'born' and the living enzymes which will serve to break the organism back into elements when it is no longer alive. When food is cooked or otherwise 'denatured,' these enzymes are destroyed and the dinner must be digested and absorbed using energy from the diner. But if 'life energy'

2 Meher Baba, *The Everything and the Nothing,* (Berkeley, CA: The Beguine Library, 1963), 1.

is retained in the food, it will not only digest itself but infuse the body with energy, enhancing health and peace, which then ripples out into the environment.

♥ Humanity was given the most amazing bodies, whose natural state is joyful health and unbounded energy.

Capable of creating magnificent works, many humans seem content, even eager to dwell in fear, violence, and illness. From a glorious world of unlimited natural resources, mankind has produced want, disorder, and disconnectedness. Our bodies have latent mental powers whose possibilities are immeasurable. They also have creative ability which enables mastery of all things.

♥ When the energy flow is disturbed, congested, or cut off in any part of an organism, disease invades the tissues and the body struggles to correct the disruption.

Disease and discomfort mean a part of us is not in alignment with our true nature—divine love. These blocks have many characteristics and intensities. They are responsible for all diseases and mental states. Belief and intent are strong conductors, as well as blockers of energy. The body perfectly and truthfully reflects these. The energy might be blocked with:

- Physical toxic debris from food and other sources
- Mental fearful anguish caused by errors in thinking

♥ When an animal dies, the cells begin to quickly break down, aided by intrinsic enzymes; while plants retain life force energy for varying amounts of time.

Under ordinary circumstances, seeds of plants can be viable for many years, even centuries after the plant is compost, which is not true of animals whose 'seed' dies soon after the animal. When breath is withdrawn (death), the physical structure is returned to its elemental building blocks—compost—by carnivores, insects and teeming microbial life. Bacteria are drawn to the dead and dying tissue to begin the composting process. This is their function in nature. Saying "bacteria cause disease" is like saying "flies cause garbage!"

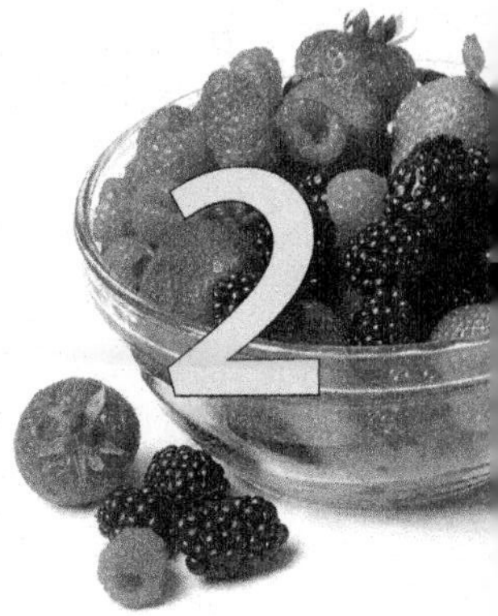

Spiritual Effects of Live Food (S.E.L.F.)—The Study

I feel like I could do anything, I am incredibly motivated and inspired!
— S.E.L.F. study participant

As I studied alternative treatments in depth, it was clear to me that most healing theories are valid, whether they begin with the body, mind, or spirit. (See cure versus healing in chapter 7.) Each person just needs to integrate and balance them for herself. Balance is the key. I have noticed that people who live in their 'spiritual self' often break their ankles and suffer diseases of the flesh. People who work-out while focused on physical beauty and fitness, as well as those obsessed with expensive material 'toys,' are often lacking in spiritual awareness. Emotional needs seem to be neglected by the overly responsible, logical, and rational intellectual. When drama and emotional upset dominate a person's life, she is most likely unaware of her intuitive wisdom. The truth is the body is *just* as important as the mind, and emotional issues need to be resolved before pure spiritual bliss can occur.

*The truth is the body is **just** as important as the mind, and emotional issues need to be resolved before pure spiritual bliss can occur.*

It also became clear that a healing plan must be evaluated both rationally as well as intuitively for short term effects, versus ultimate benefit or damage—the bottom line cost and reward. Conventional medical interventions often have serious long term consequences.

The negative 'side effects' from adopting a complete, local, organic, vegan, exquisite, and raw (CLOVER) diet pale in comparison.

When the time came to write my dissertation for a Doctor of Philosophy in Holistic Wellness at Sancta Sophia Seminary Oklahoma, it was obvious that the Spiritual Effects of Live Food would be the topic because of the amazing benefits I had witnessed. Since the Ph.D. requirements included conducting an original research project, I would need to find a way to control the diet of my subjects for a time. Fortunately, an ideal residential raw food program called Creative Health Institute (CHI) was close enough for me to access.

ANECDOTAL COMMENTS FROM PRELIMINARY SURVEY

A random survey of people already practicing some version of a raw food diet was done before the prospective study. They were found at CHI, raw restaurants, potlucks, and other raw gatherings and asked about their perception of changes after adopting a raw diet. Their comments are summarized here:

♥ Changes in Physical Health

- Skin tans instead of burning
- Sinus infection went away
- Lung tumor gone
- Tendonitis gone
- No awakening to urinate
- Feet no longer purple
- Parkinson's better
- Sight and hearing better
- No longer allergic to cats
- Incredibly energized
- Still crave bagels & cream cheese
- Nail fungus gone
- Blood pressure lower
- I feel better
- Steroid use lower
- Skin tone improved
- Hair thicker
- Adrenal gland recovering
- My health is now great
- Restless leg syndrome gone
- No menopause symptoms
- Dropped eighty-five pounds
- My colon felt better after twenty-four hours

♥ Changes in Emotional Health

- Much calmer
- More loving
- More at peace
- This diet releases old emotions
- I have a more positive attitude
- I got weepy once on the raw diet
- Emotional ups and downs
- Learned perseverance
- Learned to live and let live
- Trouble staying raw
- Depression better
- Take fewer [mood altering] medications
- I knew that many layers [of feelings] were being peeled like an onion
- I feel like I could do anything, I am incredibly motivated and inspired!
- I think my emotional problems were actually caused by the drugs [I was taking]

♥ Changes in Mental Health

- Very positive now
- I am more organized
- I am not sure how much of my symptoms are from "normal aging," electromagnetic and other frequency pollutions, toxins, mind control, and intentional social dilemmas
- My mind is sharper

♥ Changes in Spiritual Health

- I feel more open [to life]
- I have a deeper sense of peace
- My relationship with God is better
- I look forward to the afterlife
- I feel I am led to certain people and places
- I have greater awareness
- I have improved sensitivity
- I am more open to a spiritual relationship
- I could equate health with love
- It also became hard to kill insects
- It's the best thing since meditation!
- Easier to meditate—I feel I get connected faster
- Natural food is a step toward greater awareness and oneness

- The body is a vehicle and part of the trinity: Body, Mind and Spirit
- I think the higher percent raw I am the more spiritual I feel
- I understand that eating [raw food] comforts me and I don't feel so lonely [separate] from God, Spirit, The Divine

CASE STUDY—PHILIP

To illustrate the profound impact changing to a raw vegan diet can have on one's whole life, I tell (with permission) this story. Philip was 'too raw' to qualify for the study when he arrived at Creative Health Institute, but had experienced such impressive results, I wanted to use his information. He told me of his journey from 400 to 200 pounds. He was in his thirties living in Connecticut when he became acutely aware of his size after a trip to Europe where he found obesity to be a 'staring event.' Finding clothes to fit was extremely difficult, expensive, and emotional. He was forced to give up $150 tickets to a show in Las Vegas because he did not fit in the seats. He had a hard time breathing, had sleep issues, and got winded easily. He tried sixteen different ways to lose the weight, including hypnosis, fasting, and weight lifting, and even contemplated bypass surgery. Philip learned about the raw food diet from a website and he slowly adopted the raw lifestyle with the goal to be "half the man I used to be." At the time I interviewed him, he had lost 85 pounds and a year later had lost 140 pounds. He now writes of the transition to a raw lifestyle:

> *"At times I felt like I was living someone else's life. Like, why am I eating this way, but then I thought, why not? It is not so much as me feeling like I am someone else, but rather actually discovering who I always was, and just slowly removing the layers of the world from my eyes so I can re-discover the original me that was always there—just hidden."*

Philip began to notice that many people's taste buds and bodies are stimulated and distorted by things like soda, potato chips, meat, and milk products. As a result, folks tend to shy away from the fruit and veggies that children naturally love. They become addicted to coffee, burgers, and fries. He loves to tell of his experience of living the raw food lifestyle. One example was how he responded to kidding about bringing his own food to a buffet. "Yup," he says, opening his bag of raw avocado, seeds and dressing.

CREATIVE HEALTH INSTITUTE

Creative Health Institute (CHI)[3] is a raw food residential program which met my criteria of being relatively certain the diet of the students was pure because all meals were provided. The school was close enough to allow a visit every week for conducting the study. They readily gave written permission to conduct the study there and a release for me to disseminate the information in whatever way I could.

A few months before the study began, in order to understand the experience of the students, I enrolled and completed the two week program at CHI. The program was offered in a modest building by the side of a busy road in a tiny town with the unlikely name of Hodunk. Upon arrival, the students entered the two story building through a sunny porch with comfortable couches, TV, books and videos. The porch led up a few steps into the main dining hall where there was one long table and several smaller tables. In the same room, separated by a divider, was a large carpeted area with video players for exercise and classes. The kitchen (no stove) opened off the classroom next to the buffet table. The place was old and had known a previous life as a tavern serving up steaks and martinis.

---

3 Creative Health Institute in Union City, MI 49094, www.creativehealthinstitute.com.

In fact, it was these very substances that founder, Don Haughey (who also ran the tavern), blames for the many illnesses that led him to Ann Wigmore (March 4, 1909–February 16, 1994), who is considered the 'mother of the modern raw vegan lifestyle.' Her live food institute was located in Boston at that time. Don tells the story of how the doctors had sent him home, basically to die, but with handfuls of pills (116 different ones) to take while he did so. Instead, he went to Boston and got well.

Ann laughed when Don told her he wanted to open another raw food center in Michigan, but he proved he was good for his word. She came many times to help him, and it opened in 1976, teaching her self-healing methods to thousands ever since. CHI had gone from serving one kind of spirits to raising another. He was thrilled with my study of the spiritual effects of the lifestyle. Don died in December of 2010 in a fire that consumed the antique mill he had made into a charming and comfortable home across the road from the institute. Ironically, he left the same way as Ann Wigmore, who died in a fire at Hippocrates Health Institute in Boston.

Don Haughey thought very few of the thousands who graduated from CHI stayed raw after they left. He said there seemed to be a powerful social hypnosis as well as an addictive quality to cooked food that caused people to paint the situation hopeless. They slip back to the familiar comfort of cooked white flour, sugar, meat, and cheese with only a bit of fruit or vegetable. I think he would be pleased if he knew of the positive impact his work has actually had on the world. Perhaps he and Ann are still watching and teaching.

He said there seemed to be a powerful social hypnosis as well as an addictive quality to cooked food that caused people to paint the situation hopeless.

THE TWO WEEK COURSE AT CHI

After getting settled into a comfortable bedroom with full bathroom, the students began the program with an exquisite live food buffet dinner. Open to the public for a love offering, this live food feast was held every Sunday. It consisted of a variety of salad greens, various sprouts (lentil and alfalfa), chopped salad ingredients such as cucumber and tomatoes, choice of raw dressings, crackers and dip, and several special items such as nutmeat loaf, burgers, pizza, or a casserole. Buckies and sunnies (shoots of buckwheat and sunflower seeds grown in nursery flats) were a staple at almost every meal. For the weekly buffet, there was always a dessert such as fruit pie, cashew cheesecake, or ice cream and cookies. In place of conventional salt and pepper, the tables had shakers of raw ground dulse (seaweed) and cayenne powder.

After the meal, the new student was then given a tour of the building and grounds where the wood-fired sauna and gardens were found a few yards away from the main building. Off the class area was a wide hall with exercise machines such as a vibrating table, slant boards, and a small trampoline. Several student rooms were entered from here as were the stairs to the rooms upstairs and the basement. Downstairs, besides private rooms, was the laundry, the colonic room (where students can receive a special high enema (colonic) from a trained therapist), and the "green room" where wheat grass, buckies, and sunnies were grown under grow lights on shelves several tiers tall. The ancient stone foundation and earth floor could be seen here with a wood stove for very cold weather. It smelled of life and the Earth. (The place and program have changed considerably from the time the study was conducted.)

On Monday began a three day semi-fast consisting of unlimited amounts of "energy soup" made with fresh organic greens and a little fruit and vegetables blended smooth. Most Standard American Diet (SAD) students found this very austere, as it began the detoxing and cleansing of the body tissues. Wheatgrass was announced with a bell at seven every morning of the program, and the students drifted sleepily into the sprout room, removed the cut wheatgrass from the refrigerator, and juiced an ounce or two for themselves or friends. When a person is very toxic the juice tastes foul, but as she begins to purify, the taste is more like new mown hay smells—very refreshing! Wheatgrass juice is considered by many to be a most important natural "toxin magnet," attracting and pulling out poison, because its composition very closely resembles that of hemoglobin in human blood, which carries oxygen, nutrients, and waste products. Many people felt it speeded their detoxification process.

Ann Wigmore conducted scientific studies with grass seeds from all over the world. Narrowing her search for the perfect chlorophyll-rich healing grass, she enlisted the expertise of a small kitten and a cocker spaniel. They both preferred the wheatgrass over the rye, timothy, broome, canary, alfalfa, and buckwheat, as did the baby chicks and rabbits.[4]

After wheatgrass, came a period of exercise either led by a staff member or a video—an eclectic blend of yoga, aerobic repetitions, or just plain stretching. This was felt to help dislodge toxic waste from the muscles and joints. Long walks, working in the garden in summer, and other exercise were encouraged, especially trampoline jumping, which is felt to awaken the cells and get the lymph system moving. The sauna was fired up several times a week.

Many naps were taken, bringing dreams with deep insight, and resulting in diaries filled with fruitful information.

Breakfast, lunch, and dinner were announced with a gong. Students usually felt weak and tired during these first three days. Many naps were taken, bringing dreams with deep insight, and resulting in diaries filled with fruitful information. The emotions of class members often flared during this time, creating stress but also truthful information about themselves, resulting in a closeness and trust for each other.

4 Ann Wigmore, *Be Your Own Doctor,* (Wayne, NJ: Avery Publishing Group, 1982), 26.

How sweet was the fourth day and the first solid food—fruit and simple salad with the divine sensation of chewing! Heavier foods containing nuts, seeds, or oil came later. After the first three days of energy soup, breakfast consisted of fruit, green smoothies (fruit and greens), and occasionally raw oatmeal with nut milk. Strength returned and the students now looked at one another as comrades after the cleansing phase. They felt clean and proud of themselves.

They felt clean and proud of themselves.

Classes were held morning, afternoon, and evening on such things as how to give oneself a simple enema, skin brushing, sprouting, and growing greens indoors. There were also many recorded testimonials and instructional videos. Food preparation is not addressed during the first three days (for obvious reasons). The intent of the program, besides cleansing the body, was to prepare the student to feel confident about continuing the healthy diet upon return home to family and 'cooked' society.

Dr. Loraine Day, an American Medical Doctor from the west coast, states that the Ann Wigmore program healed her terminal breast cancer.[5] Several of Dr. Day's tapes were shown as part of the CHI program. She had been very near death but completely recovered by following a healthy lifestyle. Other video classes were presented by Victoria Boutenko, Ann Wigmore, Bernard Jensen, Elaina Love, and Douglas Graham. The remainder of the program focused on teaching the philosophy and live food preparation as discovered by Ann Wigmore ("Dr. Ann," as she was affectionately known by students and admirers). Most classes were hands-on in the grow room, the sprout room, and the kitchen. Students learned to prepare interesting meals that use only live vegan foods and resemble the cooked version of burgers, pizza, nori rolls, and patés. Many of the classes (as well as cleaning and maintenance) were taught by students who have stayed on after their

The intent of the program, besides cleansing the body, was to prepare the student to feel confident about continuing the healthy diet upon return home to family and 'cooked' society.

5 Lorraine Day, M.D., "Sorting Through the MAZE of Alternative Medicine" videotape found on website drday.org.

two-week class for the three month energy-exchange program, where students work to pay for their room and board at the institution.

While visiting and enrolled in the Creative Health Institute program, I had the opportunity to discuss my proposed study. The staff and administration of Creative Health Institute were most supportive at every step of the investigation.

SIGNIFICANCE OF THE RESEARCH

Anecdotal evidence had suggested that consuming an all raw vegan diet may improve the physical, emotional, mental and spiritual health in some people. I believed that it often made observable and measurable differences, as well. Stories of healing while on a live food diet are myriad but not widely known, and this method of healing is not taught to (or by) most health care providers. Nutritionist and government dietary recommendations rarely discuss the *method of food preparation.* Given the soaring incidence of chronic illness and the overwhelming cost of medical care, I perceived a need to verify the 'theory' that eating only live food improves health on all levels. The information could then be made known to those wishing a self-controlled plan for improving health with a much lower cost and much less risk than conventional treatments and therapies. The goal was to document these changes by using a well-designed instrument (questionnaire) and comparing the initial findings with those of the same subject after the diet change. The research question was: "What are the physical, emotional, mental, and spiritual effects of eating exclusively live food?"

"What are the physical, emotional, mental, and spiritual effects of eating exclusively live food?"

LITERATURE SEARCH

After completing the CHI course and before devising the study, I searched and tried to absorb all available knowledge about the subject of healing with live food. For the next year I searched the literature on diets of all types, examining bibliographies to find other written material to obtain and review. Online searches were conducted for such topics as Live Food, Natural Hygiene, and Organic Produce. Over 300 books and research studies were reviewed, many of which were out of print and obscure. I loved it.

STUDY DESIGN

Another full year was spent learning how to do research and designing the study, which was titled Spiritual Effects of Live Food (with the acronym of SELF) and which became the 'seed' for this book. This is significant because spiritual growth is dependent upon improvement in physical, emotional, and mental health, and in the study each of them were explored. It is also appropriate because the goal is to find a path to exquisite holistic wellness that each individual can control herSELF. Excellent health most definitely is a do-it-yourSELF project.

This research study sought to find and document evidence that changing to a diet consisting only of minimally processed organic plants promotes wellness of body, mind, and spirit. It is the first to record how each participant experienced the transition to a CLOVER diet physically as well as mentally, emotionally, and spiritually.

It is the first to record how each participant experienced the transition to a CLOVER diet physically as well as mentally, emotionally, and spiritually.

It was a pilot study, which usually means a small one, done in an area of little previous research for the purpose of evaluating the subject, study design, and to determine the feasibility of finding enough willing participants. Since existing research on the effects of live food was extremely sparse, it is a unique pilot study and hopefully adds to the body of knowledge about diet.

The investigation was considered a prospective study, because it was designed to follow subjects over time. It was also an observational, cohort, descriptive, and analytic study. In plain English, that means the study was designed to observe events taking place in the subjects, comparing them to themselves on previous tests, describing conditions at different times, and evaluating their answers to discover possible cause and effect.

In this case, the important variable was the diet change. Information was obtained before arrival, on the first day of their stay at CHI, and at graduation two weeks later. Each participant served as his/her own control by comparing the intake response to the graduation response to each question. The collective data from all participants was also compiled and analyzed.

Experts in the areas of research, nutrition, religious studies, spiritual studies, mental health, alternative healing, and conventional medicine were consulted and assisted me at every phase. They were there for the study design, creation of the questionnaire, advising on interview techniques, tabulation and compilation of the data, evaluation of the results, and illustration of the findings. I will always be grateful.

QUESTIONNAIRE

Unable to find existing validated questionnaires on the subject (questions that are pre-tested and cross-checked for accuracy), I interviewed experts in the field of medicine, mental health, and spiritual studies. I wanted to create a set of pertinent questions to evaluate a student's status in each aspect—physical health, emotional status, mental clarity, and spiritual growth. The S.E.L.F. questions were then composed, largely based on the interviews with these professionals. For questions on the physical aspects, I asked medical doctors and nurses, for the mental and emotional sections I met with mental health therapists, and for the spiritual questions I consulted spiritual counselors.

In all, I interviewed fourteen professionals, asking them questions about what in their opinion constituted excellent health for their field of expertise. Most of them stated that they had never given any thought to what might be the signs and symptoms of excellent health, so accustomed were they to looking for negative markers. One physician stated that she would consider a patient to be in excellent health if they felt good and had a good attitude even with a terminal disease diagnosis.

The questions were mostly compiled from the interviews, but some were taken from other places such as medical, mental health, and alternative health office intake forms. The same questions were used for both samplings. Releases of information and permission to publish were included on the questionnaire and signed by the participants. The original questionnaire is found in Appendix A.

STUDY METHODOLOGY

The questionnaire asked the student to quantify the extent to which they experienced each symptom (question) or feeling: none, little, moderate, lot, or overwhelming. The difference between their answer at the beginning of the study, compared to the end was then divided into 'change-categories': resolved, improved, unchanged, and worse at graduation. The number of students who reported each change-category for each symptom was tallied to get a total. For example, the number of students who felt the constipation they reported at intake had resolved at graduation. The percentage of each change-category for each aspect (physical, emotional, mental and spiritual) were figured separately and illustrated with a pie chart (figures 1–4). Finally a total of the numbers of students that reported each change-category for all symptoms for all aspects was obtained and illustrated.

Twelve students completed the study, adequate for this very recent field. They met the criteria of being new to live food and willing to participate in the data collection process. Over a six month period several were dropped from the study for various reasons. The final subjects were eight women and four men, aged 35 to 72 from all over the world.

The students were first contacted by email or phone when they signed up for the CHI course, and the nature of the study was explained. When there was verbal agreement, I needed to determine if they were already following the live food lifestyle. (Many people return for refresher courses or a boost in motivation.) If they agreed, they were contacted again for three consecutive days to get an exact diet diary. If careful analysis of their answers determined that they were over fifty percent cooked, they were invited to participate in S.E.L.F. The identity of these courageous people is respected and the information they provided is vitally important.

I met with each qualified student before the buffet dinner on the Sunday of their arrival at CHI, explained the study, and sat with them as they filled in the questionnaire for intake baseline data. I had little contact with the subjects during their course except an occasional email of encouragement. At graduation, each participant completed the exact same questionnaire before the celebration meal where graduating students are encouraged to make comments.

STUDY RESULTS BY INDIVIDUAL STUDENT

In Appendix B you will find tables showing study results for each student participating in the study, focusing on the changes in problems as perceived by the student. They are listed according to change categories. 'Improved' meant that the student reported a problem at a higher level of severity at intake then they did at graduation. A problem that was reported at intake but not identified as an issue at all at graduation was considered 'resolved.' They might also have reported the problem as 'worse' or 'unchanged.'

Each table shows the total number of problems in each aspect (physical, emotional, mental and spiritual) present at intake. The tables also list the change-category (resolved, improved, unchanged, and worse at graduation) in each aspect (physical, emotional, mental, and spiritual) and the percent of the problems this number represents.

There is a short description of each student before each table.

STUDY RESULTS BY GROUP

In Appendix C you will find tables illustrating collective data for all twelve students as a group. Each change-category in each aspect was calculated separately as found in Table 13–Physical Aspect, Table 14–Emotional Aspect, Table 15–Mental Aspect, and Table 16–Spiritual Aspect. The results recorded in these four collective tables represent all categories of problems, including "new at graduation."

The following pie charts for physical, emotional, mental and spiritual aspects show the most important findings of the study. They were constructed by using the data from the tables, eliminating the change-category of problems that were new at graduation. Working only with problems present at intake (when the students began the live food diet) the pie charts show the percentage of each change-category (resolved, improved, unchanged, and worse) that occurred by the end of the course for the whole group of students collectively. This is the true experimental data of the entire study, comparing the same group before and after the change to a live food lifestyle.

COLLECTIVE DATA

The total percentages from these tables are used in the pie charts, excluding the "new at graduation" category, demonstrating the difference in self-reported change in symptoms from intake to graduation only. Thus these percentages are different from those displayed in the tables. The pie charts are dramatic illustrations of the power of the live food diet even for just two weeks. The areas that were reported as worse could possibly be detoxification symptoms that appeared during the course. These did not prove to be significant. Imagine a drug that promised such a result!

Imagine a drug that promised such a result!

Physical Aspect

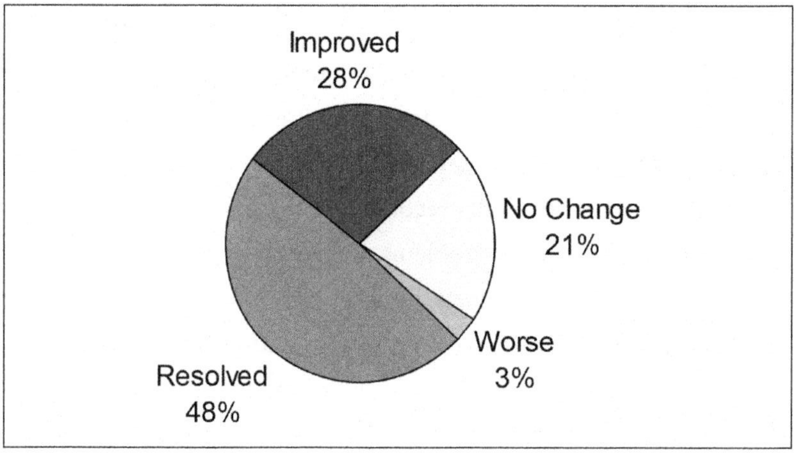

Figure 1, PHYSICAL ASPECT (Percent in each change-category of 303 problems present at intake to graduation) 48% of the physical problems students reported when they arrived at CHI were perceived as resolved at graduation.

48% of the physical problems students reported when they arrived at CHI were perceived as resolved at graduation.

Emotional Aspect

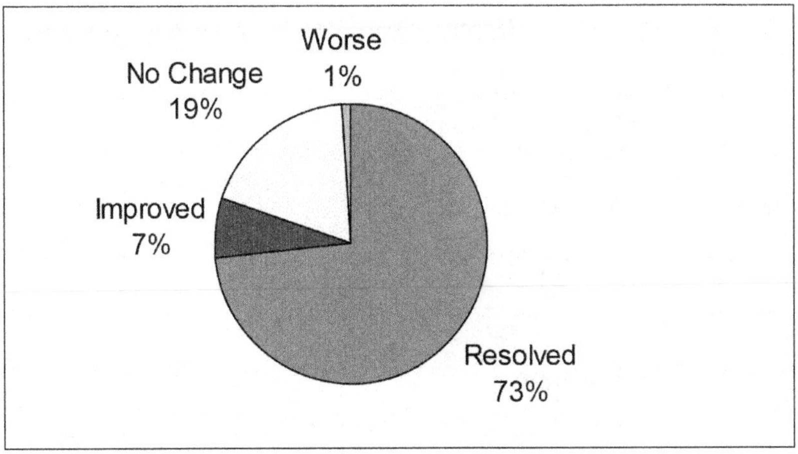

Figure 2, EMOTIONAL ASPECT (Percent in each change-category of 192 problems present at intake to graduation) 73% of the emotional problems students reported at intake were not mentioned at graduation.

73% of the emotional problems students reported at intake were not mentioned at graduation.

Mental Aspect

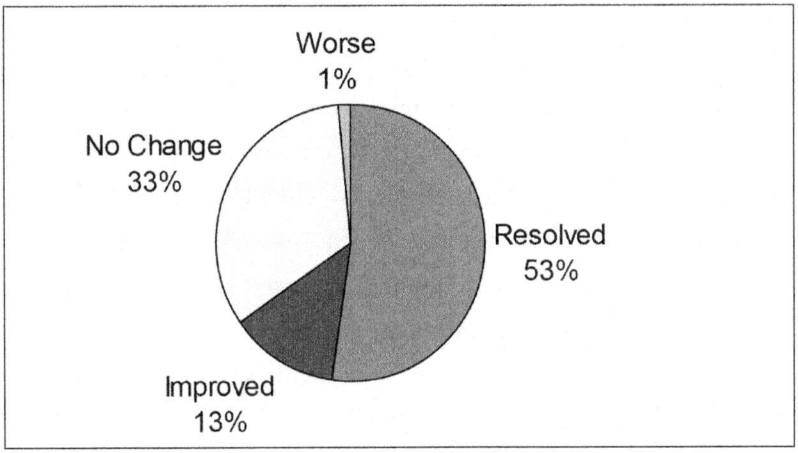

Figure 3, MENTAL ASPECT (Percent in each change-category of 234 problems present at intake to graduation) 53% of the mental problems students identified upon arrival were no longer present at graduation.

53% of the mental problems students identified upon arrival were no longer present at graduation.

Spiritual Aspect

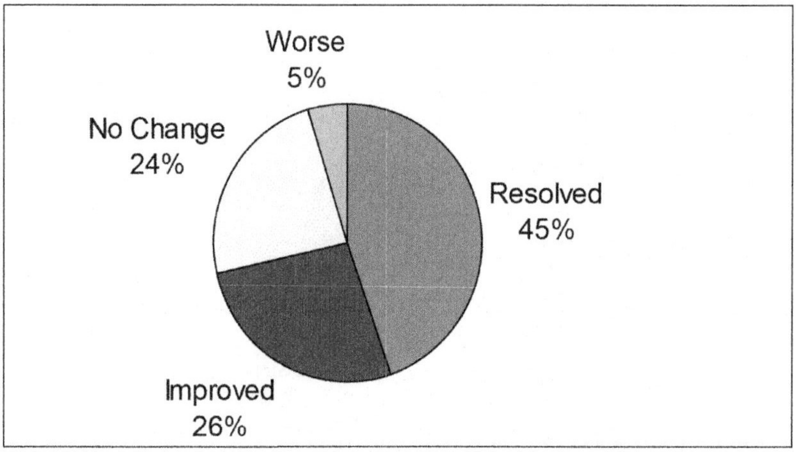

Figure 4, SPIRITUAL ASPECT (Percent in each change-category of 174 problems present at intake to graduation) 45% of the spiritual issues students felt were important at intake were no longer present at graduation.

45% of the spiritual issues students felt were important at intake were no longer present at graduation.

OVERALL STUDY RESULTS

Overall About Half of the Problems Resolved

The results of the study show that most of the subjects who agreed to participate in this study were impressed with the changes in all aspects of wellness they experienced when they changed diet and lifestyle practices. For the physical aspects, 48% were reported resolved. The emotional aspect was even more impressive in perceived relief, at 73% resolved. Mental improvement, an aspect that might be difficult to evaluate oneself, was 53%, which is highly significant. Measuring spiritual growth is an even more obscure aspect of wellness, and the results indicate that 45% of the areas they felt were issues at intake were resolved by graduation.

All Problems, All Categories

Of all problems in all categories that were reported present by all twelve students upon their arrival at Creative Health Institute, 73% were either improved or resolved after two weeks on exclusively live food. 54.75% were resolved, 18.5% were improved, 24.25% were reported as no change, and 2.5% were worse.

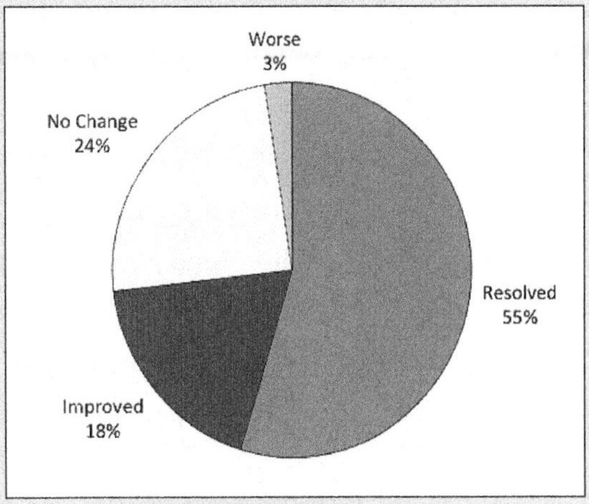

ANALYSIS OF STUDY RESULTS

The pilot study was later evaluated by research experts and found to meet basic criteria for study design. It was described as a "high-quality pilot study" by community nutrition research expert Karen Petersmarck, Michigan Department of Community Health.

Physical Implications

Adopting a live food diet lifestyle could have a positive impact on major health issues such as chronic illness, weight problems, and increasing health care costs. Considering so many diseases reverse after a raw food diet is adopted, it must be considered that many if not all physical illnesses are actually caused by toxicity. Energy or chi in the body should also be evaluated. In addition, most people begin their journey toward spiritual health by improving their physical health.

Emotional Implications

It is an interesting concept that diet can improve emotional reactions. While emotions are important tools leading to resolution of past wounds, getting stuck in those emotions is fruitless. This study (presumably) shows that by raising the energy of the body by increasing the volume of chi or energy from the sun taken in through live food, a greater proportion of positive reactions will result, perhaps by resolving the negative ones blocking the person's joy. This, according to the Law of Attraction, will enable a person to attract positive people, events and objects.

Mental Implications

Mental problems have come to be accepted as normal aging. All but one of the participants in this study might be considered 'aging.' Based on these results, it appears that assumption should be reassessed. Aging is often accompanied by poor diet and handfuls of medications. Could it be that dementia is simply 'poisoned' by medication or many years of toxic build-up from food?

These study results bring to mind the learning problems we see in our schools, not to mention discipline problems and lack of motivation in students. If more people in the society could think clearly, could we vote for better leaders? The possibilities are endless.

Spiritual Implications

A raw, organic, vegan diet is a wonderful tool to assist humans to clear the path to the Light. Being more tolerant of others, finding it easier to meditate, love and forgiveness for oneself would make this world a better place. Could we finally respect each other and live in a peaceful world? Would we respect the Earth and the animals?

WEAKNESSES OF THE STUDY

This study has plenty of weaknesses. The number of participants is small and the span of time covered by the study is relatively short. Because of the inexperience of the investigator, there was an attempt to gather too much data. The questionnaires were not cross-checked for accuracy. But I believe the study does break some new ground, and perhaps it will start a discussion for larger, more inclusive studies in the future.

FURTHER REFLECTION

After only two weeks on a (presumably) 100% living vegan food diet, the statistics were almost shocking. If I had not experienced the same, I would have thought there was a mistake. Although professionals in the medical community (providers and dietitians) feel that the lifestyle is "risky" and that eating a raw diet may delay a person from getting medical advice, how can eating organic apples and kale hurt?

Many, many testimonials are written by people who credit the living food lifestyle for reversal of deadly medical diagnoses. Among them are cancers of all areas of the body, heart diseases, a variety of colon problems, arthritis, fatigue issues, sleep disturbances, even mental states of distress. Most raw foodists, if they had any extra weight at all, would agree the weight just melted off while they were distracted preparing delicious food. Asthma and other respiratory diagnoses, thyroid problems, skin disruptions, diabetes and many more ailments have been reported in various media as no longer a problem, sometimes within a few days of stopping the SAD. Raw foodists seem to glow and to become younger and more flexible, physically and mentally, the longer they stay on the diet.

Many, many testimonials are written by people who credit the living food lifestyle for reversal of deadly medical diagnoses.

Raw foodists seem to glow and to become younger and more flexible, physically and mentally, the longer they stay on the diet.

It touches my 'truth-button,' as is usually the case when I turn to nature for answers. The trees come back to life in spring. Do we return also? When I cut myself, the wound heals. Can my diseased organ also regenerate? When I love my garden, it grows better. Will my body be healthier if I love it? When I eat food closer to the way nature prepared it, I feel better.

The physical body is the densest form of etheric energy and is the end point of intention—the 'proof of the pudding.' The body doesn't lie and can be used as a measuring stick to see if its owner is creating as intended. Love your body and it will love you back. Pay attention to your health or it will DEMAND your attention. Your physical body is your temple of the holy spirit—YOU!

The body doesn't lie and can be used as a measuring stick to see if its owner is creating as intended.

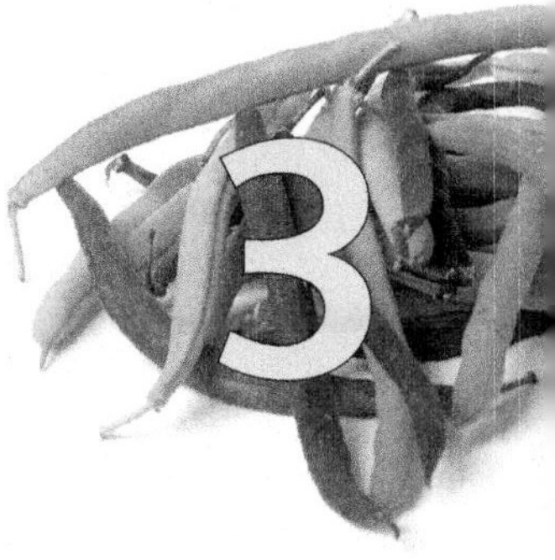

The New Age of Enlightenment

Whether or not it was written in the stars, a different age seems to be upon us...

— Marilyn Ferguson

THE TERM 'NEW AGE'

'New Age' is a figure of speech that can be emotionally charged and triggers vastly divergent attitudes. For some it is negative and terrifying and for others it means sublime spiritual anticipation. In this chapter I explore what has been written about New Age historically and why people might see it differently.

All ages are, by definition—new! "In every epoch," said scientist-philosopher, Pierre Teilhard de Chardin, "man has thought himself at a 'turning point in history.' And...as he is advancing on a rising spiral...this impression of transformation...is particularly justified... [in] our contemporary existences."[6]

The following words from the musical *Hair* stirred the soul of many a happy 'hippie' in the 1960s: "When the moon is in the Seventh House and Jupiter aligns with Mars. Then peace will guide the planets, and love will steer the stars. This is the dawning of the Age of Aquarius." But they were, according to journalist Neil Spencer, merely poetic license. He refers to them as 'astrological gibberish' because

6 Pierre Teilhard de Chardin, *The Phenomenon of Man,* (New York, NY: Perennial Library, Harper and Row, 1959), 213.

Jupiter aligns with Mars several times a year and the Moon is in the seventh house for about two hours every day.[7] The children of the popular culture known as 'New Age Movement' of that era believed that, even if the words were not accurate, they saw signs of a shift in energy from warlike to peaceful.

In the last century, the term New Age often did evoke a vision of these hippies, who engaged in free love, free drugs, and freeloading. Some people were offended by the term, believing it to be associated with sinister plots to take over the world. Others pointed to ambitious flower children going back to the land with long hair and a copy of *Homesteaders Handbook*.[8] Or it might evoke images of peace demonstrations and John Lennon singing "Imagine." But beyond these perceptions lies the spiritual New Age, the long awaited Golden Era when humanity is predicted to be peaceful, when even carnivores will lie down with herbivores.

Perception of a New Age is defined somewhat by the consciousness of the observer. For some, it is physical 'Earth Changes,' caused by human greed, such as depletion of resources, pollution of air and water, and soil that is contaminated and lifeless, leading to dust storms and floods. Others see these Earth Changes as a repeat of natural cycles and point to archeological data that supports such a theory. Some religious people await the coming to pass of predictions or prophecies, believing either in an end of the world or rescue to another place. For astrologers there are signs that the positions of the planets are in alignment for a major change. Historians read the predictions from centuries and decades ago and watch for them to happen. Spiritual teachers intuitively predict a new consciousness that will change our bodies as well as the way we think and treat each other and our environment. All may be correct.

Perception of a New Age is defined somewhat by the consciousness of the observer.

7 Neil Spencer, *True as the Stars Above*, (London, England: Orion, 2000), 115.

8 Rich Israel and Reny Slay, *Homesteader's Handbook*, (San Francisco, CA: Richard Israel and Reny Slay, 1973).

The coining of the term New Age, has been credited to Swedish Christian mystic Emanuel Swedenborg, Austrian philosopher Rudolf Steiner, and others living during the eighteenth and nineteenth centuries. From roots in such philosophies as Spiritualism, Theosophy, and Anthroposophy come important New Age writers including Helena Roerich, Madame Blavatsky, and Alice Bailey. In 1931, American devout Christian Edgar Cayce, known as the 'sleeping prophet,' founded a research organization in the United States called Association for Research and Enlightenment (ARE), which is still in existence and does research and education in spiritual consciousness specifically in this New Age. Many other 'arms' of the New Age movement have been quietly growing in all parts of the globe, especially in Brazil, Germany, and Russia, where they embrace seekers of all kinds.

New Age concepts and teachings have been documented in a long list of contemporary written works, including, for example: *A Course in Miracles, The Celestine Prophecy, Conversations with God,* and *Autobiography of a Yogi.* Other teachers of timeless works of light include Gary Zukav, Wayne Dyer, Deepak Chopra, Marianne Williamson, Jerry and Esther Hicks, Carol Parrish-Harra, and Ernest Holmes—all writing to empower readers to seek their own truth.

It is easy to see why some of the recent changes around the world might be seen as negative, even evil. The twentieth century, with its almost continuous armed conflict, witnessed the greatest number of human deaths caused by war than any other in recorded history![9] Besides one war after another, climate change and devastating natural events make Earth's existence seems precarious. Following humanity's increasing 'mastery' of the forces of nature, threatened Nature may be striking back. There are lots of formidable problems that humans

---

9 Eric Hobsbawm, "War and Peace in the 20th Century" in *London Review of Books,* Vol. 24, No. 4, February, 2002.

helped create, but collective human choices will also determine the future.

There are lots of formidable problems that humans helped create, but collective human choices will also determine the future.

Economic, industrial, political, military, and social issues are toppling leaders, parties, and governments. People are becoming restless and demanding more out of life. Many no longer allow race, age, religion, gender, sexual-orientation, life-style, geographic location, culture, physical appearance, financial, corporate, or family status, to define what they can have; or be; or do. It is becoming unacceptable to program people's minds to buy unnecessary and potentially harmful manufactured products like pesticides and drugs. There is growing compassion for animals, the Earth, and other humans which will end sending people to war or to destroy their own planet and health. The citizens of Earth are becoming aware and taking action.

The citizens of Earth are becoming aware and taking action.

"Our survival demands a change of consciousness," writes spiritual leader John White. "In addition to threats to life, are signs that the life force itself is mobilizing its resources to resist extinction."[10] Nature constantly evolves new forms of life suited to new conditions on Earth—forms of life which know how to live because their consciousness has changed and they have adapted. Genetically modified organisms, for example, have been observed to revert back to their natural (healthy) forms under the right circumstances. (More on genetic modification in Chapter 11.)

The New Age movement is giving hope to a fearful world. In the past hundred years (a minute fraction of the time that humans have apparently occupied planet Earth), profound cultural changes have made life unrecognizable (to previous generations). Real money and property have been largely replaced by commodities and debt. There has been an explosion each year of the latest 'time saving' technology, 'miracle' drugs, and 'advanced' weapons, rendering people busier,

10 John White, *The Meeting of Science and Spirit, Guidelines for a New Age,* (New York, NY: Paragon House, 1990), 17.

sicker, and more vulnerable. Vast forests have been destroyed along with three quarters of the topsoil, leaving wild animals starving and domestic animals living in deplorable conditions eating unnatural diets. The times have become dark.

There has been an explosion each year of the latest 'time saving' technology, 'miracle' drugs, and 'advanced' weapons, rendering people busier, sicker, and more vulnerable.

The New Age is a dawning of the realization that, for all the advancements of modern times, drastic changes must be made if we are to solve the formidable problems that humanity itself has unwittingly created. The concept of the whole (Holy) is now becoming more important than the instant personal gratification of the past. This is called 'enlightenment.' In response to the global emergency, millions of people are emerging more fully awake to their own inherent abilities. These times, also called the Age of Peace or the Age of Community, are bringing change to the hearts and minds of people all over the world—a move toward love for others and letting go of greed, illness, prejudice, and exclusion. It might be thought of as a 'leaderless revolution,' similar to what is occurring in governments around the world

In response to the global emergency, millions of people are emerging more fully awake to their own inherent abilities.

The New Age is a time of a new revelation of the Divine Feminine, Sophia (wisdom). It is an age of the birth of deep joy. Each human is giving birth to herself. As with most births, there will be pain, confusion, and struggle as we let go of the past and embrace the inclusive, fundamental change of consciousness in the human race. As a mother—all sweaty and shaking, crying and smiling—gazes upon the face of the new child, the fear and chaos evaporate. So it is with the emergence of enlightenment—consciousness of the ever-present truth found within. Humans are no longer seen as Newtonian automatons but as divine creatures housed in living holy temples.

Increased energy segues to the New Age with the ultimate goal of a subtle movement toward *group* enlightenment. It is 'subtle' because in this age of electronic communication, there are no corporations buying advertising time or space to blast notices of the changes...and we all profit equally. The shift is occurring quietly within each person. The New Age also brings an individual approach to spirituality as seekers learn to trust their own inner wisdom (which often agree with the basic original concepts of most religions) at an intuitive level. Attitudes are quietly changing within the hearts and minds of awakening humans and we see each other as kin, neighbors, and friends.

Increased energy segues to the New Age with the ultimate goal of a subtle movement toward group enlightenment.

PROPHESIES OF 'END TIMES'

About fifteen years ago, when I searched the Internet for information on 'Earth Changes,' there were only three websites predicting what, where, and when mass destruction would come to the planet and giving advice for survival—store food, water, guns, and ammunition (similar to the fearful 'Y2K' advice at the millennium change). Now there are pages of sites on the topic. But premonitions of transformation in this time have been recorded for ages—long before computers.

Some of the more famous historical 'seers' include Nostradamus, Edgar Cayce, and authors of the Christian Bible and other sacred texts, which give (often encoded) information about future events. Many are just now being decoded and perhaps that, too, is no accident. Strikingly similar predictions are said to be documented in the Vedas of India, Egyptian Coptic literature, writings of the Essenes, and by scribes from the civilizations of the Hopi, Aztec, and Maya in the Americas.

Prophesies found in the Christian Bible give predictions that mankind will experience Armageddon (end of the world)—flashes of lightning, earthquakes, deception, and a war between good and evil when heaven and Earth will pass away (Revelation 16:16). These concepts might refer to physical Earth changes which are certainly already happening, or maybe to the painful agony of giving birth to a new consciousness within human hearts, for this also could feel like the Earth is moving and the sky is tumbling down. A 'new heaven and a new Earth' (Revelation 21:1) might be the one clearly seen when eyes, mind, and body are purified to receive the intensifying love that is streaming toward humanity. The war *within* each human, however, is far greater than any ever fought on Earth between soldiers.

Nostradamus, a French astrologer, lived and published his works in the sixteenth century and accurately predicted Napoleon's and Hitler's rise to power. Born a Jew, raised a Roman Catholic, and trained as a doctor, he practiced an ancient method of divination to receive visions. Writing in a sort of code verse, he predicted the 'King of Terror' would appear in July of 1999. This 'antichrist' (violent, uncaring attitude that insidiously creeps into the hearts and minds of individuals and groups) called '*Mabus*' or '*Alus*' remains a mystery. John Van Auken, a student of ancient wisdom, muses that these names could be word-plays 'May-b-us' and 'All us.' They might simply mean the attitude of 'antichrist,' as well as the conflict between good and evil that depends upon 'all of us' taking responsibility for our own thoughts and actions.[11]

The war within each human, however, is far greater than any ever fought on earth between soldiers.

Some believe in the emergence of a new 'sub-race' of humans, more highly evolved. Edgar Cayce gave multiple readings to reveal an enormous amount of information over more than twenty years. He called the Aquarian Age the 'Age of the Lily,' for the purity it represents when people will be able to comprehend that awareness occurs for those who seek. He mentions several times that human body structure and chemistry will change, assisting us to become aware that we live within the presence of Life itself. Cayce writes, "Thus be more mindful

11 John Van Auken, *The End Times. Prophecies of Coming Changes*, (Virginia Beach, VA: A.R.E., 1994), 112.

of the body...that it may be a better channel for manifesting spiritual truths."[12] There is some indication that this new 'sub-race' of human will be completed somewhere around 2033–2038 CE.[13]

Carol E. Parrish-Harra, founder of Sancta Sophia Seminary, relates a message she received in 1980 telling of many fearsome earthquakes in coming years. She says the major task of 'children of light' will be to walk through the storm unafraid, knowing it is a tunnel from one time frame into another. It is not the end of the world but the end of a period, dramatically demonstrated. She says our challenge is to be both optimistic and realistic while moving into a 'group consciousness' without resistance and suspicion. "We must dare to be God, no longer the good child but now a dedicated co-creator of a new civilization."[14] Parrish-Harra believes that "humanity is to become aware of unseen life in a way unrecognizable until advanced spiritual senses evolve."[15] At some point, all will be able see the spiritual helpers who have been assisting us, presently only seen by children, animals, and sensitive people.

John Davis, director of Coptic International (a modern Christian congregation based on the philosophy of ancient Egypt), writes about the recently deciphered codes in the Bible. According to him, the book of Revelation can be summed up in verse 12:1: "A woman clothed with the sun, and the moon under her feet, and upon her head a crown of twelve stars." He interprets this verse as the age of re-empowerment of the feminine principle leading to humanity's fulfillment of its spiritual destiny.[16] This results in new freedom for

---

12 Hugh Lynn Cayce, ed., *Edgar Cayce on Diet and Health,* (New York, NY: A.R.E., 1969), 13.

13 John Van Auken, *The End Times, Prophecies of Coming Changes,* (Virginia Beach, VA: A.R.E., 1994), 92.

14 Carol E. Parrish-Harra, *Messengers of Hope, The Walk-In Phenomenon,* (Tahlequah, OK: Sparrow Hawk, 2001), 242.

15 Carol E. Parrish-Harra, Ph.D., *The New Dictionary of Spiritual Thought,* (Tahlequah, OK: Sparrow Hawk, 2002), 17.

16 John Davis, *Revelation for our Time*, (Wyoming, MI: Spiritual Unity of Nations Publishing, 1998), 16.

and unity among all people. While acknowledging that fear sells, Davis says this emergent equality of the feminine and masculine will bring peace. He writes the new world will see the image of a vengeful male God replaced with a kinder, gentler supreme divine intelligence which nurtures all creation.

Ancient and modern prophesies all over the globe agree that something powerful will be happening around now in world history. Most say that the actual happenings as well as the results depend upon human consciousness. We choose between competition and cooperation as we respond to natural changes, apparent shortages, and human technology. The mystery factor of what is going to happen in the New Age is determined by the power of our collective emotions and intent. We get to choose, collectively, and then all will live with what we have chosen.

The mystery factor of what is going to happen in the New Age is determined by the power of our collective emotions and intent.

TIME FRAME AND CYCLES

So, the concept of the 'New Age' refers less to a time period than to a state of consciousness. But there are many formulas, codes, and ways of measuring when each change of ages—during which humans experience a transition—will begin and end. Clairvoyant sources stress that the predicted events are simply 'possible' when conditions are right for them to occur. Each culture called the time divisions by a different name. The actual events themselves depend upon the level of consciousness displayed in human actions, both individually and collectively.

So, the concept of the 'New Age' refers less to a time period than to a state of consciousness.

Nature and all of life are made up of an infinite number of recurring pulses and breaths. Hearts beat predictably and rhythmically. Crickets and frogs serenade the Earth with a soothing cadence. The breath comes in and goes out. The sun comes up and goes down and the moon and the tides keep different cycles. The year is marked by shortening and lengthening days with the accompanying changes in weather and temperature. Plants come up in the spring and die or go dormant in winter. Humans are born and die; with each part of a human life more or less divided into segments where we learn physical mastery, emotional control, mental power, and finally spiritual realization. Life exists in endless cycles.

Astrological, Zodiac, or Great Ages

Life exists in endless cycles.

Beyond heartbeats and seasons of the year, time has been divided into progressively larger cycles called 'ages.' The Age of Aquarius, for example is one of the Astrological, Zodiac, or Great Ages. Probably first described by the ancient Greeks, each Astrological Age is approximately 2160 years long. We are currently leaving the great age of Pisces and entering the Aquarian Age, which is backward from the way the astrological signs appear through the year (where Aries would follow Pisces). Each zodiac age has a new framework of possibilities. These are imperceptible because each person only glimpses a relatively tiny moment in time during their own life time. In each age, latent potentials of humanity are activated, depending upon the maturity and readiness of *each member* of the population.

In each age, latent potentials of humanity are activated, depending upon the maturity and readiness of each member of the population.

Astrologers disagree widely about exact dates, and many overlap, but the following is a brief overview of the past few Great Ages. The naming system varies and is inconsistent. During the Age of Taurus (4200–2100 B.C.E.—Before Common Era), an Earth sign, farming arose and the great stone works like the pyramids of Egypt were built, demonstrating a mastery of matter that still astonishes. The fire Age of Aries followed Taurus, (2100 B.C.E.–1 C.E.) and was characterized by great empires and fighting warriors. After Aries came Pisces (1–2000 C.E.), a water sign, when Christianity was founded with its symbolism of fish, wine, and washing of feet. Pisces may be called an age of emotion and a new-found compassion and faith. When it was taken to extreme, the Piscean age was an era of religious intolerance with zealotry and absolute guidelines, "righteous violence," suffering, and guilt. The present dawning Age of Aquarius (2100–4200 C. E.), an air sign, reflects an inner shift that relates to an awakening of mind in the evolution of human consciousness. The shifting of the ages doesn't happen quickly one morning, but gradually over several centuries. Astrologers disagree about when the current age began, but there are signs that it is already happening.[17]

The Great Year or Precession of the Equinoxes

A larger measure of time is The Precession of the Equinoxes through all twelve astrological zodiac signs. One precession takes approximately 26,625 years (twelve zodiac ages of 2160 each) and is also known as a Great Year (the math is give or take a decade or two).

Yugas or World Ages

There are other divisions of time of varying lengths found in ancient Hindu documents, known as World Ages or Yugas. As with the Zodiac Ages, there is much disagreement about when each Yuga began and ended. The Golden Age in the far distant past lasted 20,000 years. It was followed by the Silver Age, which extended over a period of 15,000 years; then the Bronze Age, 10,000 years long, followed by the Iron Age which lasted 5,000 years. The Iron Age or Kali Yuga is also referred to as the Dark Age. It came to an end as long ago as 1899 when the present New Age, Satya Yuga, age of Light or Truth, began. It will last 2,500 years, half the length of Kali Yuga.[18]

Each Yuga also brings a specific quality which influences the realization of each individual self. In the Golden Age it is said humans

---

17 Ray Grasse, *Signs of the Times*, (Charlottesville, VA: Hampton Roads, 2002), 9–14.

18 Carol E. Parrish-Harra, Ph.D., *The New Dictionary of Spiritual Thought*, (Tahlequah, OK: Sparrow Hawk, 2002), 16, 195.

had greater psychic abilities such as mental telepathy, seeing and hearing spiritual energies, and communing with nature. Life spans were essentially limitless but have decreased with our plunge into darkness during the ages in between.

Gregg Braden, a computer scientist and scholar of ancient teachings, wrote in *Fractal Time* that in addition to entering the zodiac Age of Aquarius, we are also living the end of the 5,125 year long yuga. This World Age ended, according to the Mayan calendar, at the winter solstice on December 21, 2012. The close of one world age is really the beginning of the next and these transitions may be marked by war, suffering, excess, and inequality. But the transitional dark days, while necessary, appear to be brief. We can expect these changes to include physical changes to our planet as well as emotional and spiritual effects on humans. Braden compared predictions of four major traditions—Hopi, ancient India (Vedic), Aztec, and Maya. All predict cataclysm that cleanses one age and prepares the world for the next cycle. All predictions point to the time as right about now. [19]

The New Age

All predictions point to the time as right about now.

So December 21, 2012 marked the beginning of a gradual transition to a New Year (2013), a new Zodiac Age (Aquarius) of 2160 years, a new Great Year of 26,625 years, and a new Yuga (Satya) of around 2500 years, all relatively simultaneously! No wonder there are major adjustments to be made! During this transition, some believe that human perception of time will change. The Mayan calendar appears to end because of this. No one seems to know exactly how it will look. (For those interested in reading more about time cycles, *Fractal Time* by Gregg Braden contains extensive endnotes with references.)

---

19 Gregg Braden, *Fractal Time,* (Carlsbad, CA: Hay House, 2009), 1–5, 73.

PARADIGM SHIFT

New ideas are almost never widely accepted quickly because people think in concepts or paradigms—patterns of thought used for understanding and explaining certain aspects of life. A paradigm shift is a distinctly new way of thinking about old problems. In order to accept the new thought, individuals must let go of the old pattern of thought. It often comes as a "gestalt" or a flip of a switch when a person 'gets it.' The word 'gestalt' literally means 'whole' and refers to a mind-shift that occurs as new insights break through awareness, when a person suddenly perceives something from a new perspective.

According to New Age writer Marilyn Ferguson, we are now experiencing the most rapid cultural realignment in history, and it is taking place across all levels of income, education, and ages—from the humblest to the highest.[20] The participants are teachers, janitors, scientists, office workers, lawmakers, stay-home parents, nurses, artists, and millionaire celebrities. These quiet leaders are reaching for levels of fulfillment that previously seemed impossible, a way that offers a richness of choice, freedom, and human closeness without defensiveness and worry, a way to heal the hurts of the human condition and the opportunity to realign with nature. The 'gentle people' have begun a revolution that examines old assumptions and looks anew at work, relationships, religion, health, politics, goals of humanity, social power, and values.

The new understandings can come as a series of 'light bulbs' that turn on in succession down dark hallways, each illuminating the next in some mysterious way. There is a feeling of some deeper truth that eludes if pursued, yet sits at the edge of 'reality,' whispering and giggling. When a critical number of thinkers have accepted the new idea, a collective paradigm shift occurs and a new phase commences.

---

20 Marilyn Ferguson, *The Aquarian Conspiracy,* (New York, NY: Jeremy P. Tarcher/Putnam, 1980), 23–25.

When a critical number of thinkers have accepted the new idea, a collective paradigm shift occurs and a new phase commences.

Once this journey of discovery has begun in earnest, there is nothing that can dissuade, for it is engagement with 'life' itself.

New Thought, as the New Age paradigm is sometimes called, is a shift from the rational, organized, materialistic left brain to the right brain, which is intuitional, loving, and forgiving. This experience of 'cosmic consciousness' is difficult to explain and must be experienced to fully understand, much like the changes that occur when a person shifts her diet to only pure living vegetarian food.

The shift begins when an individual starts to notice where they are focusing their attention.

The shift begins when an individual starts to notice where they are focusing their attention. Often there is a trigger to this awakening—a life changing event, a loss, an illness, a chance comment that recycles through the mind until it gains the attention of the thinker. And conversely, when the mind awakens it triggers new life events and body changes. Many avoid admitting these changes in thought, because that admission would bring a responsibility for making personal changes in life style and for affecting global transformation. There is a gnawing realization that the so-called 'victim' actually has all the power and is able to change the situation themselves by shifting attention and attitude.

Perhaps the current explosion of 'mass distractions' (media-driven sensationalism) is a result of awakening souls who are frightened of being different. Awakening minds sometimes attempt to avoid the awareness with such things as drugs, alcohol, materialism, denial, sex, food, politics, religion, sports, and disease. But the murmurings of one's 'other self' are inescapable as the Yuga turns. One cannot hide from one's SELF.

CULTURAL AND ECONOMIC CHANGES

With swings in both directions, the economy changes as the attitudes of people change. People today wish for meaningful work, equal pay, and benefits. Real values—like children, education, and good health—are becoming more important than the financial 'bottom line.' There is a respect for natural resources and people are learning to share and live in ways that are kinder to the Earth. As values change, so do the choices of where to spend the energy units called 'dollars.' Recycling, valuing quality, and 'greenness' in businesses are having an impact on the money system of the world. As Americans realize that gluttony will not bring the health, peace, and joy they are seeking, waste and overconsumption are being moderated. Respect for the feelings and instincts of coworkers is changing the way decisions are made.

One cannot hide from one's SELF.

New Agers are likely to have little or no interest in pure materialism. Known as hippies or 'flower children' in the 1960s, New Agers are often interested in community living as a means to conserve resources, resolve relationship issues, and promote local self-sufficiency. They are open to explore new ideas long term and globally. New Agers began the hospice movement to provide dignity and peace as a person dies. They promote ethical investing, socially responsible journalism, and humanitarian efforts to feed the hungry of the world. They visualize a world of peace where swords are forged into garden hoes. New Agers promote nonviolent conflict resolution and the solving of the *causes* of crime, as Jesus or Gandhi or Martin Luther King would do. Hippies have given birth to self-help groups dealing with a wide range of problems and painful situations and have compassion for maligned groups and lifestyles.

New Agers are likely to have little or no interest in pure materialism.

These changes in perception have led to other cultural changes. Often drawn mysteriously to ideas previously foreign, New Agers take classes and read voraciously on energy, healing, and ancient practices, like yoga. The music developed by this group is designed to imbue the listener with peaceful, relaxed feelings to enable her to reach inside to gain perspective on emotional blocks to 'enlightenment.' The music often is meant to be used during meditation.

The realization that women are people is another mark of the cultural change.

The realization that women are people is another mark of the cultural change. It is a New Age phenomenon that married women keep their birth surname, or sometimes both partners change names. But realization is not necessarily 'real-izing,' since most women—while now employed in virtually all the major professions and increasingly assuming leadership roles—are still not paid or recognized equally to men. Some cultural changes take more time than others. But while women are busy bearing and raising children and helping men, they are quietly becoming more and more powerful. They are also learning to support each other.

Other 'minorities' (that often are actually the majority) have been given recognition from New Agers, when previously they were shunned by mainstream religions and the media. These include people of other races, religions, countries, cultures, sexual orientations, physical genders, ages, incomes, and social statuses. These groups, too, need time to achieve equality.

Green building certification, home birthing, recognition of insidious forms of abuse by anyone in a dominant position, animal rights, homeless services (such as Habitat for Humanity), and world disaster aid are a result of the New Age philosophy of compassion and inclusion. The growth of artistic recognition, self-help groups, and of course, peace movements (such the work of the Meta Peace Team and American Friends Service Committee) must be included in the list of New Age cultural developments.

ENVIRONMENTAL CONCERNS

Flower children often attempted back-to-the-land living without experience or knowledge except a copy of *Grow It,*[21] leading to

21 Richard Langer and Susan McNeill, *Grow It,* (New York, NY: Saturday Review Press, 1972).

misinterpretations about their sanity. But they were on the right track. Unconscious farming practices lead to energy and resource depletion. Petroleum, which is dwindling, is used extensively (especially in conventional agriculture) for growing, processing, transporting, and packaging our food. The perception of the Earth as a living entity has led to development of the organic (living) agriculture regulations that offer consumers more choice in the level of chemicals used in the production and preparation of their food. All explorations of New Age thought must include projecting love for the planet and advocating for restoration and preservation of her natural resources and beauty. A preference for chemical-free, heirloom (open-pollinated), and whole, unprocessed foods is a fast growing market trend.

Biodynamic agriculture, originated by Rudolf Steiner, takes environmentally friendly agriculture practices to yet a higher level, incorporating a sort of homeopathic principle whereby substances prepared from plants and animal parts are placed on the land or in compost piles to imbue the soil with the vibrational energy of that plant or animal. Both organic and biodynamic practices use no genetically modified substances and far less toxins than conventional farming, which protects not only the consumer but farm workers as well.

All explorations of New Age thought must include projecting love for the planet and advocating for restoration and preservation of her natural resources and beauty.

Energy prices as well as compassion for the Earth have stirred a revolution in the methods and materials used for new 'green' building construction. Tending toward less toxic and more insulating substances, New Agers strive to do less harm to manufacturing personnel as well as people who inhabit the structures. This revolution also aims to utilize natural energy from sun, wind, and Earth to heat and cool without burning precious fuel. Composting toilets, gray water wetlands, and the conservation of household and rain water have seen growing acceptance. (Read more on environmental issues in Chapter 11).

NEW SCIENCE AND OTHER PHENOMENA

English physicist Sir Isaac Newton (1642-1727), wrote the laws of classical mechanics regarding motion of physical objects. But there has been a perceived clash of science and spirit when bits of data refused to fit into the Newtonian 'machine' scheme, which sent scientists scrambling for new explanations. Einstein's Special Theory of Relativity formed a new paradigm of nature and opened doors for new exploration and the development of quantum theory.

According to American spiritual teacher Gary Zukav, the new science of quantum mechanics resulted from the study of the subatomic realm and is a major discovery about nature. It reveals that, "not only do we influence our reality, but, in some degree, we actually *create* it."[22] The new physics shows clearly that it is not possible to observe reality without changing it. Zukav writes, "The new physics sounds very much like old Eastern Mysticism."[23] *We* are creating the universe. Since we are part of the universe, that makes the universe (and us) self-actualizing.

The new physics shows clearly that it is not possible to observe reality without changing it.

Many 'paranormal' phenomena are associated with the New Age. Crop circles, for example, are controversial, intricate designs that are mysteriously made by the flattening of sections of crops in fields such as corn and other grain, leaving the grain unharmed. They appeared in the media in the 1970s but were reported much before that, mostly in southwest England. Some say they are hoaxes, but others say that calling them a hoax is itself a hoax. Many say they are evidence of visits from beings more intelligent than humans.

Another New Age phenomenon is increased sightings of Unidentified Flying Objects (UFOs)—previously called "flying saucers," which have been reported many times in history. The subject of UFOs has been widely investigated, hotly debated, and watched by many. Even though modern people of the Earth seem to have become

22 Gary Zukav, *The Dancing WuLi Masters,* (New York, NY: William Morrow, 1979), 53–54.

23 Gary Zukav, *The Dancing WuLi Masters,* (New York, NY: William Morrow, 1979), 96.

quite egocentric, it makes sense that there might be civilizations more advanced than ours throughout the cosmos. There might be other planets, other dimensions, or hidden places on and in the Earth which could be inhabited by these cousins and if so, they may want to visit us for some reason. Our attitude toward these 'starfolk' of advanced technology is important, for they surely will reflect our own attitude back to us. They are also sacred.

HOLISTIC HEALTH AND HEALING

The term 'holistic' (whole-istic) means the whole organism has been considered—mind, body, and soul—instead of focusing upon disease symptoms alone. Beyond that, it implies that *everything* is sacred or *holy*—(holy-istic). Holistic healing means to assist in making the many parts unified, to complete not only the physical self but the emotional, mental, and spiritual self, as well. It brings attention to the patient's interpretation of events and symptoms, and to the patient's life situation and history. Holistic wellness is freely flowing energy through and around the physical cells unimpeded by physical toxins, negative emotions, and thoughts that conflict with the higher wisdom of the Self. It comes from the assumption that all illnesses—whether considered infectious, malignant, mental illness, and even so called 'accidents'—originate in the non-physical part of the patient. Pretty much the opposite of conventional medical thinking, holistic health says:

Holistic wellness is freely flowing energy through and around the physical cells unimpeded by physical toxins, negative emotions, and thoughts that conflict with the higher wisdom of the Self.

1. We are all basically well and illness is self-imposed
2. Return to health is a natural phenomenon when mind and body are detoxed
3. Wellness has no known limits and there is no apparent reason that we die

> Sit for a few minutes with these concepts that we are well until the energy of wellness is blocked by toxins or thoughts. Does it change your attitude toward your body?

The New Age has brought a surge of interest in alternative ways to treat conditions outside the Western medical paradigm. Modern medicine has protested alternative therapies, saying the methods are harmful, unscientifically proven, and may delay or detract patients from getting 'real medicine.' But often with the passage of time and persistent questions from patients, mainstream medical providers have increasingly incorporated therapies such as nutritional supplements into practice and invited unconventional practitioners to speak at medical and nursing conferences. Little attention, however, has been given to the harmful effects of allopathic (mainstream medical) therapies, which are in reality a leading cause of death in the United States.[24] Don't toxic pills delay or detract people from seeking the cause of the disease?

HOLISTIC TECHNIQUES FOR HEALING AND WISDOM

All native cultures practice forms of meditation, prayer, and healing while looking to Nature for answers. In spite of efforts by society to institutionalize illness, religion, and education, there have remained the seeds of longing for a simpler life and ancient spiritual traditions. Originally, much esoteric (hidden) wisdom was held secret by priests, but this New Age has seen widespread dissemination of such precious knowledge among common people. Interestingly, the wisdom teachings found in ancient documents from diverse cultures and geographically separated regions are startlingly alike. Some of these teachings focus on connecting to

---

24 Gary Null, Ph.D., Carolyn Dean, M.D., N.D., Martin Feldman, M.D., Debora Raslow, M.D., and Dorothy Smith, Ph.D., "Death by Medicine," *Life Extension,* on Website: lef.org, August, 2006.

and receiving information directly from a spirit source within the reader or seeker. Runes from Norway are 'stones' with symbols that give a message. Cards used for readings, such as the ancient tarot, come from various traditions. Horoscopes increasingly appear in mainstream literature and are used for both entertainment and serious study, assisting transformation. Dream interpretation has become of interest, either in obtaining messages from etheric guides or in reflecting upon what lies in one's own subconscious belief system. Native American lore has contributed smudging, vision quests, the medicine wheel, drumming, and the sweat lodge—all used to assist healing and enlightenment. Ancient 'Mystery Schools' found in many places (especially in Greece and Egypt) teach the concept of self-determined destiny, known today as Law of Attraction. They emphasize that each of us must "know thyself." The Egyptians taught the importance of color, shapes, and aromatherapy. From Hinduism, Buddhism, and other traditions around the world comes meditation. Yoga, very popular today, is from the Hindu tradition. The concept of Feng Shui, as well as acupuncture and herbal therapy, originated in China. From Japan comes the idea of Zen and shiatsu, and from Hawaii, the Huna tradition. The popular Kabbalah (or Qabbalah) and numerology come from Jewish mysticism. All of these holistic practices have been resurrected in the New Age.

Interestingly, the wisdom teachings found in ancient documents from diverse cultures and geographically separated regions are startlingly alike.

DIET

Good nutrition is generally considered part of the New Age consciousness and holistic wellness. It ranges from thinking that 'fine dining' food is healthier than 'fast food,' (it is not) to the practice of fruitarianism (eating mostly leaves and fruit from plants). In addition to organic food, 'health food' is another New Age notion—that "you are what you eat." Raw, vegan, and organic must have been how the first humans ate.

Since the overall health of its people is a major influence on the direction of any society, and considering the changes that are predicted in the world today, diet must be a topic of discussion in these times of increasing illness. Fasting has become more popular, and many New Age thinkers have embraced a vegetarian or vegan lifestyle for various reasons. Some are concerned about the environment. Others believe eating a slaughtered animal imbues the eater with 'negative vibes.' Compassion and a sense of connection to source energy through animals influence still others. Many spiritual teachers urge attention to diet as a way to maintain physical and mental health for the needed tasks ahead. It appears that as we evolve to a higher level of consciousness, there is a desire to transform the way we live in relation to our bodies, to animals, and to the planet—all of which point to a raw, organic vegan diet.

PHILOSOPHICAL BELIEFS

It appears that as we evolve to a higher level of consciousness, there is a desire to transform the way we live in relation to our bodies, to animals, and to the planet—all of which point to a raw, organic vegan diet.

Although there is no single universally-accepted 'doctrine' or 'sacred text,' people who embrace the New Age paradigm tend to have some common philosophical beliefs. There is generally a more loving and inclusive concept of 'creator' than is understood in many modern religions. Often there is interest in an afterlife or in the idea of reincarnation and previous lives. New Age people usually believe that there is a purpose to the life of each person (animals and plants, too) and that there are spiritual lessons to be found in what might have previously been called 'coincidences.' Called 'divine order' by some, there is often the belief that there is a common purpose moving humanity toward goodness or light.

Many New Agers perceive that there are places on Earth that are more energy charged (ley lines and vortexes) or more sacred (like Stonehenge in England) and capable of infusing a person with enhanced energy. Similarly, Earth gems and stones are thought to contain energy.

There is an individual approach to spirituality—a belief that each person contains the seeds to find 'truth,' without necessarily using a religion or religious leader as a guide. Meditation has often replaced religious sermons as important to finding truth. The power of crystals, pyramid shapes, essential oils, incense, candles, and chanting have become popular means to align with a universal intelligence. The New Age philosophy is to empower the individual to seek truth within.

The New Age philosophy is to empower the individual to seek truth within.

RELIGIONS

Though not a religion, per se, New Age concepts are basically aligned with the *original* tenets of all religions. The difference between religious teachers and New Age spiritual teachers is focus. Religious teachers focus predominantly upon the past and what it teaches, and spiritual teachers emphasize the future and how it can be improved from the present. In many ways New Age thought is the re-awakening or remembering of the ancient wisdom teachings.

Religious teachers focus predominantly upon the past and what it teaches, and spiritual teachers emphasize the future and how it can be improved from the present.

Religion can either be a deterrent or play a positive role in the spiritual growth process. New Age leader Carol Parrish-Harra taught that many people who are just beginning to discover the truth of who they really are need religion as a 'handrail'—a prescribed way to think—in order to avoid allowing the dizzying realizations to topple them off balance too much. [25]

About religion, nineteenth-century Hindu saint Ramakrishna said:

25 Carol Parrish-Harra, in many classes and talks.

> *God has made different religions to suit different aspirations, times, and countries. All doctrines are only so many paths; but a path is by no means God Himself. Indeed, one can reach God if one follows any of the paths with whole-hearted devotion.*[26]

Mahatma Gandhi said "Like the bee, gathering honey from different flowers, the wise person accepts the essence of different scriptures and sees only the good in all religions." In the same vein, religious studies scholar, Huston Smith emphasizes the importance of listening to *each other*, because understanding is the only place where peace can find a home. Understanding, then, can lead to love. But the reverse is also true.

Love brings understanding; the two are reciprocal."[27] Many New Agers would agree with Smith's synthesis of certain core concepts common among world religions throughout human history:

1. Ethics (avoid murder, thieving, lying, and adultery)
2. Virtues (humility, charity, and truth telling)[28]

New Age ideas are refreshing to members of religious institutions who have felt judged or abused by the church and have been left with a deep spiritual hunger which is now being filled by the many paths open to those with eyes to see. Churches may need to learn respect for all beings and paths in order to avoid extinction.

Some religions seek obedience through fear, which is the opposite of the Law of Attraction. Fear is illogical—it causes a drowning person to fight her rescuer. Religion can become a distraction which will prevent a person from searching for her own truth. One problem with following a religious leader unquestioningly is that they are frail humans, the same as the rest of us. They too can become drunk with material possessions or power. Each person is therefore ultimately responsible for her own sincere cleansing and spiritual growth. Each

---

26 Ramakrishna, quoted in Huston Smith, *The World's Religions*, (San Francisco, CA: HarperCollins, 1991), 74.

27 Huston Smith, *The World's Religions*, (New York, NY: HarperCollins, 1991), 390.

28 Huston Smith, *The World's Religions*, (New York, NY: HarperCollins, 1991), 387.

person also influences everyone around them, not just their family, friends or students. Unlike religions of the past, the new spirituality welcomes dissenters and no one can possibly be excommunicated or 'defrocked.'

Philosopher, Keith Akers, writes that the early Jewish Christians (Ebionites or possibly the Essenes)—the early followers of Jesus—understood what he taught.[29] They identified with the poor and espoused nonviolence, simple living, and vegetarianism. They condemned temple sacrifices and both human and animal bloodshed (you shall not kill and who kills an ox is the same as kills a man). The early Christians practiced 'laying on of hands' healing, vegetarianism, harmony with Earth forces, and were thrown to the lions for being peaceful (more on the Essenes and the Bible in Chapter 8). These early Christian ideas sound a lot like the peace demonstrators, organic farmers, and energy healers of our time. It appears that Jesus may have been a New Ager.

WHAT 'NEW AGE' IS NOT

The New Age movement is not a threat to traditional religious values or beliefs, for it embraces and incorporates them. Although there are false practitioners, New Agers who subscribe to the idea of karma do not fake paranormal phenomena or metaphysical events. They offer the gifts they receive (energy or wisdom) from their connection with spirit and charge only for their time. Conscious spiritual teachers do not ask their students to turn over all their money or to follow blindly any instructions given them, preying upon the pain and weaknesses of groups and individuals. The New Age is not a religion, a political party, or organization of any sort.

New Age thought is not about giving welfare for more than a temporary measure, but rather empowering each person to access

29 Keith Akers, *The Lost Religion of Jesus,* (New York, NY: Lantern Books, 2000), 7–40.

their own talents and get the necessary training and knowledge to support themselves. It is about personal responsibility without judgment of others. Emphasis is on teaching a person to grow a garden rather than giving her vegetables. Instead of distributing free money, resources are directed to education in order to empower and enhance self-respect and enable a person to work for her own living. Fear and dependence are counter to the New Age philosophy, which says that an equal exchange of energy is healthier than lopsided giving or taking. Money can be used as a weapon to hinder struggling people or as a tool to empower them.

The New Age is not a religion, a political party, or organization of any sort.

New Agers believe fear is the opposite of love. Fear can show up in a variety of ways, including ridicule, anger, and sarcasm. Although often misunderstood, this revolution is not about believing there is nothing wrong or evil in the world. Rather there is a belief that dark and evil are simply a result of blocking the light. In fact, those who follow a spiritual path are often subjected to ridicule and violent opposition before their statements can be accepted as self-evident. Jesus was himself crucified. The light of love is not scary, but finding the path in the darkness might be.

Money can be used as a weapon to hinder struggling people or as a tool to empower them.

WEAKNESSES OF THE NEW AGE MOVEMENT

Matthew Fox, Episcopal priest and theologian (and described by some as a 'renegade clergyman'), identified several drawbacks to joining the New Age movement.[30] One of his concerns about New Agers is they tend to get caught up in the 'all is light' view of reality and ignore the 'dark nights of the soul' (turbulent experiences on the path to higher consciousness), which he believes all of humanity is undergoing. He writes that the journey to the light involves wounds.

Another of Fox's concerns is self-centeredness, which also happens with many radical religious people. It is the "We are enlightened and

30 Matthew Fox, "Spirituality for a New Era" in Duncan S. Ferguson, *New Age Spirituality, An Assessment,* (Louisville, KY: Westminster/John Knox Press, 1993), 208–211.

you aren't" attitude, which often translates to the 'we' being people with enough money to attend seminars and learn the new 'language.' New Agers need to learn that consciousness without conscience is no way to be human, for consciousness and conscience are, like humans, meant to serve each other. He points out the danger of turning one's life over to other people, such as a 'channeler' (who receives messages from the spirit world), ignoring wiser teachers and inner guidance.

Similarly, Ken Wilber wrote in *Yoga Journal* in 1988 that "most good theorists—philosophers, psychologists, and so on—hate being called 'New Age' or being in any way associated with so-called New Age trends, because of the flakiness of so many things called New Age."[31] When setting out on any path of self-improvement, there are both emotional and mental illusions that can cloud vision. It is easy to focus upon one aspect of life to the exclusion of other ideas. Many healers have gravitated from one mode to another, always believing "this is it!" In reality it takes growth on all levels. 'Lenses' must constantly be cleaned to be able to see clearly.

Many spiritually aware people neglect their physical bodies and material orderliness. This is just as off balance as one who is overly concerned with the physical and material to the exclusion of the spiritual self. It is also the responsibility of the aspirant to search for emotional wounds and mental errors. Work, for example, can be as much as an escape as alcohol.

THE AGE OF SPIRITUAL AWAKENING

The purpose of this New Age is spiritual awakening—to realize that *everything* and *everyone* is sacred. In 1990 His Holiness the Dalai Lama wrote:

> *In today's interdependent world, individuals and nations can no longer resolve many of their problems by themselves.*

In reality it takes growth on all levels. 'Lenses' must constantly be cleaned to be able to see clearly.

31 Ken Wilber, as quoted in John White, *The Meeting of Science and Spirit: Guidelines for a New Age,* (New York, NY: Paragon House, 1990), xxii.

We need one another. It is our collective and individual responsibility to protect and nurture the global family, to support its weaker members and to preserve and tend to the environment in which we all live.[32]

Our bodies and the Earth are holy and the conditions are set in this New Age for that truth to be realized. In this—the age of peace—all are called to 'spiritualize matter,' which means becoming aware that physical and spiritual are of the same divine nature. Physical matter is simply vibrating at a slower frequency than spiritual matter. If matter and spirit are the same, then indeed—matter matters!

The purpose of this New Age is spiritual awakening—to realize that everything and everyone is sacred.

With the realization of their own divinity, humans will learn to trust their own inner voice and the benefit of positive thinking, focusing upon that which is desired. Unresolved emotional issues and negative habits of thought and action must be examined, the cause determined where possible, and the power of forgiveness utilized to purify the energy and remove blocks.

In today's interdependent world, individuals and nations can no longer resolve many of their problems by themselves. We need one another.

Alice Bailey was an important spiritual teacher who wrote in the early 19th century at the direction of a spiritual guide named Djwhal Khul (referred to as "The Tibetan"). She writes in *Treatise on White Magic:* "...so the soul in humanity is seeking contact with another divine aspect. When that contact is made...the physical plane will thereby be transformed..."[33] In her book, *The Rays and the Initiations,* Bailey claims "...for in these days many are attaining sight, and light is pouring in. The task ahead is simple. The important aspect, at this time...basic oneness underlying all forms..."[34]

If matter and spirit are the same, then indeed—matter matters!

The difference for New Agers is that there is no outside "god" to impose this upon Earth. Humans, themselves, bring it forth. John

32 *A Policy of Kindness: An Anthology of Writings by and about the Dalai Lama,* (Ithaca, NY: Snow Lion, 1990), 113–114 found in John Davis *Revelation for Our Time,* 167.

33 Alice Bailey, *A Treatise on White Magic,* (New York, NY: Lucis Publishing Company, 1979), 90.

34 Alice Bailey, *Rays and the Initiations (vol. v),* (New York, NY: Lucis Publishing Company, 1988), 300.

White writes, "We are Spirit materialized, engaged in spiritualizing matter."[35] The human being is really a human *becoming*. Self-realization *is* God-realization. When we realize who we really are, we will realize the divine within. It is more of an awakening, cell by cell, of the truth that has always been there, like the fish becoming aware of the water. The movement or 'revolution' seeks to bring about a gentler age, where all matter is made sacred by realizing that it already is. It is a global emergence in response to a global emergency. The health of the individual and that of society are fundamentally interrelated. While pain, terror, disasters, and death *can* be a path of the future, with sufficient awakening within humanity, the world can become what we all want for our children—a place of love.

The difference for New Agers is that there is no outside "god" to impose this upon earth. Humans, themselves, bring it forth.

More accurately, as humans realize that matter is already spirit and that all things are made of the same material (love), they will look at things differently. Instead of fighting each other in fear, they will realize that everyone is alike and wants the same thing—a better life for themselves and their children. Children are the essence of love, and the love a parent feels is almost overwhelming. The umbilical cord never is broken, and the baby is always a very real part of both parents. DNA links us all together. It also explains why we need two—a female and a male—to find our way into a physical body from the spirit world. This overwhelming love will grow to enfold everything and everyone.

We are all mentally connected into the river of consciousness (some call God), and in the New Age we will act without electronic computers the same way birds, fish, and other animals move in formation and never crash into each other. Intuition and telepathy will be the new Internet.

35 John White, *The Meeting of Science and Spirit,* (New York, NY: Paragon House, 1990), xiv.

Vera Stanley Alder, portrait painter and scholar of ancient wisdom, referred to the New Age as the "fifth dimension."[36] She said New Age people will:

1. First, become the perfect animal by purifying the body (she advocates fruitarian diet).
2. Secondly, become the perfect human whose creative mind can mediate between all the kingdoms of nature.
3. The third task is to align with the spiritual soul who is already an inhabitant of the Heaven world.

When these have been accomplished it begins to demonstrate 'whole life' where sharing and 'loving thy neighbor' includes the animal and plant neighbors, with the only goal being to serve each other without being exploited.

Intuition and telepathy will be the new Internet.

How could the fearful Y2K 'survivalists,' with their tanks of gasoline and stash of beans and corned beef hash (with can openers), have known that the changes would occur within themselves? For even though there may be days of dark skies, a new light is being ignited inside the hearts of humankind. Our vision and communication skills will be much better than the telescopes and Internet of this brief age of technology. The mind is the most powerful computer. The 'mind over matter' concept has been around forever; it is just a matter of believing it, using it, and acting accordingly.

The 'mind over matter' concept has been around forever; it is just a matter of believing it, using it, and acting accordingly.

The New Age movement is a conscious evolution—a healthy response to promptings from the cosmos urging us to move toward the light and grow to a higher state of being. Change is always accompanied by chaos. But there are things that a person can do to make the transition easier. One of those things is to detoxify her body by raising the energy of her diet.

A living organic vegan diet assists a person to be physically healthy and mentally alert, which leads to spiritual awareness. This is

36 Vera Stanley Alder, *The Fifth Dimension*, (York Beach, ME: Samuel Weiser, Inc, 1940), 23–24.

a good thing *at* any age and *in* any age; but during these times, at the beginning of the current new age—The Age of Light, around the turn of the second millennium CE (give or take a century or two)—it is especially important.

As it turns out, 'flower children,' while appearing to be lazy, pot smoking spoiled brats who ran to hard-working parents when they needed money, were the childlike precursors of that whom we all must become. Without the drugs, 'flower children' are maturing into responsible conscious adults. We will be peaceful, inclusive, and loving children of the universe, acknowledging that connections with each other, animals, the planet, and all life forms are what we are here to learn. There is always abundance to share if we believe it so.

The New Age movement is a conscious evolution—a healthy response to promptings from the cosmos urging us to move toward the light and grow to a higher state of being.

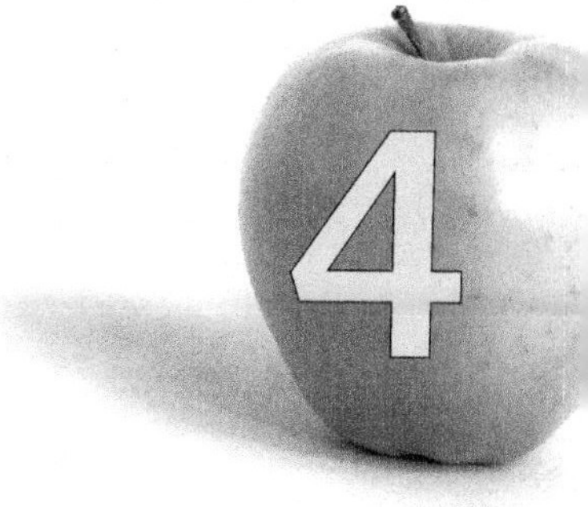

Spiritual Energy

All matter, including your body, is made up entirely of pulsating, living light-energy.

— Natalia Rose

For this chapter, prepare to look at our world in an entirely new way—a way that sees *everything* as energy. This chapter attempts to define the virtually indefinable 'substance' of the universe. Subtle spiritual energy, which ultimately creates health and peace, also forms both solid physical matter and etheric spiritual power. Matter is simply dense spiritual energy, which is why a diet of pure living vegetable food improves body-mind function, apparently by enhancing the flow of energy through the body's electrical system (discussed further in Chapter 6). Also called vibration, light, or love, spiritual energy always heals. Illusions of darkness, negative emotions, or illness are simply blocks in the flow of love-light, a kink in the 'water hose,' like cold is the absence of heat (more on this in Chapter 7).

Matter is simply dense spiritual energy, which is why a diet of pure living vegetable food improves body-mind function, apparently by enhancing the flow of energy through the body's electrical system.

Both science and spiritual study are really trying to understand what nature already knows. Science and spiritual study increasingly appear to be breaking their own laws, and by doing so, are becoming more similar to each other. According to Gary Zukav, the 20th century scientific quantum theory discovered that "it is not possible to observe reality without changing it. Not only do we influence our reality, but,

Both science and spiritual study are really trying to understand what nature already knows.

in some degree we actually *create* it."[37] This view is contrary to the Newtonian mechanical laws of old science described by Isaac Newton in the 17th century, which view the universe as a giant, predictable machine. Spiritual research finds the discovery of the enormous power of human thought, also contrary to old religious dogma, which says an external higher power is completely in charge. Physics has always been considered a science, while thoughts (or prayers) were in the spiritual domain. It now appears, however, that spirit and science are not mutually exclusive.

AN ATTEMPT TO DEFINE ENERGY

The flow of life force energy is the basic component of the universe—the substance, from which everything originates, grows, heals, and evolves, and from which the 'stuff of life' is made. Subtle spiritual energy is ultimately all there is—the matrix of the visible and the invisible world. Energy can be expressed in such forms as matter, light, electricity, will, love, money, intelligence, life, beauty, knowledge, prayer, intention, healing, or intuition. Everything is made of the same spiritual energy. All energy, whether in the form of a thought or temporarily confined to matter (like a tree, for instance), is in constant motion or 'vibrating.' Solid physical things like plants and animals simply vibrate at a slower speed than nonphysical things like love. Nothing ever remains stable, because it is always in the process of change. Not yet fully explained by science, everything from automobiles to anger has a specific vibrational energy, yet no one knows its precise nature.

Subtle spiritual energy is ultimately all there is—the matrix of the visible and the invisible world.

WHAT WE KNOW ABOUT VIBRATION

Streams of energy, constantly in motion, have individual vibrations—a tone, or quality, that influences behavior and can be

37 Gary Zukav, *The Dancing WuLi Masters, An Overview of the New Physics,* (New York, NY: Quill William Morrow, 1979), 52–56.

transmitted and shared. All energy constantly seeks its own vibration. Understanding this concept, known as the "Law of Attraction," is key to spiritual growth. It is an unbreakable law and repeats itself multiple times in nature and in history. When you are attracted to another person it is because there are similarities in your vibrations. You call in your 'similars.' For example, thoughts about a person might make them more likely to contact you.

Intentions (in the form of vibrations) participate in the creation of everything from houses to relationships, from wars to loving peace, from car accidents to glowing health. Nothing was ever created without being the vision in the mind of someone. Rich people intend to be rich and poor people expect to be poor. Energy follows the deepest intent.

Relationships do not just happen; they are the result of the vision in the minds of all involved. Sending love to a person, place, or thing in the form of a memory, a silent message, or a prayer affects the health and welfare of the recipient (and the sender). This is true even if a person has died. You cannot love genuinely without loving yourself. When you fail to forgive, you cut off the energy in your own cells.

> Next time you are waiting in line, try sensing the emotions of other people. Can you feel their anger? Their excitement? Then try sending them silent messages of 'I love you.' Can you feel their spirits lift?

Vibration tends to take on the rhythm of objects and thoughts that come to it, either by physical proximity or by the projection of consciousness from any distance. The influence of vibration is seen in the concept of 'entrainment,' like when old-fashioned wind-up clocks begin to tick-tock in unison. People living together will unconsciously adapt to each other's habits and rhythms, even their menstrual cycles. Moods and attitudes are considered 'contagious,' and sometimes a person will notice a change in attitude just from a brief encounter with a particularly joyful, or 'dark,' personality. Beliefs, attitude, and personality are simply habits of oft-repeated thoughts (which become your unconscious 'story'). We tend to gravitate to others who are like us in some respect, so if you find someone annoying or fascinating, pay close attention, and then look honestly in the mirror.

Beliefs, attitude, and personality are simply habits of oft-repeated thoughts.

SPIRIT IS ANOTHER WORD FOR ENERGY

The word "spirit" comes from the Latin word *spiritus* or "breath." Spirit is the divine spark within each soul—the breath, or essence, of Holy Spirit. [38] It is also widely used to mean all nonmaterial beings or metaphysical substance. Spirit can refer to that part of the universe AND ourselves that is not physical or part of our personality. A 'spirit' can also pertain to any nonphysical entity, but 'the spirit' (or soul) usually denotes the higher vibrational, non-physical part of a person. The term 'spiritual' has become more or less a catch-all word to mean almost anything. This is, of course, true—it does.

Universal spiritual energy, which goes by many names—life force, chi, light, love, ethers, kundalini, vital energy, and prana, for example—is the same as all other energy but vibrates at a higher (less dense or purer) level. It is always present and able to be accessed by asking, when the personality allows. The word 'spirit' can be substituted with the words 'vibration,' 'energy,' 'intelligence,' 'intent,' or even 'god.' The term 'divine' (supremely good) could be attached to any of the above words—divine spiritual energy is the basic essence. Everything is inherently a vibration and has intelligence, from the tiniest cell to the Earth as an entity—even the entire universe, too vast to comprehend. Divine spirit is the unexplained 'ghost in the machine' of Newtonian thought.

---

38 Carol E. Parrish-Harra, Ph.D.., *The New Dictionary of Spiritual Thought*, (Tahlequah, OK: Sparrow Hawk Press, 2002), 280.

The term 'spiritual' can be distinguished from 'religious' by the amount of autonomy encouraged in the individual. The New Age meaning of 'spiritual' is the allowing of each soul to reach individual understanding of truth by listening to the urgings from her own heart or spirit within. Religion is characterized by adherence to a group who follow the teachings of a particular leader, often overlooking the importance and power of each individual person. This is not to say that teachers are not important. They are most valuable; and whether or not they are aware, each person always serves as both teacher and student in every interaction. Sometimes religion is part of a soul's path and sometimes not. Both the labels 'spiritual' and 'religious' can serve as distractions, blocking energy. Both can be used as fearful weapons on fellow life-travelers.

Earlier civilizations, before modern science 'advancements,' often believed in two worlds—the physical world of nature and the unseen spirit world. Death was considered the transfer of the person's soul back into the spirit world. Special people (called healers or shamans) were believed to be able to find the energy block of a patient by contacting the spirit world, and thus improve the energy flow, sometimes using an herb or rock whose energy was beneficial. The New Age is recycling these ideas. Spirit energizes matter. Matter influences the thoughts and the energy of minds. Minds generate and direct the flow of energy.

Spirit energizes matter. Matter influences the thoughts and the energy of minds. Minds generate and direct the flow of energy.

ENERGY AND MATTER

All matter is composed of some arrangement of atomic and subatomic particles. When these particles are scientifically investigated, they behave as if they are both matter and energy, but inside each particle, only energy is found. Matter seems to be but frozen light, highly complex energy fields governed by the laws of nature. Energy in matter can be in the form of solid, liquid, or gas. Solid things like wood are vibrating at a different speed from liquids, gases, feelings, and attitudes. This is similar to water being in the form of solid ice or steam vapor, where the molecules vibrate at different speeds.

The subtle energy that comprises matter carries the information and intelligence to arrange itself into molecules, cells, and organisms, creating order and becoming the living systems of nature. There is energy and intelligence in every molecule. Matter follows the organizational instruction of energy and in nature is generally recyclable after being temporarily condensed and released, like when plants become soil again. Present bodies are actually made of material from the past, therefore, everything and everyone is connected.

ENERGY AND LIFE

The proposal in this book is that live food enlivens a living body, allowing love to flow in and around the cells, stimulating resolution of emotional blocks and thus leading to spiritual awakening. Then 'life' itself must be defined as well. The dictionary says life is an "organismic state characterized by capacity for metabolism, growth, reaction to stimuli, and reproduction."[39] Each living thing is a separate entity, although some are parasites and must live in the presence of certain other organisms. Stones and other inanimate objects contain energy of varying qualities but are not alive. Everything that is alive has energy but everything that has energy is not necessarily alive.

Living organisms contain organs—parts that function together for the good of the whole. They often produce heat and exert some sort of mobility on the Earth. Other qualities, assumed exclusive to living

39 Merriam Webster's Collegiate Dictionary, Tenth Edition, (1993), 672.

organisms, are spirit or soul and a degree of consciousness, defined by some as the capacity to love and respond to love as displayed by animals and plants. Living organisms can be the generators (creators) as well as batteries of love energy, while inanimate things can only hold energy. Life is a fine thread linking an organism with the divine whole.

Living organisms can be the generators (creators) as well as batteries of love energy, while inanimate things can only hold energy.

Living things produce other living things and lend their love to nourish and sustain new life. Bacteria and other tiny creatures in the soil, for example, enliven it and make it hospitable to plants, which nestle their roots into it. Dry sand without moisture or microbial life will grow little food. Prayers and love of a parent sustain and teach the young. Life ignites life, similar to the lighting of one candle from another.

A lack of love gives the illusion that we are somehow separate from the source of love, spawning a deep existential longing—when in fact, we are *part* of it, made of it, breathe it, and eat it every day. Feeling separated from love creates a longing and a search. The more terrible the longing, the more intense is the search. We are searching for ourselves, but we sometimes glimpse that bliss when we fall in love with another, thinking they are that for which we long. As mentioned earlier, Meher Baba, wrote about this, "To attain union is so impossibly difficult because it is impossible to become what you already are! Union is nothing other than knowledge of oneself…"[40] Living matter responds to love and dies without it.

Life ignites life, similar to the lighting of one candle from another.

Living material things often appear as a miniature image of the whole, a fractal, a hologram—like the veins of a leaf are similar to the branches of the tree (or vice versa). As above is also true below; heaven and Earth. You are a miniature mirror of the universe.

Living matter responds to love and dies without it.

40 Meher Baba, *The Everything and the Nothing,* (Berkeley, CA: The Beguine Library, 1963), 1.

THOUGHTS AND EMOTIONS ARE ENERGY, TOO

Thoughts—and the emotions those thoughts generate—are energy perceived by the matter of a human mind or body. Positive thoughts of love are of higher vibration than darker thoughts of fear, which are the result of blocking vital energy in some way, like a shadow. All positive thoughts are love and all negative thoughts are a form of fear. Love is all there is and fear is simply disallowed love. One way to determine if thoughts are in alignment with the positive vital energy of the universe is by the emotions they evoke. If a thought produces a positive emotion, it is in harmony with your higher self, but if anger or fear is felt—think again.

Love is all there is and fear is simply disallowed love.

When the sun is blocked by rain clouds it doesn't mean the sun has gone away. It is just an illusion. The same is true with emotions. We tell ourselves things that evoke negative feelings. 'Mind clouds' are just fluffy untruths we tell ourselves and each other. They block the love and give the illusion of aloneness. The sun still shines when it is raining. Love still awaits a depressed or angry person.

THREE MORE EXPRESSIONS OF SPIRITUAL ENERGY

Light

Light is another word for spiritual energy.

Light is another word for spiritual energy. Some can actually see this flow of energy radiating from and between people and objects. Indeed one can *feel* light pouring into areas of the body when healing is occurring. The light or wisdom within us attracts our attention to details that are essential to promoting the fulfillment of life's purposes. Light is the basic component from which life is made and grows.

Nature and natural things seem to have a rhythm that follows the pattern of light and darkness. There is a time of rest that (for most) correlates with night, and each morning marks a new beginning—a metaphor for the nature of life itself. The light contracts in winter but never goes completely away. In spring it emerges with increased intensity and number of daylight hours, stimulating new growth that will produce seeds for the next cycle. Each spring provides another chance to learn and complete a predetermined cycle.

The light energy of the sun is received on Earth and energizes life. Strangely, sunshine has a spotty history of being alternately utilized as a healing remedy and condemned as dangerous to health. David Wolfe, a foremost authority on raw-food nutrition, is convinced that people who detoxify their bodies on raw organic vegan food are less likely to be harmed by conscious exposure to sunshine.[41] Exposure to sunlight is as essential as touch for health and well-being and is a key in preventing serious and life threatening diseases. The energy of the sun, essential for plant and animal life, is life force energy itself, of which all plants and animals are composed.

Illness and depression occur when light energy is cut off, just as night occurs when the sun goes to the other side of the Earth. (See Chapter 7) En-'light'-en-ment occurs when thoughts of higher vibration penetrate the dark thoughts, when new truth dawns in the mind.

Love

Divine energy, also known as Lots Of Vital Energy—LOVE, is always moving toward the positive. The Biblical quote "God is love"[42] is quite literal. Love is the substance that flows through, creates, and enlivens everything. When love is flowing, there is peace and wellness. It is always there, whether one is conscious of it or not—like water to a fish. Free flow of positive energy is the cause of health and it constantly

---

41 David Wolfe, *The Sunfood Diet Success System,* (San Diego, CA: Maul Brothers Publishing, 2002), 304.

42 Holy Bible, King James Version, (Cleveland, OH and New York, NY: The World Publishing Company), I John 4:8.

churns, turning negative into positive, enlivening the blocked areas in our bodies. The love energy from the sun in living food profoundly affects the diseased parts and restores life.

Water

Water is both spirit and a most useful physical substance, literally essential to life. It has been the object of political disputes in the past and is likely to be a much greater cause of serious clashes in the future. Water is not destroyed, but humans have reduced its usefulness by contaminating and restricting the flow of rivers, changing the natural distribution of water often driven by a profit motive.

Scientifically, water has many unique and mysterious properties. Its boiling point is quite different from other oxygen compounds. It holds heat better than other related substances, moderating nearby climates of the Earth. Water is the only substance that in its frozen state becomes lighter than in the liquid state, thus allowing life to continue beneath winter's ice. Lightning and thunderstorms enhance the energy of animals and plants.

Vital in the body, water acts as both a solvent and a means of transport, detoxing and nourishing the cells. Human bodies contain essentially the same percentage of water as the surface of the Earth (approximately seventy percent). The composition of our extracellular fluids and that of ocean water is also similar. Being even a little dehydrated is a common cause of lack of energy and a possible underlying issue in physical conditions like asthma. Water conducts electricity and playing in water keeps the energies of the body clear. A shower also cleanses the body's aura or energy field, so showering at the end of the day removes the negativity encountered that day and enhances sleep. Water, made of subtle spiritual energy, is used in baptism, a purification ritual. Washing an object with water seems to restore the vital energy of the object. Associated with spiritual wisdom, it is used for healing in mineral springs, steam baths, and hot tubs.

Japanese scientist, Dr. Masaru Emoto writes, "Water is the mother of life, while also being the energy for life."[43] He took photographs of ice crystals, dramatically demonstrating changes to the water that reflected the intent or prayers of people around it. The water actually reacted to the intent of a person saying things like "thank you" or "you fool." Ice crystals, he says, are closely and permanently linked to the human soul, because they contain the key to the mysteries of the universe. This key can unlock the consciousness required to understand the proper order of the universe and our role in it. Emoto believes that water is the same as the soul; and since the body is mostly water, from a physical and spiritual perspective, the body *is* the soul. Water is literally life force energy. He says people who are in good health are also likely in good spirits. Rain, droplets of vital life energy, is truly manna from heaven!

Water is literally life force energy.

WHERE DOES ENERGY COME FROM?

Another usage of the word 'spirit' is as a name that humans give to their highest conception of an infinite living mind, a conglomerate of all life, of which 'lower' life is an integral part. This is the core of life—the central intelligence of the universe. This core is also called god, goddess, allah, nirvana, nature, brahma, holy spirit, creator, cosmic fire, and yahweh, among others, and is found within each living thing. The name of this source of spiritual energy has been bitterly fought over and has caused much suffering and grief, war and judgment, exclusion and prejudice. Indeed, fighting over the name of spirit is like railing against nature or suing your parents for the color of your eyes. Should we try to stop the snowflakes?

---

43 Masaru Emoto, *The Hidden Messages in Water,* (Hillsboro, OR: Beyond Words Publishing, 2004), 56.

Spirit transcends our understanding, and we use the term merely that we may think and speak of 'the all', which cannot be explained or defined. Spirit is the divine intelligence which underlies all life and directs the changes that evolve all creation to ever greater degrees of wholeness and of which we are all a part. Surely none of the original teachers, upon whose teachings religions were built, intended their words to be used in violent and harmful ways. Jesus, who has been called the Prince of Peace, would surely not advocate killing those who call universal intelligence by a different name.

Spirit is the divine intelligence which underlies all life and directs the changes that evolve all creation to ever greater degrees of wholeness and of which we are all a part.

WE ARE ENERGY

Humans are made of spiritual energy as are all animals, plants, and minerals in the universe. The nature of the energy in and around human bodies as well as how these energies relate to health will be discussed in Chapters 6 and 7. The body has levels of energy—physical matter, as well as emotional and mental vibrations. Past emotions are lodged in the tissues of the physical body.

Enzymes are vibrational components of the physical body—some say they are pure spiritual energy—and will be discussed in Chapter 8. Enzymes are mysterious strings of living proteins that direct the subtle life force in basic biochemical and metabolic processes of the body, even helping to repair DNA (the genetic blueprint in the cell). They act as catalysts for the chemical reactions of life, such as digestion, speeding up the rates at which these processes occur. Enzymes are necessary because, if they weren't present, the reactions would not take place fast enough to support life. They represent the 'life' element, which is biologically recognized but can be measured only in terms of activity. Some say enzymes *are* life itself, prana made physical.

Some say enzymes are life itself, prana made physical.

THE ENERGY OF THE EARTH

The Earth is an enormous energy field in a sea of an infinite number of heavenly bodies. The subtle energy in and around the Earth is arranged into a complex web of energy lines, vortices and a grid-like lattice. These energy patterns (called ley lines) are known by native people and contain both positive and negative energy spots. Sensitive people are able to detect these energy lines intuitively, sometimes by using 'dousing' techniques where questions are answered from the inner self using an instrument, such as wires which move in revealing ways. Water beneath the Earth's surface can be detected by silently asking to be guided to a source of water. Holding the wires loosely in both hands and walking over the land, the wires will 'magically' move when water is accessible beneath the spot.

Sacred sites with powerful positive energy can be enormously healing, facilitating the resolution of deep negative emotional and physical energy congestion and depletion. Sensitive people can detect these energies readily but everyone is unconsciously drawn or repelled by them. The geomagnetic field of the Earth's core stimulates the life that thrives upon her skin. Churches and other structures are often located on intersections of energy lines. Some of humanity's troubles may be due to our attempt to live detached from nature and the energies of the Earth in tall steel and concrete buildings that change and restrict the flow of Earth energies.

The geomagnetic field of the Earth's core stimulates the life that thrives upon her skin.

Subtle energies on the Earth are affected by the moon, the sun, rainstorms, and other planets. They are also affected by human inventions like those powered by electricity, the power lines that drape across the land, and the electromagnetic fields created by using electric and electronic appliances, which alter the natural energy and rhythms of the Earth. They also have a subtle negative effect on people and other living things. Therefore, it is good to keep power lines, cell phones, televisions, even clocks, away from the body, particularly while sleeping.

ENERGY FROM OBJECTS AFFECTS US

Intelligent living organisms (plants and animals) generate new energies, while nonliving material and objects serve as a reservoir or battery.

Intelligent living organisms (plants and animals) generate new energies, while nonliving material and objects serve as a reservoir or battery. Objects inherently contain vibrational energy and, like living things, have the potential to absorb and store energy from other objects and beings around them. There are people who can give accurate information about the person who last touched or who owns an object by sensing its energy. The vibration of an object is altered by the intent of the user. A knife that is used to chop vegetables would have a different energy from the same type of knife used with intent to harm an animal.

Even the placement of objects in the environment affects our energy. Feng Shui is the Chinese study of the flow of energy (or 'chi') in a space and how it can be enhanced to create harmony and balance. Subtle reaction to placement, structure, decor, and arrangement of a home or business affects the energy of occupants.

A room retains energy after an argument or fearful encounter (or loving exchange). All people, if aware enough, are able to detect this energy. Events can also be sensed before they occur in order to move to safety. Conversely, people are often found congregating where the energy feels good. The energy emanating from another person is a form of exchanging energy, and it is possible to tell if there is malevolent or benevolent intent even without words. It becomes a matter of trusting what you have innately detected. Mediums are skilled at this and are sometimes consulted in solving mysteries.

Many people save money by shopping for clothing at recycle shops. When your attention is attracted to a garment and after checking the fiber content (natural fibers are of a higher vibration than plastic fibers), it is a good idea to 'check the energy' to see what feelings are evoked when you put it on or hold it close. Sensitive people might get the feelings of the previous owner or shop workers who recently handled it. If it feels good or if you feel the energy can be enhanced by washing or blessing, then buy it—if not, leave it.

Crystals, rocks, and magnets reflect energy that affects all life forms—animals, plants, and humans. They are believed by many to have inherent healing properties and protective rays. After absorbing negativity, the energy of a gemstone can be cleansed with running water, sunlight, or by intentionally blessing it, which restores its ability to absorb negativity around itself again.

Plant vibration is often beneficial for animals and can be collected and sold in distilled form called 'essential oils.' The energy and fragrance of plants are used to balance a person's mood, enhance energy, dispel blocks causing negative emotions, and stimulate tissue healing. Essential oils are believed to encourage the oxygenation and opening of the cells to receive life force energy. They have been used for centuries to protect from diseases and raise vibration.

In the book *Anastasia* (Book One), Anastasia gives advice for enhancing the ability of a plant to facilitate human healing.[44] She instructs the gardener to hold a few seeds in her mouth and then between the palms of her hands while standing barefoot in the garden. Then present the seeds with open hand to the heavens before planting without watering right away. In this way the seed takes information from the gardener's body that will later assist in healing as well as slowing what is considered the 'aging process.' The energies of human bodies, living plant seeds and the love of the universe all cooperate in healing each other.

44 Vladimir Megre, *Anastasia, The Ringing Cedar Series, Book One,* (Kahului, HI: Ringing Cedars Press, 2008), 78.

Homeopathy is a vibrational alternative medicine based on the 'law of similars' used to treat a variety of symptoms by administration of essences that will produce symptoms similar to those of the patient. The preparations are made by diluting (usually with water) a substance (such as an herb), often until there is none scientifically detectable. These essences are thought to contain the powerful etheric field of the substance, which reacts with the energetic flow of the body to aid in healing.

The biodynamic farming movement, inaugurated in 1924 by Austrian scientist Rudolf Steiner, might be compared to homeopathic philosophy. Naturally occurring plant and animal materials are prepared in prescribed ways and left for a period of time to absorb energy. Then small amounts of the aged preparations are added to a compost pile or sprayed over the land after stirring in water. The idea is to give the organizing energy of the original substance (such as a dandelion) to the soil, which ultimately strengthens the animal that eats the enhanced plant grown on that soil. It also heals the Earth herself.[45]

If objects around us can have such a profound effect, imagine what the energy of food moving right through the core of your body can do to the vibration of your cells. If food is cooked or 'killed' in other ways, the living body must 're-energize' it in order to digest and assimilate its nutrients. What a joy to the little cells of the body when the original, vibrant energy of living plants moves in such close proximity in the digestive tract!

THE SEVEN RAYS

Teachers of ancient wisdom explain that pure life force energy is divided, moderated, and dispersed before it reaches our solar system

---

45 Sherry Wildfeuer, "An Introduction to Biodynamic Agriculture," *Stella Natura*, 1995.

or it would destroy the known human world. This energy, which builds everything seen and unseen, is arranged in streams or rays of different qualities that guide and control nature in specific ways. These universal streams of energy are called the Seven Rays and are divided into seven primary rays and seven sub-rays, sometimes compared to the colors of the rainbow or the colors refracted when sunlight is passed through a prism or crystal. Each ray has its own special attributes and qualities, and functions in a constantly striving field of energy which is never static, because the incoming energies continually vary and change, evoking new conditions. Each ray can be said to carry both positive and negative qualities, which will be individually manifested by the will of human intention. Like an astrological sign, a person's ray influence is more or less permanent, but only describes tendencies.

If objects around us can have such a profound effect, imagine what the energy of food moving right through the core of your body can do to the vibration of your cells.

Ray One is known as masculine will and power while Ray Two is love and wisdom—feminine characteristics. The Third Ray is active intelligence; the Fourth depicts harmony through conflict. The Fifth Ray is concrete knowledge and science, and the Sixth is devotion and idealism. Finally, the Seventh Ray represents order and ceremony. These qualities have influenced mankind throughout the ages. Each person (mostly unconsciously) chooses from a tapestry of qualities within their ray energies when making life choices.

Spiritual student Michael Eastcott writes that in the New Age we are moving away from the influence of the paternalistic Sixth Ray which represents undeviating devotion, unquestioning obedience, and belief in a chosen ideal, which has led to a tendency to exaggerate and intensify. Sixth Ray people tend to be either militant or unquestioning servers. Both mystics and fanatics come from this ray of great illumination and cruelty. The New Age is influenced by Ray Seven, the ray of law and order, which is already working with the Sixth Ray of the last age to bring in spiritual life forces and anchor them upon Earth to spiritualize matter.[46]

This New Age of Ray Seven will oversee right use of world resources, unity and connectedness of all people, right use of organization, and recognition of the animal 'kindom' (all are kin). Seventh Ray people pay attention to detail and create beauty with music, words, dance, and architecture, with links to the mineral kindom. They can also be over-organized and purist in nature. As with the influence of all the rays, Ray Seven people must strive for balance. The shift of ray influence is in addition to the increased spiritual energies influencing the Earth's family at this time.

Humanity is presently under the power of increased cosmic loving energies, which are impacting the rhythms and cycles of the earth and all her inhabitants.

ENERGIES ARE INCREASING IN THE NEW AGE

Humanity is presently under the power of increased cosmic loving energies, which are impacting the rhythms and cycles of the Earth and all her inhabitants. This higher vibratory frequency, from the higher intelligence of another dimension of which humans have little memory, is being sent to assist humanity and the planet during this tremendous energy shift to greater consciousness and will have a vast impact upon all. According to Alice Bailey, this pouring out of love upon the masses is leading to the emergence of the New Age. She predicts that humanity will eventually decide upon right action, saying, "In the wars raging today between conflicting ideas, only the voices of intelligent thinkers of goodwill can save the world from chaos."[47] Intelligent, awakened people do not harm each other!

Intelligent, awakened people do not harm each other!

These changes are not a form of chastisement from a 'god,' but merely the natural laws of Karma (direct effect of a cause) and are according to the Divine Master Plan (of which we are all a part).

46 Michal J. Eastcott, *The Seven Rays of Energy* (Kent, England: Sundial House Group, 1980), 52–54, 79.

47 Alice Bailey (The Tibetan), *The Rays and The Initiations,* (New York, NY: Lucis Publishing Company, 1960), 641.

Although each human can affect the course of events within the elements of her personal life, the overall destination, like the seasons of the year, cannot be modified by an individual alone. That takes the intent of humanity working as a collective.

The New Age energetic conditions make a breakthrough of human consciousness not only possible but necessary. Along with the new technologies and scientific discoveries of our time, there are areas of our brains that are changing in preparation for the future, when the concepts built on the five senses will no longer be adequate. Current technology and manipulations by science will be enhanced and sometimes rendered unnecessary by advanced, innate senses. In fact, technology might seem painfully slow, as humans acquire the ability to communicate and heal the body by changing genetic material, identifying and repairing errors in the energy field of themselves, each other, and the Earth.

Effects of This New Energy on Humans

Many believe the new energy will change physical structures, and affect emotions and mental functioning as well. There will naturally be chaotic emotional feelings, confusion, and fear; but there are 'helpers' sending nurturance and guidance to assist. Sleep cycles, food preferences, and even minor illnesses may be a part of these changes, and many will complain of feeling peculiar for a while.

Individual humans adapt in various ways to the new pressures. Some may develop mental or physical illness and disappear into the medical system. Others lower their heads and run with determination, eyes closed, stupefied with fear. And a third group is called "super-sane" by neuropsychiatrist Shafica Karagulla—humans with "higher sense perception."[48] These people may be the beginning of humans

48 Shafica Karagulla, MD, *Breakthrough to Creativity,* (Marina del Rey, CA: DeVorss & Co, 1967), 22, 31.

evolving the ability to observe and experience dimensions of environment, of which most are not currently aware. These super-sane people tune into the vibration of things, places, and the thoughts and physical sensations of others.

The powerful new subtle energies are already having an impact upon our bodies. It is believed that many 'new' diagnoses such as some autoimmune diseases could possibly be the result of asking for spiritual enlightenment in a receiver that is too congested and polluted to hold the impact. It is not the energies 'causing' the 'disease' but a result of the impurities found in the physical tissues. The increase of mental/emotional conditions and other illnesses, particularly the ones that seem to disappear on the live vegan diet, might be connected with the new energies.

These super-sane people tune into the vibration of things, places, and the thoughts and physical sensations of others.

Care must be taken to remember that the path is different for each person and each will need to adjust as she travels toward her truth and light. What meets the needs of a person at one vibratory level will be wrong at another vibration. It is not for another to judge where a person is on their personal journey or what they need to experience along the way.

How Can Humans Adjust to the New Energies?

The higher vibration of the new energies is not in harmony with the energies of the majority of toxic bodies in present day society. The new energies will cause problems in a polluted body—like using too much voltage to supply a faulty or too small appliance (one with a short circuit, for example). The massive flow of electricity coming in cannot be handled by the appliance, resulting in 'fried components' probably overheating, and causing a fire. It is like lightning hitting an unprotected computer. Similarly, the stepped up energy intensity of the New Age leads to problems in the human 'electrical system,' which affects us physically, mentally, emotionally, and therefore spiritually. The beautiful light of these New Age energies cannot be appreciated or effectively utilized in the dense darkness of a polluted, short-circuited body.

The beautiful light of these New Age energies cannot be appreciated or effectively utilized in the dense darkness of a polluted, short-circuited body.

In order for the 'new human' to be born, it is important to accept responsibility for the health of one's own body. What a person thinks and does affects her body, as well as the thoughts of others and the whole of our collective life experience. If negative, fearful thoughts are created, they will lead to negative emotions which over time will disrupt the balance of health and be lodged in the tissue of the body. These negative emotions can be physically felt as pain and lumps within the tissue and eventually fester into diseases. Being actively conscious can prevent problems. Already established energy blockages can be removed by adopting an open mind and conscious intent for health and good will. Actions are loudly expressed intentions, and diet choices reflect that intent. Energy healers, both heavenly and in the flesh, can also be of great assistance in this process.

Suffering was never intended and can be avoided by becoming increasingly conscious of thoughts, quality of food, toxins, sleep and rest, and exercise. Deliberately find the time for quiet communing with nature herself. In the midst of frantic human drama, it is possible; no, it is essential, to be still and know that we all are of divine nature and part of the divine plan.

In the midst of frantic human drama, it is possible; no, it is essential, to be still and know that we all are of divine nature and part of the divine plan.

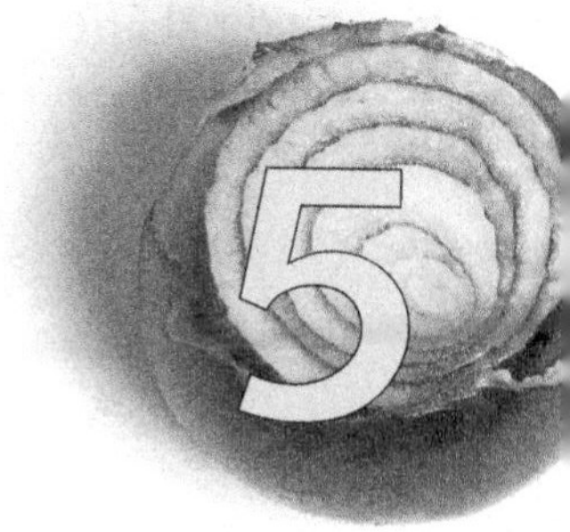

Becoming Conscious

There is no birth of consciousness without pain.

— Carl Jung

In ordinary language, 'conscious' simply means 'awake,' like after anesthesia; but in this chapter, the word is used to mean much more than that. This is a discussion about higher consciousness, a sort of 'super-consciousness,' if you will; a profoundly keener awareness known as 'spiritual consciousness.' The 'super-sane' described by Karagulla (see Chapter 4) are people who have a comprehension beyond mere understanding. It is like taking a course in psychology with a good score on the test—but then years later you *really* 'get it.' Everyone is capable of spiritual awareness all their life, not just 'gifted' people. Similar to the phases of mastery a child grows through on her way to adulthood, spiritual knowing entails progressively deeper perceptions of the various *dimensions* of the commonly known world.

Like plants, humans need to dig deeper into *hidden* dimensions in order to grow higher toward the light. These dimensions, all sacred and vitally important, include:

1. Physical matter—the intelligence of the body and its Earth and sky environment
2. Emotions and the information they deliver
3. Mental processes and their control over awareness at other levels

4. Spiritual aspects of self, other people, and helpers from the unseen spiritual dimension

Physical, emotional, mental and spiritual aspects intermingle and interact to move individuals toward ultimate 'enlightenment.' Consciousness is the result of the interaction between spirit and matter awakening the reasoning mind to deeper knowing. Higher consciousness, then, is the recognition of all dimensions in both tiny and profound ways.

LEVELS OF CONSCIOUSNESS

Conventionally, the mind is divided into three levels of awareness:

Higher consciousness, then, is the recognition of all dimensions in both tiny and profound ways.

1. Conscious mind—the readily aware and alert level, controlled by the owner
2. Unconscious mind—the level of semi-awareness
3. Subconscious mind—the level of which the owner is not normally aware

The term 'unconscious' is used in normal language to mean the inability to respond, such as in a coma or under anesthesia. It can also refer to a habit that becomes automatic, like driving to work unaware of the turns. Another use for the term is when something occurs that hints of a belief that is normally buried in the subconscious as in a 'slip of the tongue' or revelation in a dream. The unconscious lies between conscious awareness and the out-of-reach subconscious, occasionally glimpsed by the conscious mind.

The unconscious lies between conscious awareness and the out-of-reach subconscious, occasionally glimpsed by the conscious mind.

The subconscious is the largest part of the proverbial mental 'iceberg' buried under the observable, comprehending mind above the water and just beneath the unconscious, found at the 'waterline.' People do not directly experience their subconscious—an important part of their own mind—yet it has vast consequences in their lives. It logs and catalogs all past experiences as well as the reaction to and beliefs about them. This is the part of consciousness that is programmed in childhood and subtly but firmly incorporated into the personality. It becomes what is often referred to as the 'inner child' or low self.

People do not directly experience their subconscious—an important part of their own mind—yet it has vast consequences in their lives.

> Next time you get a 'deja vu' feeling or other unexpected emotions, stop and let it take you to the memory or feeling. It could help you heal something.

Medically, consciousness is measured by what *appears* to be a patient's awareness of the physical world and things in it. Different states are measured by the difficulty of getting a person to respond, which *theoretically* is the outward manifestation of the brain function. However, people who are under anesthesia or temporarily clinically dead, have accurately reported the activity in the room at the time of 'death.' There are obviously 'other' awarenesses!

In some schools of ancient wisdom such as Huna, from Hawaii, there are considered to be three 'selves.'[49]

1. 'High' self—divine healing self, super-conscious; holds profound universal wisdom
2. 'Middle' self—conscious, decision-making, aware rational mind that thinks and feels
3. 'Low' self—the half-hidden unconscious and the hidden subconscious or inner child

There are obviously 'other' awarenesses!

The 'middle' self-governs mental function, which guides and directs day-to-day activities and makes the decisions that determine the direction and nature of one's life. This is the adult-you. The thinking 'middle' mind *can* attain information from both the other selves. The perceiving middle self can choose to have access to the

49 Max Freedom Long, *What Jesus Taught in Secret,* (Marina del Rey, CA: DeVorss & Company, 1983).

'high' self, which is in close contact with higher realms of universal intelligence/wisdom, and it can watch for 'clues' from the 'low' self.

The 'high' self is the older, wiser, parental part which is peaceful and utterly trustworthy. It is the loving, forgiving place of deep meditation. High self is intuition, inspiration, and the loving 'angel' part of each of us. It teaches us to love ourselves as well as care for others. It gives us the best answer, which is always the fear-free choice.

Known as the 'inner child,' the 'low' self is the silently suffering, just-out-of-reach part of consciousness which is sometimes thought to actually *be the physical body* itself. If the subconscious mind and the body are the same, then health issues are a huge clue to the content of the subconscious mind. The information-processing 'middle' self has significant influence over the 'low' self, which harbors beliefs and emotions from 'secret' early experiences. This is because it is the rational mind that interprets for the inner child. For example, the same event, like a divorce, might be judged 'tragic' or 'normal' depending upon a person's attitude toward it. It is important to be aware of jokes, complaints, and expressions like "blows my mind," for the inner self takes it literally. Dreams are thought to have aspects of all three parts of ourselves.

> *If the subconscious mind and the body are the same, then health issues are a huge clue to the content of the subconscious mind.*

The consciousness level at any given time is related to will. We will ourselves to pay attention, but we don't always pay attention to what we are thinking about. Subconscious expectations creep in and begin to direct thoughts and actions. It is easy to see the physical results of an injury but not so easy to determine how the accident matches the person's previous thoughts. Being aware of thoughts and the environment is a matter of choice—you can focus upon the fragrance of the rose, the thorns that pierce the skin while picking it, or ignore the rose all together. It takes effort and resolve, but we *do* choose what to allow into our awareness each moment—whether to be superconscious or 'ignore-ant.'

Personal spiritual energy is divided into four parts. The physical body (low) is the densest self and the place where 'blocks'—both physical toxins and the 'issues' in the subconscious—show up as illness. The next densest 'self' is the emotional 'body' or feeling part, created by thoughts in the mental (middle) body. Emotions are perceived in the dense physical body but are the result of mental activity. This is followed by the mental self where all decisions are made and physical activity is directed. The physical body has 'knowing' and memory of events and beliefs held in the emotional unconscious and the childlike subconscious. When these deeper levels are explored and cleared, the spiritual or higher self can more easily be accessed. That is why purifying the dense body is good for spiritual growth.

The consciousness level at any given time is related to will.

ACCESSING THE SUBCONSCIOUS

Buried subconscious beliefs show up in 'clues.' It is easy to be blind to the subconscious influences which may have different intentions from the conscious mind. No one consciously trips and falls, but somehow the inner child 'sets us up' to trip, possibly to avoid some other threat. It takes extraordinary courage to face and resolve one's own fears (it is much easier to figure out other people's problems)!

Buried subconscious beliefs show up in 'clues.'

Emotions with no apparent explanation might be clues to subconscious 'issues.' Negative emotions are a result of a thought or belief that is out of vibration with divine love (high self). Beliefs are simply repeated thoughts. People can choose to pay attention, pull on that particular 'emotion-string,' bring those buried energy blocks into the focus of conscious examination, and look at them under the light of the higher self. When false beliefs are discovered, the underlying issue or event sometimes can be found (usually not what you would have guessed). After open-minded inspection, many of these notions can be analyzed and dispelled as errors in perception or survival tactics developed during childhood. The 'adult you' must calm the fear of the 'child you.'

> Talk to your baby-you and your child-you. Tell her what her infantile mind could never have understood like the circumstances of the abuse. Tell her you understand her fear. Then explain how things are different now and ask her to forgive and release the fear that is still in your body.

Exploring one's selves is an *ongoing* and *fascinating* process. Clearing the 'clouds' in the lower levels brightens the light of higher levels.

EMOTIONS

There are basically only two emotions, fear and love.

1. Fear and all related, 'negative' emotions—disgust, anger, hate, rage, frustration, sarcasm, cynicism, panic—the so-called 'hard feelings'
2. Love and all related, 'positive' emotions—affection, compassion, forgiveness, contentment, peace-of-mind, joy—the so-called happy 'soft, fuzzy feelings'

There are basically only two emotions, fear and love.

Fear occurs when there is a lack of love like dark and cold occur when there is a lack of light and heat. When love is blocked, some form of fear dominates the organism. When the conscious mind *sincerely* tells the low self that all is well, some shade of love is felt. When the inner child believes there is a threat, fear shows up in one form or another. Subconscious perceptions (beliefs) are formed by repeatedly telling ourselves that something is wrong. Pay attention to emotions because a subconscious belief is covertly lurking behind it.

Beliefs, perceptions, conclusions, oaths, and vows creep into thoughts and behavior.

An emotion always follows the thought that produced it. Think about terrible things that could happen and fear results. Conversely, choose to feel safe, take the necessary steps to *convince* the low self, and the result will be a positive emotion. Each reaction and perception is a choice in the moment. A negative emotion always indicates that the previous thought was out of alignment with the high self. Anger, for example, means events are not consistent with expectations and the person needs to decide if the expectations are not realistic or action needs to be taken to bring the physical situation into alignment with spiritual knowing. Spiritual consciousness is, therefore, learning to interpret with *new eyes*, to really *see* the rose, to smell it and drink it into your soul, and stay in positive alignment. It is a choice to look at a face (even our own) and *see* the angel shining behind those fearful eyes.

An emotion always follows the thought that produced it.

> If you feel anger, detach yourself from it and look at the situation. Do you need to change your expectations or make a change in your life? Ask for what you want and seek a balance.

SPIRITUAL CONSCIOUSNESS

Raising consciousness involves a willingness to see or accept the spiritual nature of everyone. Each person is born with a kind of spiritual 'radio receiver' installed, but the mind has control of the knob. It is a mystery whether, and when, a person will turn their radio on or to what station they will tune it. Most stay hidden in the shadow, clinging in fear to old teachings, often numbed by drugs and junk food, and preoccupied by other distractions.

Raising consciousness involves a willingness to see or accept the spiritual nature of everyone.

An individual's choice to awaken sometimes appears to be controlled from outside when seemingly cosmic events like weather, accidents, or the actions of other people jar perceptions of reality. These so-called tragedies—like death of a loved one, an auto accident, or a tornado—are really attracted by our subconscious asking and longing for truth. Adversity can make a person mean and bitter or forgiving and resourceful. Death can be a wake-up call for those left behind. A physical assault is more likely if the victim's body language signals "I am trash." The energy we expend to avoid being aware can be greater than the courage we need to walk the 'valley of the shadow' and examine our own inner motives.

Enlightenment occurs on this, the matter side of the veil, but involves urging and coaching from the higher vibration side. Raising one's level of consciousness is an awesome and constantly unfolding experience. Just when it seems clear that a lesson has been learned, another cosmic 'finger' taps and more awareness seeps in, like an enchanting, infectious dance melody or the constantly undulating, mesmerizing waves of the ocean. It is scary, painful, and profoundly satisfying at the same time.

Part of being spiritually conscious is being able to *see* illusions that have trapped the mind in emotional pain and physical illness. It is seeing through and beyond the impressions we were given in childhood, such as feeling either 'obliged' to give or 'entitled' to receive more than others. Becoming aware of programming instilled by society, family, and institutions, enables deliberate choices about what is right for us at the time, regardless of cynical or sarcastic (fear) reactions from others. Conscious people feel free to tell the truth and to ask for what they want, simply because they *are* holy and precious.

Part of being spiritually conscious is being able to see illusions that have trapped the mind in emotional pain and physical illness.

ASPIRANTS

An aspirant, sometimes called an initiate, is one who aspires or seeks to consciously walk a spiritual path, to walk in the light. Everyone yearns, whether aware of it or not, for higher consciousness—to know the answers to age-old existential questions. Spiritual yearning often begins with a desire to be healthier, slimmer, or for some other physical change. This makes sense because physical problems result from blocks in vital energy. With each new expansion of awareness comes the disconcerting reality that previously held beliefs are untrue. Often considered initially to be unpleasant intrusions into comfortable lifestyles, spiritual awareness leads to much greater peace. Some believe that mental illness, substance addictions, and various forms of 'antisocial behavior' can be a reaction to enhanced sensitivity to the falseness of modern life in an attempt to dull awareness.

An aspirant, sometimes called an initiate, is one who aspires or seeks to consciously walk a spiritual path, to walk in the light.

Light-workers struggle to believe in their higher wisdom within, to trust their own intuition, and work to clear negativity in whatever way they can. Sometimes this entails changing jobs, partners, or locations. The self-selected aspirant often never feels she belongs anywhere—never really fits in with any group or even individual. She is usually content to share parts of her thoughts with different people. This can be lonely but also exhilarating! Universal spirit speaking through the heart will lead with gentle enticements toward light which dispels darkness. Eventually the struggle with old beliefs ceases, and the aspirant becomes open to further spiritual growth, even if it is uncomfortable or painful. You are never alone!

BLOCKS TO CONSCIOUSNESS

You are never alone!

The modern world is filled with what many wise observers have called 'weapons of mass distraction'—those ubiquitous carnival-barkers called commercials, electronic gadgets, automobiles, and incessant noises that distract and divert peaceful knowing. None of the distracters are inherently bad. It is not money that is the root of all evil; it is focusing excessively upon it that distracts from family, spirit-within, and love of our own sacred body-temples.

Almost any aspect of life can be (or be used as) a distraction—a job or career, cleaning house, volunteer work, sugar or other 'comfort' food, for example. When distracted, the mind is not conscious and may slip into 'automatic' (subconscious) thinking, which usually means the attitudes instilled by parents and society.

Loyalty to a religion or other organization can be an unconscious routine—reminiscent of cheering for the home team in high school. It tends to become an 'us' and 'them' war, a 'mob mentality' that causes individuals to cease examining the beliefs and actions of the group and to harshly judge 'outsiders.' Teachings of all religions promote peace, and yet churches often dehumanize the 'enemy' and promote war.

Fear kills.

Searching for a good movie with a message of peace—even for a seven-year old—is difficult. Movie producers, however, make films to please the people who patronize them, just as leaders must reflect the wishes of those who vote for them. It is a vicious circle, literally. Violent and scary movies instill fear—a block to spiritual love. Buying a ticket ensures that more will be made. Fear kills. Corporations who sponsor violent TV shows have no conscience or consciousness; they exist solely to make money for shareholders. Choosing how you spend your money is a vote for how you want the world to be.

Choosing how you spend your money is a vote for how you want the world to be.

Authority figures of science (doctors), religion (clergy), law (attorneys), finance (advisors), education (teachers), government (elected officials), and industry (corporate CEO's advertisements) have been the policy makers of minds. They dwell on bad news and promote fear, placing distractions along the road. Because education is often supported by corporate money, those in lab coats, clergy collars, and tailored suits often unconsciously support corporate financial interests. New Age spiritual initiates strive to rise above these 'weapons of mass distraction' and see with clear eyes.

DIET AND CONSCIOUSNESS

In this chapter on consciousness, it must be pointed out that processed food is a major physical and mental distraction, not only because of advertisements, but because whatever pollutes the body clouds the mind. It is impossible to explain how important this is to SAD (Standard American Diet) eaters, because people who are the least aware tend to live mainly on white flour, sugar, and flesh. But the quick, easy, chemically-flavored food, offered by corporations at low prices, is addictive. A pure diet makes the mind clearer. It puts the person back in her right mind and puts the 'middle' self back in control. A living diet becomes the conscious choice when one realizes that matter intensely matters! Eating meat is not only toxic to the body but requires the eater to deaden her mind to the suffering of the living animal the burger used to be. Most people who change to a raw vegan diet mention clarity of thought as a benefit. (There is much more on the effects of diet on physical, mental and spiritual energy in Chapters 6, 7, and 8).

A pure diet makes the mind clearer.

The theory that diet affects all aspects of a person was explored in the study Spiritual Effects of Live Food (S.E.L.F.), conducted by the author (discussed earlier in Chapter 2). The subjects were asked to rate twenty-seven mental areas, such as: trouble concentrating, forgetfulness, and lack of discipline before and after two weeks on living organic vegan food. The study revealed the students themselves felt the raw vegan diet significantly improved their mind function. Of the mental issues reported as problems at the beginning of the study,

A living diet becomes the conscious choice when one realizes that matter intensely matters!

53% were resolved, 13% were improved, 33% unchanged, and only 1% were perceived as worse at the end of the course. This shows there probably is a connection between diet and mental clarity.

Since mental habits and emotions are so closely linked to each other, diet must be considered in a discussion of both of them. People who change to an all raw vegan diet also talk about initial surging emotions and then ultimately—emotional well-being. The S.E.L.F. study illustrated this as well. In the early days of the course, while actively detoxing, the students often snapped at each other and the staff. But later a feeling of closeness developed.

Of the emotional issues (such as guilt, out-of-proportion anger, and depression) reported by the students when they arrived, 73% were perceived as resolved at the end of two weeks eating all raw vegan. Another 7% were improved, 19% unchanged, and only 1% were worse. Compare that to the studies on mood-altering drugs. It is not a panacea but perhaps clearing toxins from the physical body frees inner fears to more quickly express and dissolve. (There is much more on the effects of diet later.)

TEACHERS

Aspirants attract teachers and often experience spirit guides (unseen teachers such as angels). No one attains enlightenment alone—for each emits a 'radio vibration' that affects others. Light/love is stronger than dark/fear. Assistance on the path to super-consciousness can come in a variety of surprising messages from people in conversation, lectures, or written material from a formal teacher or a member of the family. It could be an event, book, animal, or intuitive inner whisper. It might even be a lying, cheating boyfriend!

Awakening is a willful choice of each person to listen to the message. This choice is then made even more powerful, because with every firm decision comes the assistance of a host of guides. Helpers are from the light, either as unseen etheric beings or in-the-flesh spiritual teachers.

Eventually the student will become the teacher. At some point the seeker realizes that she has learned enough to know that she already knew everything a teacher can teach her. This is when she gives back 'service' by shining a light for others on the consciousness path. But a teacher cannot *do* the spiritual work of clearing the energy blocks *for* the student no matter how much they love or want to help, because no one knows the path another person has to travel or for what purpose. A teacher can 'walk beside' the aspirant, send light and love to enhance the energy, and be there for advice (if asked).

Eventually the student will become the teacher.

An aspirant, intoxicated on her first sip of divine love, follows an individual path and teachers hold a responsibility to allow this. As with parenting, there are fine lines between protecting, encouraging, guiding, and controlling. Sometimes all a teacher or healer needs to do is simply to sit quietly, and hold a space, serving as a 'battery' for divine light to flow to the student in crisis, who must walk alone in the 'valley of the shadow.' We are here to empower and enhance each other. We must choose our teachers wisely, sensing with our inner wisdom if their energy will enhance our own.

Devoted spiritual teachers do not ask for adoration. They encourage students to follow their own higher self. But all giving and no getting is as destructive as always taking. Teachers understand that money is simply another exchange of energy (gifts of spirit are free) and can be requested only for the teacher's time and expenses. Lopsided relationships result in resentment on both sides, so it is good to seek an equal energy exchange that is fair for all.

But all giving and no getting is as destructive as always taking.

Enlightenment is a do-it-yourself project and the best that can be hoped for is a good role model or two. There are no servants and no masters—only mutually beneficial relationships (even painful ones). The real story about past 'miracles' and 'masters' is not that they were human like us, but that we also are gods and miracle workers—like them! Divine spirit lives as a potential miracle within each person, just waiting to be noticed.

SPIRITUAL GROWTH

'Spiritual growth' is actually clearing the physical, emotional, and mental clouds that hide the truth of existence from our awareness. When the fog of erroneous thought is cleared on this, the physical side of the veil, divine love is waiting patiently to wrap the soul in light and kudos. It is a journey, an ever-ongoing process. Whatever assists us to find the causes of the negative energy (errors or blocks) in and around us, leads to higher consciousness and growth toward the spiritual light. We do not forget what has been truly learned.

We do not forget what has been truly learned.

When we grow toward the spiritual light, we become more sensitive and aware of subtle life—energy forms that are unrecognizable until advanced senses evolve. Becoming conscious is being aware of spirit (whatever name is chosen) in every circumstance of life—thoughts, words, deeds, communications, and aspirations. It is realizing that everything and everyone *is* spirit. We heal ourselves by seeing the loving intelligence in each face—human, lobster, cow, puppy, or sand hill crane. We heal the world by seeing the hand of Sophia (feminine aspect of that called "God") in each tree and flower.

When one has embarked on the healing journey there may be a time of chaos, confusion, and discomfort. When a healthier diet is started, there will be physical detoxification withdrawal symptoms, which may be uncomfortable and seem like an illness, similar to withdrawal from heavy alcohol use. This is one kind of 'healing crisis.' When spiritual studies are begun there may also be emotionally

When one has embarked on the healing journey there may be a time of chaos, confusion, and discomfort.

uncomfortable times. Trust the heart to decide whom to consult. As with housework, the road to cleaning body and mind entails removing garbage and clutter, plus changing life-habits—some of which were familiar, comfortable—and destructive!

ANCIENT WISDOM

Teachers from years and ages past communicate with the words they left behind, or sometimes they speak through living 'volunteer authors.' These truths are called 'ancient' or 'ageless' wisdom. Ancient wisdom, or esoteric (hidden) laws, contain the secrets of the ever-pulsating living energies of the universe and serve as a guide for aspirants. It is not a religion; they are truths available to any spiritual aspirant who seeks to understand the relationship between humanity and the rest of the universe. Each soul, consciously or unconsciously, evokes the truth for which she is ready.

In the past, the mass of people were not allowed to know these ancient wisdom secrets, for knowledge of them has sometimes been used selfishly or carelessly, creating pain and destruction. But this New Age is the time for these wonderful secrets to be revealed to all so everyone can choose health, positive attitude, and long life. People need to know loving universal energy is always working toward good and is itself, protection from danger.

"Humans are divine," say the ancient sages; and human thoughts and intentions direct energy, giving each individual a share in the collective outcome. As evolution proceeds and humans become less dense and better conductors of light, conscious loving individuals will dispel the darkness of collective fear. An unknown indigenous elder once said, "If you are coming to help me, you are wasting your time. But if you are coming because your liberation is bound up with mine, then let us work together."

"Humans are divine," say the ancient sages; and human thoughts and intentions direct energy, giving each individual a share in the collective outcome.

Hermes Trismegistus, a very wise Egyptian and contemporary of the biblical Abraham, originated the laws known as the Hermetic philosophy, a collection of principles or statements of truth handed down verbally. It is said that all other spiritual teachings are based on these principles. The first law of Hermes is "All is mind."[50] The great work of influencing one's environment is accomplished by mental power, for we are all a part of the universal mind in which we live and move and have our being. This is the first Hermetic principle—it also reveals that physical matter is composed of spiritual energies.

Ancient wisdom reveals what is known as the Law of Attraction. In his book *Bridges,* Aart Jurriaanse offers clear interpretations of the extensive work of Alice Bailey, one of the 'volunteer authors' of ancient wisdom, saying:

> *"Could man but be convinced of the fantastic powers at his command when thoughts are correctly motivated and controlled! The creating entity generates energy in direct proportion to the intensity of his thinking, and its quality will be determined by the theme of the thought. 'Energy follows thought'."*[51]

INTENT AND THE LAW OF ATTRACTION

We each control our own lives by our attention and intention. Energy follows intent.

You move and the universe rushes to assist. This *is* the Law of Attraction, also found in many other well-known phrases—self-fulfilling prophecy, power of prayer, what goes around comes around, as a man thinketh in his heart, reap what you sow, or "the master key." However it is described, it is a matter of deliberate intent. *We* each control our own lives by our attention and intention. Energy follows intent. Our job is to *allow* its unimpeded flow to

50 Three Initiates, *The Kybalion, Hermetic Philosophy,* (Chicago, IL: Yogi Publication Society, 1940), 26.

51 Aart Jurriaanse, *Bridges*, Copyright: This book is dedicated to Humanity without reservation. Man's versions of the Truth should not be offered with restrictions, (Johannesburg, South Africa, 1986), 320.

wholeness—to holiness. The road to *heaven* (not hell) is paved with good intentions.

The Law of Attraction says: what we most often choose to dwell upon will come to us. Therefore, conscious intent needs to be more powerful than social conditioning. The goal is to stay in higher mind. Which mind is dominating in the moment is revealed by the emotions being evoked in that moment.

Everything begins with a thought and we have control of that. Every word and deed begins in the mind. Words are simply loud thoughts and actions are loud words, so all action began with a mental notion. When conscious awareness dawns, with it comes a deliberateness of action and keen observation of results. The universe gives choices and those choices can be taken away only with our permission.

Everything begins with a thought and we have control of that.

"The focused human mind is the most powerful instrument in the universe," says Jill Bolte Taylor.[52] She was a young Harvard neuroanatomist (brain scientist) who observed her own mind completely deteriorate when she experienced a massive stroke on the left side of her brain (the rational, grounded side) at age 37. In order to heal, she learned to pay attention to her self-talk and to discipline her conscious mind. She shares her spiritual insight that we actively choose how we perceive personal experience like "tending the garden of the mind." The peanut-sized "negative story-teller" part of our brain must be disciplined sharply by the conscious mind. She says, "Our desire for peace must be stronger than our attachment to our misery." These are lessons all humanity is learning in these new times. Energy follows intent.

Many people are discovering the Law of Attraction or the first law of Hermes via popular films like *The Secret* and *What the Bleep*

52 Jill Bolte Taylor, Ph.D., *My Stroke of Insight,* (New York, NY: Penguin Group, 2006), 157.

do we Know? The same principle is taught in a set of popular tapes and books by Esther and Jerry Hicks, who channel a group of entities known as 'Abraham.' They say, "you are attracting the essence of whatever you are choosing to give your attention to—whether wanted or unwanted."[53] Deep inside, everyone from Hermes to a present day school child knows people have the power to change situations that are not wanted. Everything is attracted by the protagonist in the "story of your life"—you, the person in the mirror.

Consciousness is being aware of the impact of both your action and your neglect.

Consciousness is being aware of the impact of both your action and your neglect. Being a steward of the Earth is often another early step on the spiritual path. Choices change when a human awakens to previously hidden realities, such as the suffering of animals, the futility of materialism, war, and revenge, or the folly of the 'race to the top.' These choices cover all parts of life, like clothing, food, household products, building materials, and mode of transportation. Certainly, as we move toward a critical mass of thinkers who are focused upon love instead of fear, the Earth has a better chance for survival, too.

Thoughts change the vibration of the thinker and attract more of that same energy, whether desired or not.

Thoughts change the vibration of the thinker and attract more of that same energy, whether desired or not. To a certain extent, thoughts affect others, too. The "100th monkey syndrome" is a term coined when one Japanese monkey learned to wash sweet potatoes before eating and taught it to others. At a critical number, all the monkeys, even those on islands with whom the potato-washing monkeys had no contact, also began to wash their food.[54] The same is true of humans. When a critical mass of minds has discovered the light, the darkness will dissipate. Each person affects the energy of humanity. What a responsibility; what an honor!

---

53 Esther Hicks channeling Abraham, "A Twelve Point Synopsis of Abraham-Hicks Teachings" in *The Science of Deliberate Creation*, Vol. 23, Jan, Feb, Mar, 2003, 18.

54 Ken Keyes, Jr., *The Hundredth Monkey*, (Coos Bay, OR: Vision Books, 1983), 11–16.

Steps To Using The Law Of Attraction

The steps to using the Law of Attraction are simple but not easy:

1. Honestly become aware of what currently *is*, both "good" and "bad." It might be easier to see what is wanted if we briefly look at what is currently here that is not wanted. Observe conditions or objects which are causing anger, frustration, or other negative emotion. Abraham-Hicks calls this "contrast."

2. (Maybe the hardest.) Decide what is wanted in place of the unwanted situation. Visualize health, money, or a loyal, loving, supportive partner until it already feels real, complete with joyful emotions.

3. (The easy one.) Ask for what is wanted – ask a person to do something, ask the universe to bring something, ask for the raise, enlightenment, health, or peace on Earth. Be aware that when one asks sincerely and then allows (expects) the wish to be fulfilled, it must happen.

4. Then make physical preparations for it to be made manifest. This can be anything from deciding how to spend the lottery money, to clearing the body of toxins in preparation for enlightenment, or getting rid of closet clutter for the new love to move in. If asking for a pony, start taking riding lessons.

5. The final step in the process of the Law of Attraction is gratitude. Allow the eagerness and giddiness of a child on Christmas. Welcome the desired events, objects, and conditions with glee and great celebration. Feel the love flowing through mind and tissues and give thanks. Let this love flow to the gift and slather it on those around it. Bless and say "thank you" as often as you can.

If asking for a pony, start taking riding lessons.

SPIRITUAL INITIATIONS

The *steps* involved in expansion of consciousness have been numbered in various ways by different spiritual writers when referring to the progress of the soul on its quest to return to the ultimate light experience of its far distant past. These steps are called 'spiritual initiations.' References are found in mystery schools, Theosophy, Christian mysticism, Hinduism, Buddhism, yoga, and many other traditions. The Christian version is often depicted by episodes in the life of Jesus, or Stations of the Cross. Every major religion identifies specific stages of development marked with rituals and symbols with varying rules and requirements for the milestones with guideposts along the way. Like new ages, each initiation brings a fresh stage of life with new challenges and delights.

Human souls are in the process of progressive "at-one-ment" and each stage must be preceded by a burning or destruction of the inner veil that shields the mind and flesh from experiences for which they are not yet ready. To dwell in the high self, the low self must be understood. The path is begun when the person turns their back on many human activities and takes the first hesitant steps toward the spiritual 'kin-dom'—the joining with all others as 'kin.' There are three stages of initiation common to many traditions:

1. It is usually considered the *first initiation* when some measure of control is won over the physical vehicle. Gluttony, drunkenness and other excesses are now brought under conscious control of the will. Usually, there is an effort to become fit, healthier, or engaged in alternative healing. It can be a long, tedious, and difficult struggle to discipline one's physical self. Most of humanity is at this level.
2. The *second initiation* occurs when the individual has attained reasonable control over her emotions, eventually stilling

those turbulent waters. This is not to say that so called 'negative emotions' like anger and fear are bad, for they are clues and can lead to change. They just cease to constantly rule the thoughts and actions of the aspirant. During this time acute emotional distresses of the past are allowed to come up for examination ushering in a time of inner turmoil and uncertainty, serious self-examination, periods of deep subjective discontent, and often major changes in life conditions. It is sometimes referred to as the "dark night of the soul" and joyfully leads (if the shadow is traversed), to a relatively calm world where the meaning of spiritual love can be 'real-ized.' Forgiveness occurs at this level—forgiveness of parents, perpetrators, and most importantly, self. There are no alternatives, no bridges over, and our path cannot be walked by another no matter how great the love or money.

3. The *third major initiation* comes when fear has subsided and the initiate learns mental control over thought-matter. At this time the spiritual higher self becomes the dominating force of the personality. More and more the suffering caused by the glamour and illusion of the material 'dream' world humans collectively agree to inhabit, is overcome.

There are, of course, still greater realms of thought and being, which are as yet far beyond human conception and comprehension. The path of spiritual evolution is never-ending. When the summit of each spiritual 'mountain' is reached, there appears yet another path—upwards!

The path of spiritual evolution is never-ending.

ENLIGHTENMENT

The realization that everything is made of divine energy is called enlightenment and is the goal of spiritual life. This realization is beyond a rational, mental understanding of the word. It is an ever-evolving awareness of the universe as a unified living entity of which each is a part. Enlightenment is a measure of confidence that all is moving toward good. It is a childlike trust in a loving universe, a deep, peaceful feeling that all is really, *really* well; or if not perfect at the moment, that it will ultimately turn out for the highest good of all. It doesn't mean we stop striving, growing, or helping our siblings. We learn to do these things without the angst. Enlightenment is a deep acceptance that all is in divine order.

People are in each other's lives both to comfort and confront.

The consciousness of the universe is made up of the consciousness of each member of the 'circle of life.' Each awakening mind, therefore, matters to every other. Enlightenment is a group project, all moving toward the light. Together we explore the messages from physical, emotional, mental, and spiritual dimensions and become 'light-workers.' Being super-conscious means overcoming subconscious beliefs.

Enlightenment or cosmic consciousness occurs when the energy flows smoothly in and around the mind and body. This love-light then sparks the candle of the next person like a Christmas Eve service. In this New Age, groups work, study, and learn together, enabling members to advance faster, speeding up enlightenment for humanity. Members will recognize 'soul-mates' and groups will be comprised of initiates at various levels of development—teachers and students all. The process must be walked alone, but can be cheered on by others. People are in each other's lives both to comfort and confront.

Enlightenment is a deep acceptance that all is in divine order.

Spirit is the fiery ball of collective intelligent love-energy, and all entities are a spark of this cosmic fire. Evolutionary progress finds those dense human sparks attracted back to the magnetic glow of which they are a part, like moths to a flame. They are assisted by spiritual beings, some closer to the light and some nearer the physical world of matter. Spiritual enlightenment means to become aware that *matter matters.*

John White calls enlightenment "the realization of the truth of Being." He says the answer to what many seek is none other than what we already are. "We are manifestations of Being, but like the cosmos itself, we are also in the process of becoming and growing into higher states."[55] We are 'human becomings!' Buddha and Christ are both titles which denote a person who has achieved 'enlightenment' or a state of profound peace. Both taught that everyone could achieve that state. Everyone can walk in the light.

Spiritual enlightenment means to become aware that matter matters.

Spiritual consciousness is being at one with the universe (at-one-ment or a-tone-ment) and it is easier to achieve when the body is healthy so that it does not distract. Blocks in energy can be at the mental, emotional, or physical level. The live food diet seems to assist healing of issues that need to resolve instead of becoming lodged in the tissues. It allows them, to come into the light of consciousness and resolve, which reveals spiritual peace like sunshine after the storm.

---

55 John White, *The Meeting of Science and Spirit, Guidelines for a New Age,* (New York, NY: Paragon, 1990), 203.

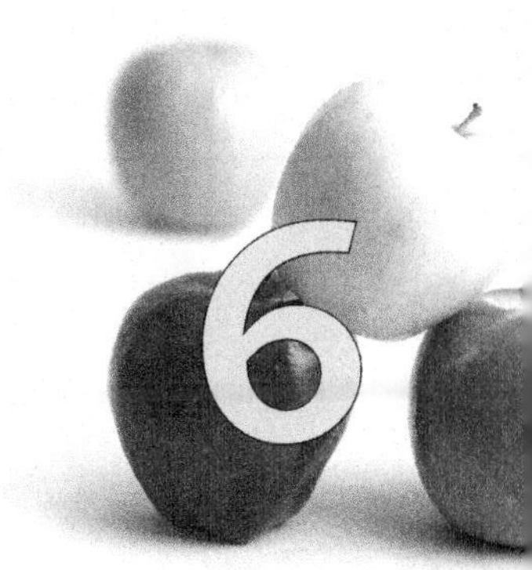

Our Amazing Body Temples

As above, so below.

— Ina Crawford

In *A Guide to the Mysteries,* spiritual writer Ina Crawford writes: "As children of the universe, our energy fields are copies—in minute form—of the Universe: as above so below; the macrocosm and the microcosm."[56] Each microcosm (you) contains the blueprint, the wisdom and secrets of the macrocosm. In each human cell therefore, is the intelligence of the universe. Each cell knows what it needs to heal, grow, and thrive. Mental power of each person begins the process by making a decision to be healthy, and when loved and nourished with food alive from the sun, the cells of our divine body temples heal and flourish.

In each human cell therefore, is the intelligence of the universe.

BIOFIELDS

Since everything is made of spiritual energy, human bodies must also be spirit. Indeed, many have described seeing spiritual fields of life, "biofields," or "auras" in and around living organisms. Some people report seeing beautifully colored light around people, animals and other things from nature, and these colors have been captured with special photography equipment. Eventually, all humans will probably be able to see these 'rainbows of energy'; but even if one

56 Ina Crawford, *Guide to the Mysteries,* (London, England: The Lucis Trust, 1990), 19.

has not realized this talent yet, it is still possible to sense another person's energy using 'inner knowing' to read their feelings and intent. Everyone has sensors, like radio tuners, in all parts of the body, especially in the head and hands, to receive energies that others are transmitting.

These energy sensing body parts also can transmit energy and some energy is always given off by living animals like body heat. Thought signals are also generated by a person and can be received at any distance. We just need to learn to pay attention to these 'radio waves.'

But the physical body itself is built and organized by biofield scaffolds just outside the flesh. Spirit and matter are of the same energy which becomes physical at the skin the same way water vapor condenses into liquid and solid ice. Steam is still water but in different form. Physical substance is built *from* and *by* a complex network of interwoven fields of light-energy. Cellular matter inside the body is then organized and nourished by the same subtle energetic prana (a Sanskrit term for 'life force'), which continues to coordinate the energy in the body after it becomes physical.

The biofield, located just outside the dense physical body, forms an etheric (unseen, but meant to be found) body-double which gives warmth, motion, and sensitivity to the physical apparatus and acts as a connector to incoming energies from other entities and from the Cosmos. Etheric anatomy is the study of the design and flow of this prana in and around the body. Richard Gerber, a medical doctor who has extensively studied subtle energy and how it functions in the human body, calls it the "organizing bioenergetic field," which interpenetrates the cellular matrix of the physical body.[57] Our physical body actually comes from the etheric body which surrounds and interpenetrates it.

---

57 Richard Gerber, M.D., *Vibrational Medicine* Third edition, (Rochester, VT: Bear & Company, 2001), 59.

Matter is frozen light energy. It is physical because the particles are moving slower, like water molecules move slower in ice form. Humans are microcosms of the universe just as a drop of water is a miniature version of the ocean. Prana comes into the body from the Earth's magnetic field, radiation of the cosmos, oxygen in the breath, sunbeams, love from others, food, and water. Physical bodies as well as life sustaining love are both made of prana.

Our physical body actually comes from the etheric body which surrounds and interpenetrates it.

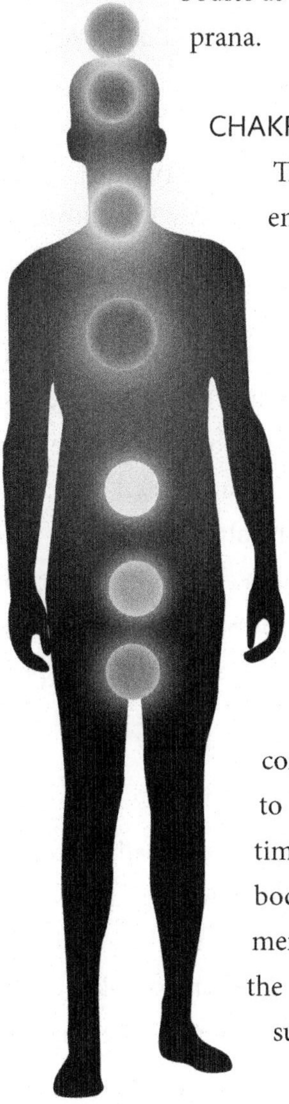

CHAKRAS

The biofield energizes everything. Fiery energies of the universe have been stepped down through unseen levels of vibration and literally become the major centers of the body, which are called chakras or vortices. Each chakra, or "wheel of spinning energy," organizes the prana into organs, glands, and other structures which function together to make the digestive, circulatory, musculoskeletal and other systems. Our bodies are divine miracles.

Physical bodies as well as life sustaining love are both made of prana.

Chakras are multi-dimensional because each one represents a level of consciousness from physical on the lower levels to spiritual on the higher ones. At the same time, each chakra also vibrates on the physical body dimension but also at the emotional, mental, and spiritual dimensions. For example, the root chakra is basically about physical survival and yet it also connects the physical

Our bodies are divine miracles.

to spiritual energy. Blocks and congestion can occur at any level and at any dimension. Chakras can be thought of like the electrical box in a house where the 'juice' comes in and is directed to all areas of the building.

There are seven main identified chakras each associated with various body parts, emotional states, and colors. At the lower end of the spine is found the base or root chakra (red), which is involved with survival and grounding, sense of smell, the reproductive organs, and fear. About in the middle of the abdomen is the sacral chakra (orange), the center of relationships, urinary system, emotions, sense of taste, and intimacy. The solar plexus chakra (yellow), found just below the sternum, is well known as the center of will power, awareness, digestive system, sight, anger and self-control. The heart chakra (green) is where it would be expected—mid-chest; it controls the cardiovascular system, and of course, is associated with touch, love, and forgiveness. The throat chakra (blue) is the center of creativity, speech, communication, and the sense of hearing. The ajna or third eye chakra (indigo), the seat of intuition and vision, is located just above and between the eyebrows. It controls the endocrine and autonomic nervous systems. The crown chakra (violet), at the top of the head, is linked with spiritual consciousness, thinking, wisdom, DNA, and the central nervous system. Chakras are where spirit becomes matter.

Chakras are where spirit becomes matter.

ENERGY PATHWAYS

All living things sparkle with energy centers, pathways and points—each a miniature constellation.

All living things sparkle with energy centers, pathways and points—each a miniature constellation. Inside what is known as the 'physical body,' life-power is delivered to each cell by a pathway, like wiring in a house or roads on a map. These pathways, known as meridians, connect big and little centers located everywhere in the body. When light-energy flows, so do the fluids and impulses in the lymphatic, circulatory, and neurological systems. Besides the chakras, there are major centers in the palms of the hands, spleen, and the soles of the feet. It is the Einsteinian principle that explains how the networks of energy fields can interface with physical system of cells: *energy equals matter*. Since these energies are intelligent, they can find the places where there is an energy deficiency and fill it. When the current is vibrantly flowing, it leads to a healthy body, happy thoughts, and a strong connection with the universe. Vitally glowing people then influence others who are ready to see and be seen.

Enzymes are discussed in detail in Chapter 8, but they need to be mentioned as part of the energy system of the body. The mysterious substances called enzymes are also part of the energy network, as well as being involved in innumerable tasks such as digestion. In fact, enzymes are sometimes described as the essence of bioenergy—life itself. They play a vital role in keeping the entire system working efficiently. Every (raw) food naturally contains the exact enzyme to digest itself and thereby enhance the chi of the cells of the body. Cooking destroys those enzymes, forcing the body to make new ones, which depletes vitality.

When the body is congested with dead and toxic foreign matter, prana has more difficulty flowing.

Energy flows best where the channels are kept pure and free of debris. When the body is congested with dead and toxic foreign matter, prana has more difficulty flowing. The vital current is short circuited. In a house or car this can cause a fire. Perhaps this is where "inflammation" comes from? Many people take less care of their bodies than they do their automobiles, using the correct type of fuel, keeping the fluids topped off, and changing the oil properly to remove irritants in their cars. Our bodies need maintenance, too.

In other words we become what we live, think, and eat.

Richard Gerber writes: "These unique energy systems are powerfully affected by our emotions and level of spiritual balance as well as by nutritional and environmental factors."[58] In other words we become what we live, think, and eat.

HUMANS AS CRYSTALS

Gabriel Cousens, a medical doctor and spiritual teacher who advocates live vegan food, says the assimilation of energy into physical bodies is through a series of synchronous, interacting, crystal structures. Each organ, gland, cell, and fluid, contains salt which has some degree of crystalline function. The body has the ability to convert vibrational energy, such as sound or light, into electromagnetic and electric energy just as crystals can absorb, store, amplify, transduce, and transmit energy waves. The bone structure acts as an internal antenna for incoming vibratory energy and information, including direct thought-form energy. "We are indeed precious gems."[59] Human bodies are solar-powered and infinitely rechargeable.

Human bodies are solar-powered and infinitely rechargeable.

KUNDALINI

Kundalini, is a Sanskrit term literally meaning "circular power." It is primal energy, lying coiled in potential form at the base of each human spine. Kundalini rises with spiritual growth to initiate enlightenment—a shift in the very energy balance of the atoms. When kundalini energy is awakened, humans become aware of their true nature—their greatness. It is the force latent in matter itself and its work is only with matter. Once kundalini has been awakened and raised, it destroys the enfolding, protective etheric webs which lie between the chakras, thus allowing the freer flow of energies within the body. [60] It is also said to be the basis of the medical symbol, the Caduceus.

---

58 Richard Gerber, M.D., *Vibrational Medicine* Third Edition, (Rochester, VT: Bear & Company, 2001), 43.

59 Gabriel Cousens, M.D., *Spiritual Nutrition,* (Berkeley, CA: North Atlantic Books, 2005), 141–150.

60 Ina Crawford, *A Guide to the Mysteries,* (London, England: Lucis Press, 1990), 51.

Gabriel Cousens writes that after the body has been purified, it is easier for kundalini energy to rise and spiritualize the matter of the body. Eating in a healthy, harmonious way results in a greater ability to attune and commune with the divine. If food containing life force is consumed, the kundalini channel is more energized. Watery fruits and vegetables, in their natural form, because of their higher conductivity and their structured water energy, enhance this divine connection. The closer food is to pure prana, the easier it is for its nourishment to be drawn into the body energy fields.

The closer food is to pure prana, the easier it is for its nourishment to be drawn into the body energy fields.

SACRED TEMPLES

As a young woman, Ann Wigmore, mother of the modern raw vegan movement, was directed to "become a minister and build My temples."[61] At first she thought that meant brick buildings called churches. But later she realized the 'temples' were human bodies, considered in many spiritual traditions to be holy temples, the home of the soul. She writes, "The spiritual needs and the physical natural laws which permit the spark of God to dwell comfortably in that temple are closely interwoven." She vowed to do her utmost to rehabilitate temples of flesh and blood!

Bodies are spirit in a more dense form, just as teeth and bones are denser than the eyeball or the brain. Each cell, infused with divine energy, has intelligence to perform a function or lots of functions without our specific conscious direction. The creation and operation of the human body or 'Earth space suit,' donned by the individual soul for the journey into the dense world, occurs at many levels—spiritual, mental, emotional, and physical. Energy is received as unseen etheric spiritual substance and then becomes flesh and bone according to the sacred blueprint found in the genetic material which alters itself according to internal and external conditions.

Energy is received as unseen etheric spiritual substance and then becomes flesh and bone according to the sacred blueprint found in the genetic material which alters itself according to internal and external conditions.

61 Ann Wigmore, *Why Suffer?*, (Wayne, NJ: Avery Publishing, 1985), 91.

SELF-CLEANING ORGANISM

At the physical level, the body can survive assaults of impact, toxic materials, temperature, and other abuse. The miracle is that anyone survives any time at all in the modern world. Constantly vigilant and cunningly clever, the body uses what it can to expel or hide offensive matter in nonessential places, such as fat cells and joints where they won't kill the person, at least not immediately. Most, if not all, of what are termed 'symptoms' are efforts by the physical body to remove harmful substances. Some of these are fever, runny nose, sweating, diarrhea, bad breath, skin rash, cough, and even pimples and gray hair. They are evidence of natural 'garbage removal.'

Most, if not all, of what are termed 'symptoms' are efforts by the physical body to remove harmful substances.

The toxins in the Standard American Diet (SAD) have increased with each generation, and they show up as physical disease, mental fogginess, and inability to find the spiritual light. Toxic foreign substances are introduced into the food chain in agriculture with genetic modification, hybridization, pesticides, and chemical 'fertilizers.' During food preparation artificial colors, flavors, preservatives, plastic containers, sweeteners, high heat, microwaving, and other methods of embalming food add to the toxic mess. Poisonous environmental cleaning products, manufacturing chemicals, and other noxious substances are found nearly everywhere in modern life. It takes effort to avoid potent toxins in today's world.

It takes effort to avoid potent toxins in today's world.

The good news is this body of flesh that we inhabit during our trip to Earth is equipped with efficient mechanisms to get rid of that which is not life-giving. Holy temples are not only beautiful and amazing but are self-cleaning organisms. Toxins are expelled in feces, urine, sweat, through the skin, phlegm from the lungs and throat, ear wax, nose secretions, tears, breath, and probably via many other methods that have escaped observation as of yet.

When our temples have symptoms such as cough, we have been told this means we are sick. In reality, the symptom is actually evidence that there is enough life force energy in the physical body and enough will in the mind to make an effort to expel the offending substance. The same is true for vomiting, diarrhea, vaginal discharge, and bleeding if the skin is violated followed by a protective scab. But 'illness' is a good excuse to stay quiet in bed for a day, which is probably a good idea. It cleanses the body-mind and reconnects us to spirit.

There are examples of self-healing everywhere. Broken bones knit back together. Skin lacerations heal. Bodies that have grievous injuries miraculously survive, even if it seems unlikely. Divine energy and will power account for survival, as well as for blooming health.

There are examples of self-healing everywhere.

THE PHENOMENON OF VITAL ADAPTATION

According to the obscure Law of Vital Adaptation the physical body is most able to withstand the effects of a toxic substance when it is saturated with that substance and possibly in a dangerously weakened state. These toxins can be pesticides, preservatives, or other chemicals foreign to the body. This seems the opposite of what is logical, but it is why people who seem 'healthy' will suddenly be found to be full of cancer or suffer a major heart attack. They are not as healthy as they seem. Toxic bodies are working hard to stay alive; hence the escalation of chronic illness in this day of processed food. To put it another way, the purer the body, the less able it is to tolerate toxins.

According to the obscure Law of Vital Adaptation the physical body is most able to withstand the effects of a toxic substance when it is saturated with that substance and possibly in a dangerously weakened state.

> It is well known that an alcoholic can drink more liquor without effects than can a total abstainer. It is an example of the Law of Vital Adaption. Tolerance is built up by the drinker trying to get a 'buzz" by increasing her intake. The damage increases with the greater alcohol but the drunk is unaware.

Vital Adaptation can be seen in the well-known story of the frog in the pot of water that is steadily heated. The frog continues to adapt to the higher temperature until she "suddenly" becomes cooked. People, too, are unaware of the insidious danger.

Professor Hilton Hotema, from the mid-twentieth century, writes of Vital Adjustment or Vital Accommodation as a riddle that puzzles doctors.

> *As a hostile environment is not capable of adjusting itself to the stature, shape, and requirements of the human body, the adjustment must be made to prevent sudden death; it is made by the body itself, at the expense of its vitality. Thus the body constantly grows weaker as it strives to live where it is not made to live. Death creeps upon the unsuspecting victim by slow degrees, dying by steps and stages of 'disease' while paying the doctor thru the years to do what you think he can do, but what he knows he can't do.*[62]

It is a paradox that the body, in a weakened condition, will tolerate more and endure longer in a toxic environment than a more vitally alive one. But for the Law of Vital Adaptation, the race would have perished ages ago, as toxins were introduced into diets and environments. But poisons have taken their subtle toll. Instead of dying when a lower 'dose' of a toxin is first encountered, the general vitality of human bodies has gradually degenerated with the pollutants, and through the ages this has reduced the average life-span of mankind from hundreds of years in Biblical times, to less than eighty in modern times. Instead of dropping dead, one dies by inches, and in the process of dying slowly, suffers chronic ailments until the body can endure no more.

No chemical substance has the ability to act in and of itself—its apparent 'effect' is merely the body's reaction to the chemical—an aspirin in a dead body does nothing.

No chemical substance has the ability to act in and of itself—its apparent 'effect' is merely the body's *reaction* to the chemical—*an*

62 Professor Hilton Hotema, *Man's Higher Consciousness,* (Mokelumne Hill, CA: Health Research 1962 revised edition—first appeared in 1952 under the title *Man's Miraculous Unused Powers,* using the pseudonym Kenyon Klamonti), 21–26.

aspirin in a dead body does nothing. A raw foodist might react more strongly to medications, because her body is not 'adapted' to them. Conversely, the body nourished with only raw vegan food and thus enhanced with chi, seems to recover from trauma more quickly and completely, with less need for pain medications. It just seems 'unfair' somehow that a clean raw vegan can't indulge herself occasionally without suffering illness symptoms!

Just as the experience of spiritual awakening makes it difficult to live in a cacophony of negative energy, ironically, once the transition to a predominantly raw organic vegetarian diet has been made, one becomes more susceptible to physical toxins. All evidence shows that the more vital the organism, the more quickly it succumbs to harmful conditions. Conversely, the amount of toxins a body can tolerate without effect is actually a measure of its current toxicity level, not a sign of health!

Conversely, the amount of toxins a body can tolerate without effect is actually a measure of its current toxicity level, not a sign of health!

Every living thing is dedicated to survival, to prolonging life to the maximum, and will do its best to adjust to any change in environment for this purpose. This can be observed in a dandelion growing in the crack in the concrete, the rabbit changing the color of its fur with the changing seasons, or a burdock burr clinging to a horse's tail to seed a new place. Disease-like symptoms are nothing but the body's effort to survive. One gets to decide if a slow suicide is better than going through a detoxification withdrawal process to revitalize the body. Precious bodies are dedicated to the survival of the owner who decides its fate.

The best way to detox the body is to quit "toxing" it!!

The best way to detox the body is to quit "toxing" it!!

PHYSICAL EXPELLING OF EMOTIONAL TOXINS

Tears are always cleansing, both physically and emotionally. When disrespect, abuse, rejection, or other emotional wounds are

Tears are always cleansing, both physically and emotionally.

perceived, tears are a natural release. Carol Parrish-Harra says that tears are cleansing, whether for happy or sad reasons.[63] They clear the energy system and the physical body at the same time. When a person has a reason to cry, it is not usually thought of as a chance to heal, but it is—both for the adult and for her inner child. Crying should be encouraged to continue until the hurt is drained away. Of course, this can potentially become habitual, holding a person in the perceived 'glamour' of the crying and illness (and the attention it draws), rather than moving on in a more healthy way. Your inner wisdom will reveal when the pain is drained.

Skin rashes are said to represent emotional cleansing as well; and if possible, it is best to let them do their work without toxic medications. Focus instead upon getting in touch with the emotional issues underlying the symptom. They can be identified and resolved by techniques that ask the inner child what the present situation is triggering from the past. This is *real* healing. "Just like children, emotions heal when they are heard and validated," writes Jill Bolte Taylor.[64] Any physical symptom is an opportunity to examine the subconscious cause.

WILL

People *can* control their thoughts. Choosing not to monitor your thoughts is also a choice of the will. We will ourselves to think and to act. No one else can *really* control that but us. Positive thoughts and emotions encourage the flow of energy in the body and in the universe. This may be the most important information in healing and consciousness—it is the Law of Attraction in action (as discussed in Chapter 5). That which is dwelt upon will grow, whether it is something that is desired or not. That is why it is best to focus upon

63 Carol E. Parrish-Harra, many personal communications.

64 Jill Bolte Taylor, Ph.D., *My Stroke of Insight, A Brain Scientist's Personal Journey,* (New York, NY: Viking, Penguin Group, 2006), 156.

the beautiful dreams and ideals of your soul. It is important that we honestly wish each other well and ask for prayers and loving thoughts. Energy follows intent.

It is will that determines what thoughts occupy your mind at any specific time. We will ourselves to be happy, to accept others decisions, to follow a healthy lifestyle. We are able to resist advertising, social pressures, and the remarks of others only by exercising our own will to have, to be, or to do what we have thoughtfully decided is best for ourselves, our family, and the planet. Will is the moment-to-moment decision that we make every waking instant. Shakespeare put it perfectly in Othello, "Our bodies are gardens to which our wills are gardeners." Whatever the mind plants, weeds, loves, waters, and fertilizes determines what will come to 'harvest.' It all lies in the power of the will. Each chooses, whether aware of it or not, her own health and connection with universal spirit.

Energy follows intent.

RENEWAL

Purifying the holy body temple removes distractions that block or distort healthy functioning like ice on a windshield blocks clear vision. When the physical blocks of disease and fatigue and the mental blocks of depression and illusion are removed, one is free to observe clearly what was there all along—spiritual truth. Vital energy can then flow freely.

Each chooses, whether aware of it or not, her own health and connection with universal spirit.

Sleep is nature's way of reconnecting individual souls with the collective soul. It is a time for etheric helpers to come calling because the conscious mind is not watching. Clues are revealed about subconscious emotional issues during sleep, so it is a good idea to keep a paper and pencil by the bed to write them down to ponder later. Many artistic compositions and practical inventions have been born during sleep. Insights often dawn with the sunrise about what is causing negative emotions or unreasonable actions.

Life energy is constantly renewed in the body by various means. Scientists know that breathing in and out replenishes oxygen and removes gaseous waste bringing vital life to the cells of the body. Water is essential to the lymph, urinary, and circulatory systems involved in the physical removal of toxins. Its energy can be enhanced or diminished by the human attitude displayed toward it before consumption. Blessing it, for example, enhances water. Water and oxygen are potent carriers of prana.

Oblivious of science, nature blooms around us and heals body and soul. Food represents light from the sun; air and water are love from heaven. Eyes absorb the energy of the blues and greens of the sky and the Earth, splashed with the fuchsias and oranges of flowers—a feast for the soul. Music and the sound of frogs and crickets carry heavenly love to our bones and heart. Silence can be filled with an inner dialog of peace and gratitude. Nature is constantly in a state of renewal and we are part of nature—awakening humanity in the New Age.

Without this renewal of nature, the body struggles, choking from a lack of life force, and becomes ill and crippled. The direction of nature is always toward life. Minerals are absorbed by and become plants, plants are eaten and become part of animals, and animals die and become soil once again. Even death promotes renewal, because it moves the physical body back into compost and the spirit, enhanced from a lifetime of learning, back into the river of life.

Living organisms have consciousness and generate love energy. Animals have loved and sacrificed not only for their own young, but for humans as well. Making a decision to love one's self, renews the tissues of the body just as hugging a child nourishes her and stimulates growth. Love-light ripples out until it meets a block, like the sun shines until something casts a shadow. Removing the clouds, allowing light to flow *is* spiritual healing.

Removing the clouds, allowing light to flow is spiritual healing.

NUTRITION AND SPIRITUAL HEALTH

Gabriel Cousens writes that when people eat in a healthy, harmonious way, they intensify their communion with the divine. Proper nutrition is best understood as a support for spiritual evolution. Cousens promotes a diet of vegan, organic, live food, naturally highly mineralized and low in concentrated sugar, individualized and eaten in moderate amounts. He also recommends keeping well hydrated with pure living water and fasting periodically to enhance the energies of the body. This diet is filled with living chi—life force energy that will sustain the physical structure much better while it transitions, in these new times. The oxygen that is taken from living plants is a source of high-electron energy from the sun.[65] If the Standard American Diet is continued, the body is forced to function less optimally on unbalanced nutrients and work harder to survive, leaving little energy for spiritual growth.

Human hunger is actually for divine essence not physical food.

Human hunger is actually for divine essence not physical food. There are stories of humans called 'breatharians,' who currently or in the past have not eaten any physical food at all for extended periods of times, and who thrive on receiving 'manna' from the streams of Life Force Energy. Predictions are that after the New Age transition, the need for food will dramatically change. But even if a person is not ready to absorb life exclusively from the air and has a belief that food is necessary, sugar and dead flesh are probably not good ways to honor the body temple. Fresh fruit, green leafy and other fresh raw vegetables supplemented with a small amount of sprouted grains, seeds, and soaked nuts will be much more harmonious with the body's

---

65 Gabriel Cousens, M.D., *Spiritual Nutrition,* (Berkeley, CA: North Atlantic Books, 2005), xix, 13.

progressively lighter vibration. The rate of transition toward physical as well as spiritual health is up to the individual.

PHYSICAL DEATH

There is no such thing as spiritual death, only physical death of the body.

There is no such thing as spiritual death, only physical death of the body. The etheric body is formed immediately before birth and becomes the architect of the physical body. This subtle body assists in cleansing the blocks to spiritual consciousness, and it lives on after the death of the physical body. The light is turned off in the body and flows into the ocean of light. The body is then like a room with the light off, but the light that is the essence of a person lives on.

Science has been unable to find an identifiable 'longevity button' that predetermines the length of a life. Since each of us changes our genetic material by our choice of inner and outer environment, none of us can blame our parents. (See next section and DNA and epigenetics in Chapter 12.) Germs are only attracted to dead matter, so they are not to blame either. (See section on bacteria in Chapter 7.) That leaves only the Chief Executive Officer (CEO) of the structure—the conscious mind or ego—either by intent or default. Just like the CEO of a company, the conscious mind is ultimately responsible for the most critical decisions of life or death. The struggle before death can be long and painful or quick and easy, *but it is a choice.* So we cannot blame god (by any name), germs or genes for our death! The mind itself directs longevity.

The mind itself directs longevity.

Death occurs when the will is gone to pull in enough energy to overcome the toxins, emotional challenges, and other blocks in the energy flow. When the physical body is overwhelmed with toxins and the body's attempts to clear the machinery have failed, cancers, clogged blood vessels, diabetes, and other life threatening diseases develop. Paradoxically, disease and death are spiritual for they, too, are healing. They either awaken the owner to the truth of troubling issues or return the organism to a holy space and even greater learning. The light of the soul temporarily lives in a body and recycles after the body's physical death. Death may be just the beginning of the journey, like a snowperson melting into the lawn and becoming part of a mighty river.

Abraham-Hicks has implied that all death is suicide. "We promise you, the timing of your death is always chosen by you."[66] If that premise is accepted, then perhaps the staggering number of years people were purported to live according to early Bible teachings might not have been metaphor. People might actually have lived hundreds of years in a different time. Some believe life can be extended forever. There appears to be no apparent reason for the length of a life except for the belief in the myth of entropy—a titillating thought at least.

EFFECT OF NEW AGE ENERGIES ON BODIES AND DNA

Virginia Essene is a teacher, grief counselor, channel, and metaphysical writer. In *New Cells, New Bodies, New Life!*, compiled and edited by Essene, she discloses the striking similarity of twelve different participating authors, sensitive to the intelligence and wisdom of their spiritual guides on the topic of DNA. They all wrote that there is a powerful energy shift occurring which will affect every part of human life. The genes of our bodies are changing to allow the cells to be able to receive more light. The two helix strands of human DNA are expanding into twelve, the state of enlightenment. People will retain a physical body, but it will be greatly transformed into a being of light. The spiritual guides give advice for Earth-dwellers. They suggest that one should focus upon maintaining positive thinking, emotional stability, and a healthy body during this extraordinary time. They all emphasized the importance of

The genes of our bodies are changing to allow the cells to be able to receive more light.

66 Esther Hicks, Excerpted from the workshop in Chicago, IL—Sat. September 7, 2002. Found on website www.abraham-hicks.com/lawofattractionsource/journal.PHP?eid=154.

affirming positive thoughts, for this will heal the body and assist the new energies bringing 'God' into matter. Some suggest that we have conversations with our body parts and ask them what they like and want, instead of ignoring them or resisting their messages. Some of the writers said we should minimize the use of alternating current appliances. Many mentioned food, suggesting that our bodies will love raw and organic fruits and vegetables, soaked nuts, and sprouted seeds, which hold the greatest natural light.[67]

José Trigueirinho Netto, a spiritual researcher and teacher in South America who emphasizes a pure food diet, writes that the Earth is taking a unique step in its evolution, and as a result, the human genetic code which contains a blueprint for the state of consciousness of the organism is being changed. DNA is also an instrument for the Plan of Evolution to guide humans toward the energy pattern they are destined to express.[68] Humanity is now undergoing unimaginable changes facilitated by the implantation of a new genetic code. The planet is becoming progressively more spiritualized, and therefore our bodies will become more subtle. This new code draws cosmic patterns of life down to the Earth and will release humans from the old structure of heredity and karma. They will lose their aggressiveness and will understand that all goods belong to everyone and not only to a few. Bodies will be purer and know that they are part of a harmony that integrates them.

Trigueirinho's contacts in the metaphysical world explain how spiritual aspirants are invited to rejoice in what they have achieved and to aspire to cooperate with humanity's evolution toward the fire of love. He writes that human healers should live in such a way that their vehicles may be continually transformed and purified to the maximum so that the new atoms coming from the spirit world may

---

67 Virginia Essene (ed), *New Cells, New Bodies, NEW LIFE!, You're Becoming a Fountain of Youth,* (Santa Clara, CA: S.E.E. Publishing Company, 1991), 60.

68 José Trigueirinho Netto, *Calling Humanity,* (Tahlequah, OK: Sparrow Hawk Press, 2002), 75-79.

flow through them. Diet should be individual, but he believes that eating meat hinders the refinement of the material body.

In *You are Becoming a Galactic Human,* we are told that sometime in our past, humans lost the original 12-helix DNA strands, which meant they also lost the mental recollection of their history and their former psychic abilities, such as mental telepathy—seeing and hearing spiritual energy, communing with nature, and the truth of who they really are. Virginia Essene says humans are already undergoing a great degree of genetic alteration, which may explain the seeming increase in physical ailments that often leave as quietly as they come. In this New Age there is an unknown chapter awaiting discovery and a sublimely exciting future.[69] There is more on DNA in Chapter 12.

THE TIME IS NOW

It is essential to heal humans already on the planet so that physical bodies can be maintained while the genetic structure and body cells achieve higher vibration. A powerful healthy body can heal, maintain itself in joy, and will know intuitively what is good for it in any given moment.

Humans have but two choices—join in and participate in the new flow of love or resist the flow with fear and toxins. Joining will bring as yet unimaginable miracles and ultimate grace. Resisting will bring the opposite. If one looks upon the changes as an imposition, life will be very trying. Love is the healer and the balm to soothe mind and body. Do it now while in your physical body.

Humans have but two choices—join in and participate in the new flow of love or resist the flow with fear and toxins.

> *If you don't break your ropes while you are alive, do you think ghosts will do it after? If you make love with the divine now, in the next life you will have the face of satisfied desire.*
>
> — *Kabir (6.24)*[70]

---

69 Virginia Essene and Sheldon Nidle, *You are Becoming a Galactic Human,* (Santa Clara, CA: S.E.E. Publishing, 1994), 2.

70 Kabir, cited in Robert Bly, *The Kabir Book,* (Beacon Press, 1977) found in Matthew Fox, *Original Blessings,* (Santa Fe, NM: Bear and Company, 1983), 103.

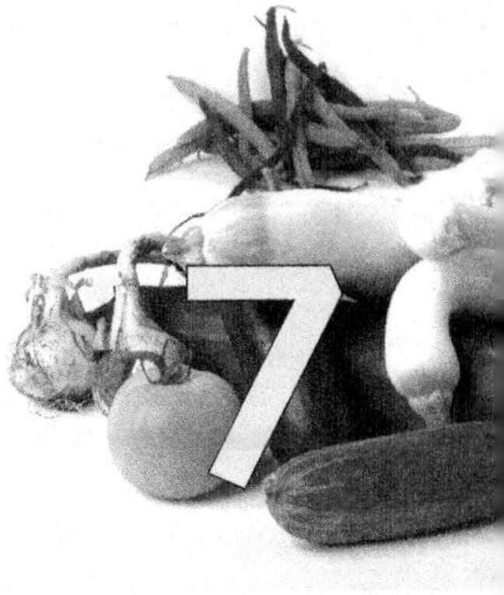

Blocked Energy is Illness

All disease is the result of inhibited soul life.

— Alice Bailey

If everything—from physical matter, to thoughts, emotions, and spirit is made of life force energy, then it makes sense that a disruption in the flow of this energy would cause a problem of some sort. These blockages or distortions of the flow of energy can occur in many ways at any level—physical, emotional, or mental, and from almost unlimited sources. From the physical aspect, blockages can be caused by such things as accumulation of toxins, constrictions from build-up of excess substances, or other impediments to the free flow of fluids and energy in the body.

If everything—from physical matter, to thoughts, emotions, and spirit is made of life force energy, then it makes sense that a disruption in the flow of this energy would cause a problem of some sort.

> Think of what happens when you put a tight rubber band around a finger; it doesn't take long before it turns blue and hurts. This is similar to what happens with any block in your body's chi.

Some blockages are mental—such as a persistent belief that stifles a person's growth. If you don't believe you can sing—then you can't! Other constrictions are of an emotional nature—for example, perceived insults, fears, and betrayals that are difficult to release. If you almost drowned once you might have an 'unreasonable' fear of water.

To further complicate the process, blockages at all these levels interact. Physical blocks affect emotions. Emotions impact thought habits. Thoughts precede every physical action that either helps or hinders the flow of energy. It is impossible to consider them as separate topics and yet, to explain each aspect they must be discussed independently. The result of any block is some sort of discomfort in body, mind, or soul—a lack of ease, or dis-ease. Whatever removes toxins or restores energy flow will benefit the physical body and mental/emotional state in a positive way. This could include changing one's diet, exercising, or drinking water. Any time you can change your attitude, forgive, or see a situation through a more loving lens, it will improve your health and also the health of people around you. Physical blocks affect mental and emotional well-being, mental blocks affect emotional and physical health, and emotional blocks affect mental and physical energy.

All this, of course, suggests that the owner of the body is in control of the decisions that determine which life conditions will appear. If this sounds like blaming the victim, *it is*, for it is the 'victim' who decided to be a victim instead of a hero. *But* with blame comes hope of change. If I caused this disease, then I can darn well clear it from my life! We know people do that all the time, but conventional experts are mystified by these 'unusual' cases that take a different course than science has predicted. We should study and learn from them—the ones who have healed *themselves.*

Whatever removes toxins or restores energy flow will benefit the physical body and mental/emotional state in a positive way.

Contrast *self*-healing with thinking all disease 'invades' your body from germs, genes, or gods. Even worse is the thought that disease automatically accompanies aging. Wouldn't you rather be in control? According to the Law of Attraction, when you make a decision to be well, the germs, genes, and gods assist you in your quest. When you empower yourself, the angels also empower you. This takes practice, so aging then becomes a really, really good thing!

THE CAUSE OF ALL DIS-EASE

According to the Law of Attraction, when you make a decision to be well, the germs, genes, and gods assist you in your quest.

Pain, disease, and anguish are simply blocked energy—Self Inflicted Nonsense (SIN). Alice Bailey wrote, "All disease is the result of inhibited soul life. The art of the healer consists in releasing the soul so that its life can flow through the aggregate of organisms which constitute any particular form."[71] In other words, the cause of all disease is the disruption of the flow of life energy either physically or mentally/emotionally. What happens in the mind ultimately shows up in the body. Conversely, the environment and the condition of the body affect the mind.

Djwhal Khul, the Tibetan who spoke through Alice Bailey, made these points:

In other words, the cause of all dis-ease is the disruption of the flow of life energy either physically or mentally/emotionally.

- ♥ "The dense physical body is the response apparatus of the indwelling spiritual man and serves to put that spiritual entity en rapport with the...Life in which we live and move and have our being."
- ♥ "All disease (and this is a platitude) is caused by a lack of harmony—a disharmony to be found existing between the form aspect and the life."
- ♥ "All these conditions, however, can be regarded as purificatory in their effects, and must be so regarded by humanity if the right attitude towards disease is to be assumed."
- ♥ "When human thought reverses the usual ideas as to disease, and accepts disease as a fact in nature, man will begin to work with . . . right thought, leading to nonresistance."

71 Alice A. Bailey, *Esoteric Healing,* (New York, NY: Lucis Publishing Company, 1993), 532.

♥ "From one angle, disease is a process of liberation, and the enemy of that which is static and crystallized."[72]

PHYSICAL DISRUPTIONS IN THE FLOW OF LIFE ENERGY

Exposing the body-mind to things like toxic food, air, water, or drugs obstructs the physical flow of vital energy. The amazing body sorts out what it can use (pure water, nutrients, and vital energy) from the decayed molecules, toxic additives, and other corrosive and noxious substances in the digestive tract, airways, skin, and inner veins and ducts. It does its best to expel these unnecessary materials; but if there is no way to do this, it stashes them in non-vital areas like the pouches of the colon, joints, fat cells and other 'hiding places' to preserve the survival of the organism (you). The toxins accumulate over the years that a person continues to 'tox' her body. This theory explains why malnourished people can be fat (fat cells are needed for garbage storage), why 'degenerative diseases' tend to appear later in life (accumulation), and how a person can keep moving in a severely toxic body.

The toxins accumulate over the years that a person continues to 'tox' her body.

These toxins harm their 'store rooms' in two ways. They pollute the area, which hinders the normal function, and they add to the already existing blockage that prevents vital energy from flowing through the part. As the toxins build up, the conditions are exacerbated. Adding another toxin to the body to cover the symptom adds to the dilemma of the garbage removal process. Surgically removing the toxic part serves to temporarily restore function, but it does nothing to address the underlying cause of the problem and the body keeps trying to find 'hiding places.' That is why liposuction needs to be done again. Skin needs to breathe and sweat; joints need clear lubricated 'swing room' to flex; lungs need to be able to expand to clear membranes of toxins.

They pollute the area, which hinders the normal function, and they add to the already existing blockage that prevents vital energy from flowing through the part. As the toxins build up, the conditions are exacerbated.

---

72 Alice A. Bailey, *Esoteric Healing*, (New York, NY: Lucis Publishing Company, 1993), 2–14.

Constriction and toxic pollution of any part hampers nature at work and destroys life.

MENTAL DISRUPTIONS IN THE FLOW OF LIFE ENERGY

Errors in thinking obstruct, hinder, and divert the flow of vital life force. Thoughts (like rivers) run deep or shallow, can cut deep channels, and have many ways to be diverted. In nature, rocks and trees obstruct rivers and humans divert the flow of water with back hoes. People block the flow of chi with erroneous thoughts and dig neuropathway canals in their brains by repeating the error over and over. The character of the 'thought-error' determines the body part affected and the nature of the disease that ensues. It is like telling a part of the body it is not OK. These thoughts become deeply embedded and automatic, resulting in subconscious beliefs.

Thoughts are affected by physical circumstances—living in a diseased physical body, for example. Errors in thinking can result from past emotional trauma, real or imagined. It might be a loathing for a certain body part—like the breasts, for instance. Or the error can be in neglecting one's self or body. Louise Hay, a popular metaphysical teacher, writes that breast problems are caused by "A refusal to nourish the self. Putting everyone else first."[73] Self-Inflicted Nonsense (SIN) is an erroneous belief such as, "I don't deserve (money, love, health, respect)," but the human owner of the thought *can* forge a new neuropathway channel by a conscious change in habits of thought.

Thoughts are affected by physical circumstances—living in a diseased physical body, for example.

Thoughts cause illness and illness alters thought. So, like the parable of the tomato (Which came first, the fruit or the seed?), do we begin purifying and detoxifying at the physical level, the emotional level, or the mental thought level? The answer is "yes." Since most people find it difficult to simply change their thoughts, physical habits

Thoughts cause illness and illness alters thought.

73 Louise L. Hay, *Heal Your Body,* (Carson, CA: Hay House, 1988), 21.

might be an easier place to start. However, it takes a thought to change an action, and most of us remain stuck in the circle, becoming ill by default, never making a clear choice. This is, of course, a decision in itself.

What is focused upon will grow and the intensity of emotion that accompanies the thought will speed it into actualizing. (See Law of Attraction in Chapter 5.) It does not matter if thoughts are positive or negative. Negative thoughts simply attract what is *not* wanted—often referred to as 'self-fulfilling prophecy.' Deep subconscious attitudes or beliefs are very powerful attractors. It might be thrilling to dramatically ponder death; but if a great deal of energy is expended towards dying, it will hasten the event. Placing the body in a toxic position is a choice. Focus instead upon what *is* wanted, behave accordingly, and more of what is desired will come. The CEO of the body is the decider. It may seem like a very strong statement, but all suffering, illness, or disease on every level is self-inflicted in some way. The universe supports your ultimate intent even if it is subconscious. Change your intent and you will change your status because your body and subconscious mind believe every word you say or think.

It may seem like a very strong statement, but all suffering, illness, or disease on every level is self-inflicted in some way.

EMOTIONAL ENERGY BLOCKS ARE ALL SOME FORM OF FEAR

Light bearers and energy healers agree that the fundamental cause of disease is the blockage and imbalance of chi or prana—life force energy as it surges through the electrical system of the etheric and physical bodies. At the root of emotional blockages is always some variation of fear, such as anger, shame, or guilt. Negative emotions are all outward manifestations of being afraid of something—punishment, losing something important like love or self-respect, physical harm, or being exposed, for example. These emotions often lead to poor habits of eating, thinking, and immoderate living, in an effort to cope with the disturbing emotion. That leads to further blocks in the flow of energy through the body cells, causing what then becomes identified as cancer, arthritis, or thousands of other diagnoses. However—if it is self-inflicted, it *can* self-heal.

Fear is a natural emotion and most likely felt by our early human ancestors, because there were environmental conditions with which a human had to contend (being a creature with no fur, fangs, or claws). At a distinct physical disadvantage, she needed to outsmart such things as beasts and snow. Times have changed and what *was* healthy fear has degenerated into war, oppressive religions, tyrannical governments, senseless crimes, and widespread anxiety. What humans as a species dwell upon is what they will collectively attract. It will take both brains and will to figure it out.

However—if it is self-inflicted, it can self-heal.

Fear shows up as sarcasm, rage, disgust, jealousy, closed-mindedness, law suits, and an overwhelming need to control others and grab power. It distorts the mental barrier between physical matter and spirit. Modern humans often live in fear of crime, financial lack, relationship friction, disease, and failure (in its many forms). Our social systems fuel the fear. Teachers correct mistakes, doctors search for disease and focus on risk factors, preachers remind congregations of sins and inadequacies, and parents berate. Even the media thinks the public is stupid and will buy hundreds of useless products if they appeal to our fear of not being popular, smelling bad, or not being able to sleep.

Our social systems fuel the fear.

Then the individual takes over the 'fear talk' and whispers disparaging words to herself. We pick up where our parents left off. People deliberately choose fear by patronizing violent movies, video games, and sports. Fear is physical as well as mental and emotional; it lodges in the cells of the body.

Fear is physical as well as mental and emotional; it lodges in the cells of the body.

CLEANSE THE BODY AND REDUCE THE FEAR

There are many ways to lower the fear level. Some people have found that cleansing the physical body by switching to an organic live vegan diet seems to somehow lower the amplitude of fear. The energy systems of most humans are 'gummed up' like an unmaintained automobile burning the wrong fuel, leading to depressing thoughts. Conversely, errors in thought result in bad choices and toxic diet. These physical toxins collect in the tissues and along with negative emotions serve as barricades to block the energy in the etheric web that weaves through the physical body, causing untold suffering on all levels. Food is a main source of the toxins that collect in the 'corners' of the body and overwhelm the natural defenses that are trying to eliminate them. The body can remove these toxins by itself if the insults are stopped.

The body can remove these toxins by itself if the insults are stopped.

David Wolfe, a raw food proponent, writes that it takes about three years for the lymph system to remove this silt and clear the circulatory system after a SAD person adopts the live organic vegan diet.[74] Others say it takes a month to recover from each SAD year. Still others maintain there is a progression from physical cleansing, followed by mental and emotional releasing, and finally contact with Spirit.

But life is not a pass-fail curriculum. It is a self-study program with a progressive series of lessons, automatically adjusted by a personalized 'computer' which inputs every 'thought-vote.' If a lesson comes our way again, it is because it has not yet been fully learned. We are eternal beings; we cannot fail and we cannot drop out. Even dying won't get a person expelled from Universal University!

We are eternal beings; we cannot fail and we cannot drop out.

MASS DISTRACTION AND ILLNESS

Since illness ultimately begins in the mental arena, things that affect thought, inflict disease. People today often dash through life in

74 David Wolfe, *The Sunfood Diet Success System,* (San Diego, CA: Maul Brothers Publishing, 2002), 143.

'frantic mode,' distracted by rules and threats. These weapons of mass distraction can cause a person to forget who she really is, and instill thoughts of fear. Modern citizens are bombarded with hard-to-ignore authorities and offers.

These weapons of mass distraction can cause a person to forget who she really is, and instill thoughts of fear.

Mass media is a major distraction for most Americans, who seem to be continuously hooked electronically to drama. It can be fictionalized violence, shrieking talk shows, or loud canned laughter on sitcoms. Advertisements are intended to create the illusion of lack in a person's life, enticing them to spend money to fill it. An astonishing number of ads are for toxic drugs, hoping for more addicts who will buy the poisons for the rest of their lives. Corporations, whose sole purpose is to make money for stockholders, do their best to convince folks that food comes in plastic containers and is quickly microwavable. Companies have no conscience or responsibility to assist humans to awaken to their real selves—in fact they have a stake in each human feeling as bad as possible, so they can sell remedies. Even video games and a lot of music are off-putting for the delicate soul on a quest for peace, love, and wisdom.

It is difficult to find a movie that is not intended to instill unnecessary fear in the viewer, even those made for children. Uplifting movies are often described as 'feel-good,' as if that is somehow a bad thing. Dark drama produces adrenaline rushes that are addicting, and *fear sells*. Cooked food, pills, and weapons of mass distraction arouse fear, but love and compassion remove and transmute fear and all its cousins.

TOXIC RELIGION

While religion can be a valuable guide to spiritual freedom, it too can also be a major distraction from truth. While some religious leaders encourage responsibility, compassion, and self-love, these influential people could do more to teach about energy flow, the law of attraction, and the power of love. They could encourage self-love, inclusion, and tolerance. Religious people are mostly good-hearted and well-intentioned—many of them, however, are simply uninformed. They, like doctors, are unaware of the flow of energy and the natural laws which could heal and bring peace.

Conscious aspirants embrace others on different journeys without coercion or judgment—they seek common ground with new people. They look for similarities instead of differences. OK, so your skin is a different shade or you attend a different religious service; do you like raspberries like I do?

ILLNESS AND MEDICINE

The medical community, sometimes erroneously referred to as a 'health care system,' is part of the cycle of rewarding illness. So, too, are the systems known as drug and insurance companies. Health care providers usually look for what is wrong; not what is right. They focus mainly upon classifying symptoms and labeling syndromes. While this is interesting to scientists, it is not of much help to patients. Many diagnoses, which are often found together, are declared to be causing one another. Obesity and diabetes, for example are often found together; but both are signs of toxic overload and nutrient starvation—and not a matter of cause and effect.

The medical community, sometimes erroneously referred to as a 'health care system,' is part of the cycle of rewarding illness.

Most people leave a medical office holding a slip of paper with the name of a chemical substance written on it. It might be to disguise a symptom or complaint, intended to aid sleep, calm a person, or block pain. It could even be a vitamin pill. Sometimes people feel better after taking the prescribed medication, sometimes not. Studies show that around a third of the time, improvement may actually be attributed to what is called the 'placebo effect.' This is a term used when an inert substance or 'fake' treatment appears to help the patient in some way. The placebo effect shows that the change was not the result of the therapy, but probably from an illusion held by the patient, the provider, or both. The point is, it often works as well as 'real medicine,' opening the possibility of therapy without pills (and no toxic side effects).

Most medications do not address the underlying cause of symptoms. Illnesses are not caused by a deficiency of drugs. Besides creating new illnesses, toxic medication often leads to addiction and new even more serious physical problems. Medications are fear-based; they clog the physical apparatus, cloud mental functioning, and block the light from divine source. Taking pain and sleeping pills will not detect and resolve subconscious fears. Denial and oblivion are not the same as resolution and health.

Illnesses are not caused by a deficiency of drugs.

According to Gary Null and colleagues, medical treatment is a leading cause of death in the U. S.[75] Medical science can prolong life and marvelously repair damaged body parts surgically, but cures almost nothing. Physically, drugs poison the body and radiation interferes with the energy system. Everyone then assumes the patient died of the disease and not from the treatments *or* from the expectations of the patient or those around her.

Denial and oblivion are not the same as resolution and health.

Allopathy is a term coined in the early 19th century to describe treatments used by mainstream practitioners which are, by definition, intended to create a new symptom that directly opposes the complaint of the patient. Metaphysical practitioners say that in addition to the original disease, the body then needs to overcome the effects of the toxin, as well as find a way to expel the drug. For example, if a person is suffering from diarrhea, presumably because the body wisdom is trying to rid the body of something, the bowel then has to overcome the constipating effect of the drug. Drugs have no inherent 'action.'

75 Gary Null, Ph.D., Carolyn Dean, M.D., N.D., Martin Feldman, M.D., Debora Raslow, M.D., and Dorothy Smith, Ph.D., "Death by Medicine," *Life Extension,* on Website: lef.org, August, 2006.

They always work by provoking the body to react in an effort to remove it, for if you give the drug to a dead body, nothing happens.

The contemporary view of illness says it is caused by genes, germs, or gamble—all out of the hands of the patient. Self-treatments like diet, avoiding toxins, smoking cessation, and exercise come after pharmaceutical profit. Gene and germ theories, believed by contemporary medical providers, promote a 'not-my-fault' attitude which discourages patients from searching for causes within themselves and accepting responsibility for their illness.

But some scientists now suggest that genes can be altered by beliefs and habits (see Chapters 6 and 12). Both beliefs and habits can be changed by the owner. It has also been suggested by many that germs are attracted to tissue that lacks life energy (see section on bacteria below) which gives a different perspective on 'infection.' Science is slowly becoming 'spiritual' by seeing that thoughts, intent, and energy are the cause of disease instead of some outside 'attacker' or the fateful roll of the 'genetic dice.'

Science is slowly becoming 'spiritual' by seeing that thoughts, intent, and energy are the cause of disease instead of some outside 'attacker' or the fateful roll of the 'genetic dice.'

NARROW VISION

Humans tend to pick one particular point of view or theory and fail to explore others. For example, many in the field of medicine seem fixated on the Newtonian world of 'body as a machine.' Spiritual energy, patient beliefs, and the power of thought are usually ignored by mainstream allopathic medical practitioners. Modern medicine considers the body a closed system, a sort of mechanism. Physical sciences operate mainly at the physical level, so there is often a feeling of failure when a patient does not respond.

Conversely, aspirants and students of religious and metaphysical studies can become fixated at the spiritual level and tend to ignore the physical. Worse yet, they demonize the physical, perhaps a result of the influence of the some of the early Gnostics, who felt the body was inherently evil. Spiritual people in physical pain often turn to allopathic medicine for a cure, ignoring the Law of Attraction. Healing, however, must occur at all levels and it is important to accept responsibility for self-healing. Spiritual energy is to be integrated with the physical in this New Age and suffering on any level is not necessary; it is simply the result of error.

Healing, however, must occur at all levels and it is important to accept responsibility for self-healing.

ADDICTION vs. HABIT vs. BODY NEEDS

An aspirant in transition from cooked to fresh organic vegan food may have difficulty determining whether a longing for a certain food is an addiction, a long term comfortable habit, or her body actually craving needed nutrients. The truth can come only from watching one's own reactions over time to any food after it is consumed to see if it enhances or depresses well-being. Sometimes a craving occurs when the body reaches a particular substance in its cleaning program, like finding an old memory in a dusty scrap book, which creates a longing for it.

An aspirant in transition from cooked to fresh organic vegan food may have difficulty determining whether a longing for a certain food is an addiction, a long term comfortable habit, or her body actually craving needed nutrients.

When Victoria Boutenko was a student of the raw food lifestyle before she began to teach and speak extensively on the subject, she asked Don Haughey, the founder of Creative Health Institute, how many of the students actually stay raw after they leave the school. She was astonished when he estimated only about two percent stayed on the healthy diet. It was a mystery to her why people would revert back when they reported feeling so much better on raw food. Then a friend invited her to an Alcoholics Anonymous meeting and during the talk, she realized the attachment to cooked food is in the same category with alcohol and drugs craved by AA members. She believes that cooked food is a legal addiction stronger and harder to break than any other addiction. She makes the comparison to coffee or cigarettes, which most of us found repulsive at first and then eventually some learned to 'like' (babies spit out cooked food at first, too).[76] Boutenko maintains that the cooked food addiction is on all levels: physical, emotional, mental, and spiritual. Most contemporary mothers served us cooked food, which has come to mean 'comfort' on many levels.

In studies done at Princeton University, researchers found that when addictive drugs such as morphine are stopped, there are characteristic effects on both the behavior and the brain. They found these same signs in animals that consumed sugar and then stopped, leading the scientists to suggest that they had become sugar dependent.[77] Many people say in jest that they are 'addicted' to things such as chocolate and cheese, but it may actually be true. "Cooked flesh is powerfully addictive," says Elizabeth Baker, who studied food consumed by humans as recorded in the Bible.[78]

Many writers wonder why the simple truth about live food is not generally known by scientists. Wolfe (et al.) writes that science tends to ignore the facts because "humanity is addicted to cooked food and addiction has blinded everybody."[79] This means that scientists and physicians are also addicted to the SAD and can therefore hardly be expected to advocate a raw, vegan diet. From his experience prescribing raw foods to patients, Dr. John Douglass found that common addictions like alcohol and cigarettes seem to lose their potency on a diet of raw foods.[80]

Dead food is seductive. If something seems to be calling, the only way to decide is to eat some, then watch the reaction on physical,

Dead food is seductive.

---

76 Victoria Boutenko, *12 Steps to Raw Food,* (Ashland, OR: Raw Family Publishing, 2002), 56–60.

77 Kelly Brownell, *Food Fight,* (New York, NY: McGraw-Hill, 2004), 34.

78 Elizabeth Baker, *Does The Bible Teach Nutrition?,* (Mukilteo, WA: Winepress Publishing, 1997), 19.

79 Arlin, Dini, and Wolfe, *Nature's First Law,* (San Diego, CA: Maul Brothers, 2003), 15.

80 Arlin, Dini, and Wolfe, *Nature's First Law,* (San Diego, CA: Maul Brothers, 2003), 215.

emotional, and mental levels for the next few days. The 'hangover' might come immediately, the next morning, or it could take a few days. People react with different 'symptoms' to various foods, and it might take days or weeks to tell. Watch for body aches, energy level changes, gastrointestinal symptoms, enthusiasm shifts, level of stress, and sleep patterns. Willpower, like a muscle, strengthens when it is exercised. The mind decides—is the hangover worth the taste? More than likely the same flavor and texture can be created in a raw version without 'side effects.'

Willpower, like a muscle, strengthens when it is exercised.

DISEASE DEFINED

'Dis-ease' is a lack of 'ease'—suffering in some way. Conventional medicine defines illness as "a condition that impairs normal function." But there is no real definition of 'normal' or 'wellness,' since most medical studies are done on chronically-toxic SAD people. The metaphysical definition of disease is a condition where the body is in disharmony with the love energy it naturally wants to conduct. The physical body is a sum result of subconscious beliefs, thoughts, social drama, diet, and general lifestyle—a veritable snapshot of your life. The body does not lie.

'Dis-ease' is a lack of 'ease'—suffering in some way.

John Sanford, a psychologist and priest, defines illness as something that results in a malfunctioning of consciousness—the part of us that sets our morality. He says "The center of consciousness is the *ego*, the 'I' part of us that does the willing, suffering, and choosing in life; the part of us of which we are most immediately aware [mental, adult, or middle self]. If this part is not able to function, it seems that we are ill." This could be either physically or psychologically. Sanford writes, "There is a force within us that always works to heal by bringing things into the light."[81] I believe he is referring to the high self here.

The body does not lie.

81 John Sanford, *Healing and Wholeness*, (New York, NY: Paulist Press, 1977), 5-6.

According to the Second Law of Thermodynamics, it is the natural order of things to break down as they age, like the rusting of iron. This is called *entropy* and most professionals believe this. The truth, however, is the process of entropy does not apply to pure vital organisms. Living organisms *generate* healing energy, while objects merely have and absorb energy. Vital bodies constantly work to clear energy blocks and toxic accumulation in the safest and most life-preserving way. Energy creates matter, not the other way around. Nutrients found in living food, oxygen, and water activate the life force in animals directly, which is contrary to the law of entropy.

The truth, however, is the process of entropy does not apply to pure vital organisms.

THE PURPOSE OF ILLNESS

It is difficult to accept at first glance that disease might serve a spiritual purpose. Indeed, sickness has many healing functions, as do other so-called 'bad' things, like rain and flies. Illness focuses attention on the problem, where the energy block is occurring, and where the error of thought finds its physical counterpart. As long as there is no suffering of any kind, where is the motivation to change or to look deeper? Even things like accidents, assaults, and supposed tragedies provide rips in the armor around our subconscious selves and allow cracks of light to penetrate, bringing hints about our issues into conscious awareness. Perhaps the purpose of everything is to lure a person to look deeper into what 'seems to be.' A sufferer can choose to remain in the place of darkness, of course, but there comes a turning point where illness either brings an end to the current life, or a decision to rise into the light.

Illness focuses attention on the problem, where the energy block is occurring, and where the error of thought finds its physical counterpart.

Illness is not a punishment, and suffering is not necessary for enlightenment. There is no glory in suffering; it is not part of the Divine plan. Suffering is simply a mistake, a SIN, an error in thought. Disease helps identify and define that mistake and moves to help purify the energy blocks in the precious holy physical body, propelling it toward wellness. The living physical vehicle is constantly purifying itself. Illness often brings us to the bottom line, helps clarify life's purpose, and guides a person to what is really important. A couple days in bed with the flu (which forces fasting in some cases) can be exactly the clarifying experience needed to make better decisions about an individual path of life. Like meditation, illness causes a person to slow down, quit the chatter and rushing of everyday life, and get down into the bowels where important answers are found.

The symptom alerts one that the inner, psychological balance has been lost—that something is wrong.

Spiritual psychologists Thorwald Dethlefsen and Rudiger Dahlke, have written that an illness and a symptom are not the same thing. They suggest that when a symptom manifests in a person's body, it interrupts life's continuity and demands our attention. The symptom alerts one that the inner, psychological balance has been lost—that something is wrong. When a warning light comes on in the car, it would be annoying, even perhaps deadly, if the mechanic simply unscrewed the bulb without searching for the underlying problem. Allopathic medicine often equates symptom with illness, applying enormous resources and skills to eliminating the symptom—but rarely looks at the *person* who is ill. In effect, they 'unscrew the light bulb.' Instead of the great enemy, symptoms can be honest teachers and guides to true healing. Illness is a path to perfection.[82]

Instead of the great enemy, symptoms can be honest teachers and guides to true healing. Illness is a path to perfection.

Florence Nightingale herself wrote in the mid-1800s, "all disease…is more or less a reparative process…an effort of nature to remedy a process of poisoning or of decay."[83] Disease is intended to purify the body and by survival of the fittest, the species. Sickness is a result of a block of energy but one must look at what caused the block. Illness gives a thread to tug on in order to unravel the mystery of where the block began. It is impossible to separate the spiritual

82 Thorwald Dethlefsen & Rudiger Dahlke, M.D., *The Healing Power of Illness,* (Rockport, MA: Element Books, Inc, 1991), 8–9, 91.

83 Florence Nightingale, *Notes on Nursing,* (New York, NY: Dover Publications, 1969), 7.

from the physical and mental, so they must be considered together, just as vitamins are attached to their natural companions and must be eaten together. When a body is cleansed, the mind is also purified, which leads to spiritual enlightenment. The reverse is also true. There is a physical surge of energy with a cleansing mental discovery—the legendary "ah ha!" moment.

Illness not only points out errors in thought, it purifies the vehicle with such things as fever, which speeds up metabolism to assist the body with purification. Vomiting and diarrhea rid the digestive tract of something the wisdom of the body knows is not desirable. Coughing clears the respiratory system. Covering symptoms with drugs causes an added strain to an already over-taxed vehicle, like putting sugar in the gas tank. Sickness demands our attention, sometimes quite abruptly. We would not be pleased with a mechanic who reached in, unscrewed the bulb, and charged $100. Why do we tolerate that behavior from health care providers? An even more profound question is why do providers not question what they are doing?

CHOICE

Illness is a choice, albeit not usually a conscious one.

Illness is a choice, albeit not usually a conscious one. It is inevitably done out of habit, imitation, or default; but the outcome is that it keeps one from participating in society, for good or for bad. Infirmity can actually be a pleasurable choice with many rewards for some. There must be a payoff, such as relieving a person from societal responsibility. Children are rewarded for illness by their mothers rocking them, or giving them special food, or allowing them to stay home from school or church. The boss actually wants you to stay home from work with the dreaded flu of the year. Depending on the severity of the illness, friends or relatives may visit, bring flowers, or pray. Often the center of attention, a patient is dismissed from everyday routine, and in some ways returned to child-status with doctor and nurse acting as parents.

Old people, often neglected and ignored by society, gain importance by letting people poke, listen to, and cut on parts of their body. Even though the touching is not always comfortable, *it is touching*—a balm to a touch-starved body. Loving attention heaped upon the ill person, often for the first time, can be seductive.

Medical corporations, with no incentive to assist people to be really healthy, reward illness by insisting that medicine is a 'right.' Medications further toxify the body and cloud mental acuity. The sickest people get the most damaging treatments. The medical system feeds upon itself and is self-perpetuating. The question is just how many non-functioning people can society afford to support?

THE ENERGY OF NEGLECT—CUTTING OFF THE FLOW OF ENERGY

Spiritual energy is free; it flows like light from cosmic fire and is only absent when it is blocked by something—denied access.

Spiritual energy is free; it flows like light from cosmic fire and is only absent when it is blocked by something—denied access. Darkness—in its many forms, comes from blocks (possibly placed in error) to the source of light. There is always the potential to make the darkness light at any time. There is only light and absence of light. We don't turn *on* a 'dark switch' when we leave a room. The power source, still there, is merely shut off. Cold is merely the absence of heat. Sadness is the blocking of joy, like shade is the blocking of sun. All negativity is a result of being cut off from our true home, our true nature.

All negativity is a result of being cut off from our true home, our true nature.

Dulling one's mind with physical toxins like cooked food and drugs, and mental distractions like TV, cut off the flow of cosmic energy to one's life. They cause us to forget who we really are. Of course, the occasional dark thought, an evening of television, or a glass of wine won't cause cancer or death; but habitual repetition of negative thoughts and actions repel the light.

It is the *removal of attention* from an aspect of one's existence that severely restricts the flow of life—the denial or withholding of love. Just like a neglected and untouched baby will likely die, even if given plenty of food and kept clean. Lack of nurturing will kill an organism or even part of an organism such as a liver. Not necessarily a bad thing, death is, therefore ultimately a form of suicide—a choice made by some part of our being, whether consciously intentional or not. It is the choice to stop nurturing our self. Your body is precious, treasure it. Pay attention to your health while you still have it. (See Physical Death section in Chapter 6.)

Not necessarily a bad thing, death is, therefore ultimately a form of suicide—a choice made by some part of our being, whether consciously intentional or not.

When Life Force Energy is withdrawn from a living body, the physical shell, containing the slower vibration, slowly decomposes back into basic elements and is reused to create new living bodies, infused with life. Germs, flies, and vultures are some of the means nature has provided to clean up dead tissue. Road kill must be returned to nature by macro means (carnivores), micro means (bacteria and enzymes), and some in-between means (worms and flies). These will break down a dead carcass, quickly returning it to rich compost, alive with micro-life, enhancing the soil, which in turn will build new plants and eventually new animal bodies. It is a beautiful circle of energy, directed by cellular intelligence which has knowledge of the laws of the universe.

When there is *withholding* of attention from an area of life *as a result of some form of fear,* that part becomes dark or negative. It might be a body part or a space in your home, but the energy there slows or ceases to flow all together. Here is another good reason to clean house—to renew the energy in an area by paying attention to it and making it more pleasing to the senses—a closet, your teeth, or the

When there is withholding of attention from an area of life as a result of some form of fear, that part becomes dark or negative.

backseat of the car. No wonder it feels good to clean (well it feels good after the cleaning is done, at least).

> Even friendships and pets need attention to thrive. Stop and visit your first-grade teacher, take her a fruit basket and thank her. Call an old friend or make the first move to make a new one. Adopt a cat from the shelter. Expand your awareness of others and parts of yourself that are neglected. Spreading love is a gift to yourself.

Money is a form of energy, too, so be conscious where you spend it. Give your tithe to someone or some organization you want to encourage. Leave a big tip for a sincere waitress that touches your heart. Instead of buying junk food, support a local organic farmer. Support yourself by putting a bouquet of flowers in your bedroom. Support causes that make society safer, healthier, and more peaceful.

> Do research on corporations and charities before donating your money. Look on the label before you buy. Find out where the company spends their money, what percent goes to administration, for example. What is the difference in the salary between the CEO and the check-out lady? To what political candidates do they donate and why? What community causes do they support? Are they mindful of the effect their products or services have on their consumers?

DIAGNOSES

When the energy flow to a part of the body is blocked with some fear-laden belief, it is like that part is 'holding its breath.' It is possible to hold the breath for a minute or so, but beyond that it begins to interfere with body function and could result in the death of the organism. The block acts as a physical 'net' which collects toxic debris. Like a dead tree restricts the river, toxins (such as animal protein)

When the energy flow to a part of the body is blocked with some fear-laden belief, it is like that part is 'holding its breath.'

block the chi that normally bathes each cell. Eventually, if the fearful thoughts and toxic substances are continued, the natural defenses of the body are overwhelmed, and the parts of the body most often bombarded will break down and at this point a medical diagnosis can be made. This diagnosis is a clue to the cause of the block, but the owner of the body must be ready to look at it that way.

Diseases often develop in alignment *with* the belief system of the person, which then blocks the flow of energy and results in collection of toxic debris in some part of the body. There are many books that discuss possible issues responsible for specific diseases in different body parts, written for those with an open heart and mind. A few of these are: J. A. Winter, *Why We Get Sick: The Origins of Illness and Anxiety*; Debbie Shapiro, *The Bodymind Workbook*; and most well-known, Louise Hay, *You Can Heal Your Life.*

Louise Hay, a battered child who healed her body of cancer with forgiveness and physical detoxification, set the golden standard for books connecting mental attitude with physical health. She says what we give out (our story), we get back in our body. Life is a mirror for what lies within our mind, and disease comes in a state of 'unforgiveness.' Whatever we believe *becomes* true for us. Various parts of the body physically represent an unseen mental attitude. Some examples are: ears represent the capacity to 'hear,' eyes are the capacity to 'see,' and throat is the ability to 'speak up' (a sore throat is unresolved anger). The heart, of course, represents love and joy, so a heart attack can mean these are blocked. The stomach digests new ideas as well as food, so problems there might lead to looking at what the mind is trying to accept that the inner wisdom is rejecting (what you are trying to 'swallow'). Cancer represents deep hurt, a secret, hatred, grief or a giving up.[84] Inflammation is listed by Hay as fear and seeing red. Skin rashes might be a 'breaking out' of repressed

---

84 Louise L. Hay, *You Can Heal Your Life,* (Carlsbad, CA: Hay House, Inc., 1987), 138.

emotions. Perhaps arthritis develops because we do not express anger, and we unconsciously stiffen up to prevent punching someone. Each person must examine her own symptoms and find the underlying cause for herself.

Fear, in one form or another, is listed by many writers as a cause of all disease. The body does not lie. A person doesn't need to speak the fear out loud to be screaming it energetically. It is the core belief, the emotional charge given to a thought, that blocks the light. Both positive and negative energy are contagious. Sometimes diseases, like cancer, actually begin before birth when the fetus feels the negative emotions of people involved with the pregnancy.

The body does not lie.

BACTERIA

Modern science teaches the 'germ theory,' which was promoted by Louis Pasteur and is generally accepted in medical thought. It claims that a fixed species of microbes from an external source invades the body and is the first cause of 'infectious' disease (each species causing a specific set of disease symptoms). This assumption has been refuted by many, however, including perhaps Pasteur himself who, according to nutritionist Nancy Appleton, admitted on his death bed, "Claude Bernard was right…the microbe is nothing, the terrain is everything."[85] (Bernard had an opposing view to Pasteur's). Appleton writes, "Because of his persistence and standing in the medical community, Pasteur's theory was adopted." It persists today as absolute fact.

Gabriel Cousens' rainbow diet is based on his belief that microorganisms are not the primary cause of disease, only opportunistic scavengers that appear when the body is weak and out of balance. He tells the story of the much publicized debate in the late 1800s between French microbiologists Louis Pasteur and Claude Bernard. When Pasteur said Bernard was right, he was admitting that the primary

85 Nancy Appleton, *Rethinking Pasteur's Germ Theory,* (Berkeley, CA: Frog, Ltd, 2002), 28–30.

underlying etiology of disease was a disruption of the "biological terrain." He goes on to specify that the *proper* terrain means:

1. Low levels of toxicity and fermentation
2. Proper range of acid/alkaline balance
3. Strong electromagnetic potential
4. High cellular oxygenation
5. A high number of pro-biotic beneficial bacteria and a low number of pathogenic microorganisms[86]

The pathogenic microorganisms Cousens refers to occur in tissues that are out of balance and lacking life force energy. They are there to compost the 'dead tissue.' Cousens asserts that his low sugar 'live food cuisine' heals the biological terrain of the body, thus preventing this activity.

Florence Nightingale also refuted the theory of germs as the outside cause of infectious diseases when she observed, "I have seen with my eyes and smelt with my nose small-pox growing up in first specimens ...where it could not by any possibility have been "caught," but must have begun." She also writes "I have seen diseases begin, grow up, and pass into...another [disease]. Now, dogs do not pass into cats."[87]

Robert O. Young, a microbiologist who has done extensive research into the causes of disease, agrees with Bernard, Cousens and Nightingale (and many others) when he writes, "Disease is a general condition of one's internal environment. Bacteria, yeast, fungus, and mold are morbid evolutions of healthy cells, caused by a disturbance in the central electromagnetic balance of the cell. Though germs don't cause disease, secondary symptoms are produced in response to their activity."[88]

86 Gabriel Cousens, M.D., *Rainbow Green Live—Food Cuisine,* (Berkeley, CA: North Atlantic Books, 2003), xiv-xv.

87 Florence Nightingale, *Notes on Nursing,* (New York, NY: Dover Publications, 1969), 32-33.

88 Robert O. Young, Ph.D., D.Sc. with Shelley Redford Young, L.M.T., *Sick and Tired?,* (Pleasant Grove, UT: Woodland Publishing, 2001), 19–22.

The originators of the 'terrain theory' of disease were Claude Bernard, Antoine Béchamp and Günther Enderlein. Their research showed that "disease is a general manifestation of a disruption to internal biological environment; and that a species of pathogens is most often a pleomorphic change in a specific growth cycle of that species."[89] They develop into bacteria associated with illness. Healthy and unhealthy forms of the microbes depend on the internal conditions of the fluids and tissues of the body and do not attack from the outside.

In reality, bacteria merely 'clean up' or purify tissue that is dead from a lack of prana. Saying bacteria cause disease is like saying 'flies cause garbage.' Finding bacteria at the scene of disease is circumstantial evidence but also a 'red herring,' for both are precipitated by a third unseen factor—blocked energy. Bacteria, like carnivores and weeds, are all good things. They break down and convert our 'garbage,' (dead organic matter such as road kill and fallen trees) to produce nutrients for the soil. Bugs, worms, and bacteria (all friends of humanity) make possible our very existence and do not deserve the bad rap given them. Together, we are part of the same cosmos—macro and micro, evolving toward good. Victoria Boutenko believes that bacteria have no harmful effect on anything still alive. She writes, "Bacteria can tell what is living and what is dead and it is only interested in dead matter."[90]

In reality, bacteria merely 'clean up' or purify tissue that is dead from a lack of prana. Saying bacteria cause disease is like saying 'flies cause garbage.'

Bacteria, vultures, and flies play their part in nature's plan to return everything to be recycled when it loses prana. Enzymes, worms, rain, and fire also purify. When toxic thoughts and physical toxins block the flow of life, the tissue becomes dead and nature will take action to reuse it. Germs show up when and where they are needed. Attitude is contagious, germs are not.

---

89 Robert O Young, Ph.D., D.Sc. with Shelley Redford Young, L.M.T., *Sick and Tired?*, (Pleasant Grove, UT: Woodland Publishing, 2001), 10.

90 Victoria Boutenko, *12 Steps to Raw Foods,* (Ashland, OR: Raw Family Publishing, 2002), 30.

The intelligence of bacteria can be seen by the increase of microscopic creatures resistant to human-made antibiotic chemicals. No sooner do scientists develop a substance that appears to kill a bacterium accused of causing a symptom, when it morphs into something else that will withstand antibiotic attack. Gardeners fight a never-ending battle with weeds. What could nature possibly be saying by putting so much importance and energy into maintaining bacteria and weeds when humans expend so much energy and money to kill them? Maybe they are here for the good of all? Humans do not yet understand all the functions of 'micro-beings' but it is quite clear that they are here to serve and are summoned by the energy of the host. (See DNA section, Chapter 12).

Attitude is contagious, germs are not.

PAIN

Pain, like death, is nature's way of getting a person to slow down and pay attention—a sort of 'cosmic baseball bat.' It forces the sufferer to figure out where she got off track with thoughts, activities, or attitude. Sometimes pain can be relieved by shifting the energies, either with the help of a healer or by focused intent.

Living in the modern world cuts us off from the healing energy naturally emanating from and to the Earth. We have filled the space with human-generated concrete and artificial energies such as high-voltage electricity grids. These negative energies can cause harm in some sensitive people and probably do not do anyone any good. Some people have found magnets seem to restore Earth energy to the body, relieving painful conditions.

Pain, like death, is nature's way of getting a person to slow down and pay attention—a sort of 'cosmic baseball bat.'

Pain is also caused by a congestion of stored physical toxins. Massage, exercise, stretching, and other forms of physical manipulation can help dislodge it. It also helps to stop the toxification. Gout is an example of how energetic and physical congestion work together. Foot problems can be caused by fear of stepping forward in life. Uric acid, the ash from consuming animal parts, needs to be deposited where it does not threaten life. Fear directs the uric acid to the feet to produce gout. Pain occurs when the body is overwhelmed with fear and toxins; it is not from a deficiency of pain-relievers!

AGING

Aging is viewed bleakly in American society. Unconscious beliefs programmed into modern minds tell us that along with advancing age comes dimmed eyesight, stiff joints, failing memory, and inevitable illness, often followed by a painful death. These beliefs come from circumstantial evidence—most people *do* get these things. These 'aging symptoms' or entropy (which does not naturally apply to living systems) are actually created by the mind and diet, as evidenced when changing these things relieves the conditions. People *expect* that if their ancestors in the genetic tree were afflicted, they will surely fall prey to the same disease as they age, too. It takes conscious effort to evaluate a symptom to see what message is contained and to 'counter-act.' Beliefs can be contagious, but only if allowed to be.

Pain occurs when the body is overwhelmed with fear and toxins; it is not by a deficiency of pain-relievers!

It is not necessary to look into the future with dread after whatever age is chosen to symbolize 'old' (for some it is 100, others choose 40). *Of course*, the body will tremble in fear and shut down if it believes aging means pain and social rejection followed by being tied to a bed with tubes and restraints, trapped like an animal caught in the steely jaws that were set earlier in life. Or aging might mean sitting in a large padded wheelchair in a brightly-lit shiny hallway, mumbling in gibberish and cursed with dull, thin grey hair, and wrinkled, awkward bodies unable to tolerate a stroll in the woods or a walk to the grocery store.

Beliefs can be contagious, but only if allowed to be.

It doesn't have to be this way! It is unknown how many of the 'signs and symptoms of aging' might be inevitable—probably none are. If a way can be found to preserve and 'youth' the body by mental and physical means, why not do it? Is the Standard American Diet of white flour, sugar, and animal parts, seared by heat and smothered with herb flavored sauce, worth the scenes in the emergency room or the long term care facility? With a flick of the attitude-switch a decision can be made to love one's body as much as a newborn child, feeding and tending it to bring about a peaceful and comfortable future.

TOXINS IN FOOD BLOCK ENERGY

Blocked energy in the body traps poisons from food, further disturbing the flow. Artificial colors, flavors, and preservatives along with pesticides might not instantly cause actual 'symptoms' in a toxic body (as they do in a detoxed body), but they are accumulating and they become lodged in non-vital areas to create ultimately dangerous conditions. Plus they combine together, especially when heated to very high temperatures to create new and unintended chemicals. These 'additives' are unnatural and unnecessary substances used to sell products and extend shelf life. They build upon each other as the fallen tree in the river catches other floating debris adding to the 'dam' effect.

Blocked energy in the body traps poisons from food, further disturbing the flow.

Cooking not only exacerbates toxicity but it dehydrates the cells of the food, destroys enzymes, and eliminates the life force energy it held from the garden. Fear, adrenaline, and negative energy of slaughtered gentle animals remain in the dinner and affect the body of the diner. The choice of food is as important as the choice of thoughts. (Much more on the effects of cooked food in Chapter 8.)

There are thousands of reports of physical healing believed to be brought about when the body is allowed to detoxify itself by discontinuing the consumption of processed, dead, and flesh food, eating only living organic vegan food. It stands to reason that if a disease reverses itself when the body is detoxified that the toxins played a major role in causing the illness. But there probably will never be a compilation beyond anecdotal stories of personal healing with live food, because that could possibly be considered a medical claim. Each person has to do her own research in her own way and then use her own body to experiment for herself.

OTHER TOXINS

Besides diet, there are many other ways that physical bodies get polluted in this century, at least in the industrialized world. These, too, become lodged in the tissues of the body and create the same energy blocks that the toxic food does, and must be discontinued before the body can clear them away. The air is often filled with poisons—from a factory or chemical crop sprays, for example. Water, too, has been contaminated with things like chlorine and fluoride. The shower is a major source of chlorine absorption, because pores in the skin are open in the warmth of the water and the chlorine released in steam is inhaled through the lungs. Chlorine and fluoride are deadly toxins.

It stands to reason that if a disease reverses itself when the body is detoxified that the toxins played a major role in causing the illness.

Products used in and on the body can also be toxic. These include soaps, shampoo, lotions, toothpaste, and laundry products containing such things as sodium lauryl sulphate. Wearing natural fibers, especially organic cotton, is mindful of both the planet and your own energy. Bug sprays, air deodorizers, perfume, aftershave, vehicle exhaust, smoke, and new carpet and furniture (the 'new car smell') carry varying amounts of harmful substances. The question is how much poison can be tolerated even by a toxic body; how sick is 'sick'? (More on environmental toxins and safe alternatives in Chapter 10.)

There are two ways mental processes are involved in physical toxins causing disease.

♥ People choose to buy and use then in and around the body. They choose to put their body in harm's way.

♥ Where in the body the toxin will get 'stuck' is determined by where vital energy is lacking. When energy is blocked, the body is unable to clear away toxins.

It is a choice, first to allow toxins into the body, and then to mentally 'block' their removal from the system because of attitude. It is not toxin alone that will end up as cancer or other disease; there is an attitude of allowing it that must be there. Humans, collectively keep corporations manufacturing unnatural, toxic substances by spending money on them. When you purchase non-organic food you choose to keep the GMO seed company, the chemical pesticide company, and chemical farms in business. We must uncover the truth as intelligent beings and make hard choices every day.

Humans, collectively keep corporations manufacturing unnatural, toxic substances by spending money on them.

GETTING WELL

Before wellness on any level can begin, an individual needs to make a private and very definite decision. This commitment requires deep introspection. What are your motives for:

1. The actions you take
2. The words you speak
3. The beliefs you hold

Before wellness on any level can begin, an individual needs to make a private and very definite decision.

People are hesitant to look deeply into the real 'gut' of their issues, but the power that is unleashed from the effort is atomic and perpetual. A decision to become better in some way is huge and produces change not only personally but for the planet.

Getting well is not so much a belief in the healing method being used but the willingness to give up the (false) belief that caused the energy block in the first place. That is why meditation is so important. It slows the constant chatter in the mind so that unseen ethereal teachers can impress loving wisdom upon human hearts, opening them to greater awareness. Even a subtle glance sends a message rippling into the air; the awesome power of a smile at a stranger might save a life, change the course of history, or reverse the cancer in the smiler or the smilee.

A decision to become better in some way is huge and produces change not only personally but for the planet.

Whenever energies are blocked—on the physical level with toxins, the emotional level by fear, or the mental level by an implanted lie—there is discomfort, a disconnection between an individual and the light of love. Removing the blocks can bring deceiving results initially, however, because the process of clearing can *temporarily* increase discomfort called detoxification symptoms. Detoxification withdrawal symptoms on the emotional and on the physical level can be perceived to be as severe as the pain of the block itself, especially since toxic food dulls the mind and people tend to ignore the symptoms of toxicity until they reach 'diagnosis' level. But detoxification leads to a resolution, where continued toxing leads to death. Consider when a house cleaning or remodeling project is undertaken—before the end result can be realized, there must be a time of chaos with furniture moving, scattered dust and trash accompanied by considerable noise, discomfort, and inconvenience. Each person travels the detoxification path alone and must discover her own personal answers.

But detoxification leads to a resolution, where continued toxing leads to death.

CURE vs. HEALING

Healing does not always result in what is normally thought of as a cure. Conversely, a cure does not always involve healing. A cure removes symptoms of illness, while healing promotes wellness and consciousness in whatever form needed by each person.

Healing encourages peace of mind, soothing of emotions, a connection with truth; it takes positive emotions to a place of prominence and greater depth than previously experienced. A person's body might remain severely ill, even die. But healing is a deep 'knowing' that will make death a moment of peace. This peace, which may not have been present until the moment before death, goes with the soul. Healing takes place on the soul level when the veil between heaven and human opens. The person recognizes herself as part of the universal energy of love and feels no longer separate. It raises consciousness above the level of suffering, above the vibration that experiences fear. Healing very often reverses physical illness, too, but in a deep multilayered way. A person is unlikely to 'relapse' after real healing.

A cure involves relief of the symptoms or signs of disease in the physical body, or the appearance of resolution of a mental or emotional issue. Cure might evoke some level of healing, and healing can produce a partial or complete cure; but they are not the same and do not always occur together. Cure implies that some outside influence was involved in the change, such as when water cures thirst. Often 'cure' is used to mean a covering of symptoms.

Medical providers do not pretend to distribute panaceas for all illnesses—body or mind. But, like mothers and teachers, they often get blamed when there is a poor outcome. Today's clergy are not usually taught healing methods, although healing was originally part of many religions. The responsibility, then, lies solely with the owner-operator of each living body. It is as important to care lovingly for one's body as it is to become a seeker of spiritual joy; and perhaps physical health is a good place to begin a spiritual journey. Moms can love to their capacity, medical intervention might relieve pain, and teachers can present material for the mind—but full spectrum healing is 'self-inflicted.'

The most efficient way to detoxify the body is always to stop "toxing" it.

Sometimes deeply awakened people remain ill or impaired in some way. Everyone has 'issues' that stem from the far distant past. Humans are compound and complex individuals. Most of us do not know ourselves, let alone know the recesses of another's mind. Perhaps it is possible that souls with a deep spiritual connection choose to remain physically afflicted to retain a connection with humanity in order to lead. Or perhaps the spiritual aspect of such a person is developed to a high degree while the physical aspect is neglected. Or a person can be a 'spiritual intellectual' and know a lot about spiritual science but have no real personal connection to the loving universe, the Law of Attraction, or her fellow travelers. Another possibility is they are busy healing others and have forgotten to include themselves, taking the myth of 'more blessed to give than receive' to extremes.

SPIRITUAL EFFECTS OF LIVE FOOD STUDY—RAW DIET AND PHYSICAL FUNCTION

One of the most common reasons for exploring a pure raw food diet is because a person has serious or annoying physical problems. Often those symptoms *do* resolve as the body detoxes itself. The students in the Spiritual Effects of Live Food study reported significant benefit from the two weeks of eating only fresh living vegan food. Of the 303 physical problems that were present at intake for all twelve students, 48 percent were resolved and another 28% were improved at the end of the program. These symptoms commonly included body odor, pain in joints, weight, sleep issues, dry skin, and food cravings.

People expect the physical issues to improve on live food because they have heard testimonials from others, but when their weight normalizes, their hair turns back to their youthful shade, and their energy surges, they are delightfully surprised. There are numerous published accounts of blood pressure normalizing along with serious illnesses such as cancer, heart disease, and diabetes resolving over varying spans of time.

Detoxification takes place on all levels and takes time.

PHYSICAL DETOXIFICATION SYMPTOMS

Some of the changes that occur physically when toxic substances are discontinued are called detoxification or withdrawal symptoms—a transition from the poisonous effects of the Standard American Diet to purification of the tissues. These symptoms that feel like illness are actually signs that the organs of the body are eliminating waste products and setting the stage for regeneration. The process is similar to what is experienced when an alcoholic or drug user is 'dried out' and can be quite uncomfortable. The most efficient way to detoxify the body is always to stop "toxing" it.

Healing the self requires listening to the guidance of intuitive inner wisdom.

Whenever steps have been taken to begin the healing process—whether by diet, energetic treatments, or other means—there is often a time of feeling worse in some way. It usually follows a period of feeling better and precedes the real healing. Evidence of the detoxification process can present in a variety of ways, unpredictable in timing and

Detoxification explains why the morning cup of coffee *seems* to stimulate and awaken a person. During sleep the body is actually fasting and beginning the process of detoxification, which will make it feel sluggish in the morning because the body has ushered 'stashed toxins' into the blood stream, attempting to sneak them out in the night. When the potent toxins in coffee such as caffeine are introduced, the body shifts into third gear to remove them, abandoning the night's work of cleansing. The coffee drinker is actually more ill but feels invigorated because the toxins in coffee promote an emergency state of alarm for the body. A quart of pure water is a much better waker-upper!

manifestation. Withdrawal symptoms are messages from the wisdom of the cells of the body and should be listened to.

When toxic foods such as cooked white flour and animal flesh are no longer consumed, the detoxification that follows can elicit a wide range of symptoms from fatigue, weakness, flu-like symptoms, or discomfort in various parts of the body as the toxins are cleaned out by the miraculous living temple called a body. This is sometimes referred to as simply 'detox,' just like a person addicted to any harmful substance. Other physical detoxification symptoms might be: skin rashes, aching, emotional changes, weakness, or bowel-habit changes. One might experience an over-full feeling, gas, bloating or increased mucous. When organs and blood become congested with debris being eliminated, one feels tired; but as it is removed from the system, energy will soar again.

As a general rule, the purer the diet, the faster the food moves through the digestive tract (bowels), removing toxic substances and increasing the percentage of the nutrients absorbed. For this book, pure food means close to being 100 percent Complete (contains all the components found in nature, especially fiber), Locally grown, Organic, Vegan, Exquisite to the senses, and Raw (not ever heated over 118°) (CLOVER). (Much more on CLOVER in Chapter 9.)

It is not just the surface of the mouth and tongue that needs water, the 'radiator reservoir' of the body must be kept full.

On the physical level it is easy to see how toxins might be stashed away in the non-essential-to-life parts of the body like fat, joints, and muscles. This accumulation tends to occur at the area that is being blocked mentally (false beliefs) and emotionally (past insults a person is unwilling to forgive). Detoxification takes place on all levels and takes time. The longer the erroneous belief or physical toxin has been present, the longer it takes to remove it, reversing the signs and symptoms it caused. Disease symptoms will often disappear in reverse order of their original appearance, uncovering hidden emotions on

A cure removes symptoms of illness, while healing promotes wellness and consciousness in whatever form needed by each person.

Healing takes place on the soul level when the veil between heaven and human opens.

the way to healing. It is a process, and patience is needed for this insider do-it-yourself program.

There might be a time, even years into the raw diet, when there will be a strange taste or smell of something familiar that is not really present at that moment. This can be the point when the body reaches some toxin inhaled or encountered in childhood and it is being removed. A craving for something such as flesh food might be that the 'clean up crew' is getting out the remains of that food which was eaten in the past.

Detoxification is a good thing—it means the body is cooperating with a mental plan to get clean and healthy. If the pains are great or uneasiness is felt, a health care provider should be consulted, but be aware that she is unlikely to be familiar with cooked food detoxification symptoms. Healing the self requires listening to the guidance of intuitive inner wisdom. Do what it takes to be at peace with it but don't ignore it.

DRINK PLENTY OF WATER

During the detoxification period it is especially important to drink an adequate amount of clear and pure water to wash away the toxins being dislodged. In general, that means about a gallon for an average adult in a 24-hour period, which is a cup an hour while awake. If some food from your personal 'contraband list' is eaten, begin soon afterward to flush with water. Symptoms (besides dry mouth and throat) that might remind a person to drink more water can be fatigue, cough, dizziness, sleepiness, back ache, headache, difficulty breathing, and even hunger. It is easy to try drinking water before resorting to pills. Drink the purest water available with no sugar, caffeine, or alcohol. Toxic drinks like these actually result in a net water loss because of the water needed to clear *them* from the body. It

Moms can love to their capacity, medical intervention might relieve pain, and teachers can present material for the mind—but full spectrum healing is 'self-inflicted.

is not just the surface of the mouth and tongue that needs water, the 'radiator reservoir' of the body must be kept full.

SPIRITUAL WELLNESS

There can be no spiritual wellness without incorporating the wisdom of the body and the cries of the inner child. Spiritual awareness and the experience of love (both giving and receiving) are intensely healing to the body. They promote the free flow of life-giving chi through and between the sacred cells, which is the basic cause of health. In this New Age it will become vital for survival to love everyone as a sibling. It begins with each individual awakening to their inherent capacity to love. Nature is always gently teaching, loving us, and waiting for us to wake up and return the favor. Your health, that of society, and the health of the planet are fundamentally interrelated.

Spiritual awareness and the experience of love (both giving and receiving) are intensely healing to the body.

Biologist Rupert Sheldrake, who has linked science and intuition, hypothesized a phenomenon he calls "morphic resonance" (feedback between forms), which suggests that self-organizing systems at all levels of complexity—including molecules, crystals, cells, tissues, organisms, and societies of organisms—are organized by morphic fields. He believes this is an inherent memory among living organisms that influences like-entities and does not diminish over distance. Genes are inherited materially but the morphic field is transferred from others, creating a sort of collective memory or instinct. When one member of a society learns a new pattern of behavior, others can learn it more quickly and easily, even without contact.[91]

Your health, that of society, and the health of the planet are fundamentally interrelated.

This is why the awakening of one person affects the consciousness of others everywhere in the universe. Masaru Emoto agrees with Sheldrake—sounds of the same frequency resonate. This can also

91 Rupert Sheldrake, *The Rebirth of Nature, Science and God,* (Rochester, VT: Park Street Press, 1994), 110–115.

be seen in human relationships. People with similar frequencies are attracted to each other. When frequencies are fundamentally incompatible they cannot resonate. Fear attracts fear. Love has the effect of raising the frequency level. Filling one's own heart with love and gratitude (by giving up fear and resentment) will attract others of the same frequency. It will also attract material and etheric assistance that resonate with that love and gratitude, generating more things for which to be grateful.[92] (More on the Law of Attraction in Chapter 5)

Society functions very much like a single organism, and what we visualize collectively will happen much quicker and with greater intensity than one person alone. This means that when many people face their personal issues and find compassion for themselves and others within, humanity as a whole moves toward peace. Living in a healthy way will thwart an epidemic faster than raising money for research. Compassion will also dispel war more effectively than 'marching against it'!

PHYSICAL CONNECTION WITH SPIRIT

Physical illness depresses the ability to feel joy and to allow joyful thoughts. For example, it is hard to meditate when distracted by physical pain. Illness gives the illusion of lack of love and this 'ill-usion' in turn makes a person ill. Spiritual light is free, but humans (in contrast to animals) tend to 'pull the shades' and block the light. Since the body is physical flesh as well as a divine structure, it acts as a light-bridge between the physical and the spiritual realms. It gets caught in the clash between a person's pure loving spirit and the toxins in the physical tissues. Illness distracts from spiritual connection—creates a diversion *from* the path. To cure the darkness, light a candle. To cure fear, love something. To cure a diseased body, fill it with light and love.

Illness gives the illusion of lack of love and this 'ill-usion' in turn makes a person ill.

92 Masaru Emoto, *The Hidden Messages in Water,* (Hillsboro, OR: Beyond Words Publishing, 2004), 48.

Physical actions and changes in lifestyle cannot directly connect one to spirit—like dialing a phone to a central operator. Diversions like illness, alcohol, and money (also known as glamours) can become addictions. But the body functioning truly comfortably and smoothly is a compelling clue that something has gone drastically right on all levels. Your body is the 'canary in the mine.' Eating a diet filled with light acts as a catalyst to clear physical, emotional, and mental blocks, which leads to connection with spirit. Physical toxins have negative, unnatural energy. Whenever food is cooked (or highly processed) it loses life force energy. Food found naturally on the planet was intended to dance with and enhance the life force energy in the sacred body.

To find spirit, follow your heart. Instructions from the heart will feel good, and there is an electric feeling of excitement and joy about a decision or path. The head confuses things by giving fearful instructions, warnings, and worry. Fear always means a disconnection from the river of spiritual love. The heart entices with a peaceful feeling of 'rightness.'

But the body functioning truly comfortably and smoothly is a compelling clue that something has gone drastically right on all levels.

NEW AGE ENERGIES AND DISEASE

Physical illnesses appear to be increasing as the spiritual energies increase in these new times. There are several categories of autoimmune and other illnesses that have not been identified before in medicine, and some have implicated the higher spiritual frequencies in causing them. Others believe that blocks found in the physical and the mental aspects of a human might make the higher frequencies more difficult to assimilate, resulting in these new diseases. Resistance of any kind to spiritual energy can produce physical and mental suffering.

The heart entices with a peaceful feeling of 'rightness.'

Illness is *not* an inevitable result of becoming spiritually conscious. Suffering is never necessary, but instead is a clue to the block or error involved. What would happen if the body could be made purer and of higher vibration to match the energies that are being summoned? It seems like it would be worth a try. As toxins are decreased, the physical Holy Temple is able to hold the energy. The time has come to be conscious about the sacredness of the physical plane.

The time has come to be conscious about the sacredness of the physical plane.

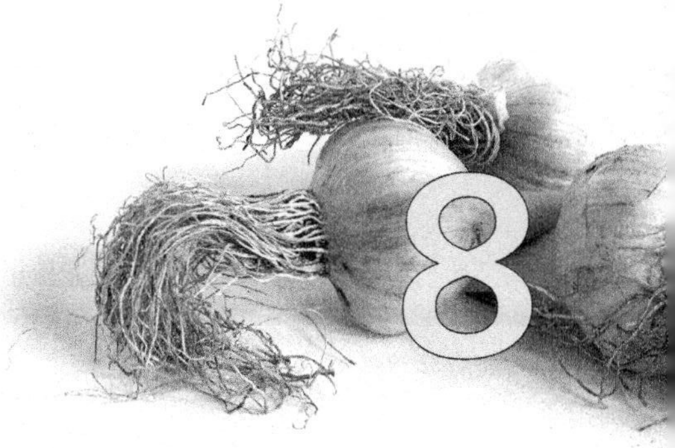

How Diet Affects Spiritual Energy

When we eat in a healthy, harmonious way, our ability to attune and commune with the Divine is enhanced.

— Gabriel Cousens

Diet profoundly affects (causes change in some way) virtually all life conditions; it is also the effect (end result) of the level of consciousness already achieved. As I have said many times diet is more personal than any other subject and people get highly emotional when discussing it—more than sex and religion. They would rather be ill than to give up something, oblivious to the immense reward awaiting them. People eat according to their level of understanding of the power of spiritual energy. Uninformed people tend to eat what everyone else eats, unaware that it is poison. No one consciously harms or destroys her body, of course. When a person is truly aware that everything is made of divine subtle energy, it becomes easier to withstand the temptations of cooked 'comfort food' and withdrawal symptoms and take care of her physical body as if it were her own newborn child.

Diet profoundly affects (causes change in some way) virtually all life conditions; it is also the effect (end result) of the level of consciousness already achieved.

As revealed in the author's study, S.E.L.F. (see Chapter 2), food affects body, mind, and emotions and thus our awareness of spirit—which in turn affects health and thoughts. Physical, emotional, and mental aspects are all inextricably connected. Everyday diet choices are the external manifestations of an inner decision to honor and respect one's body as a holy temple (or not). Giving up toxic substances as a sacrifice (to make sacred) to obtain physical health is similar to giving up toxic thoughts (forgiving) to get spiritual rewards. *Raw* is *war* backwards! *Live* is *evil* backwards! Choose living raw food and live in peace.

Like a sculptor who looks at a chunk of alabaster and sees the angel hidden within, it is possible to take one's presently inhabited body, chip away all that is not pure divine light and find the angel. It is a journey we travel alone, for almost no one can be forced to eat anything (on a regular basis). Food choices (in times of lack as well as abundance) are a manifestation of thoughts, which are changeable. Each person also serves as a role model for others, affecting food choices of those around them—especially children. Habits can be changed.

Habits can be changed.

Almost always when a person starts on a spiritual path for whatever reason, one of the first things that changes is attention to food. One becomes compassionate for farmers and for animals that are killed. Spiritual growth can be measured in several ways, and each turn on the path up the 'mountain of light' results in changes of behavior, often directed at improving physical health. Before ordering food, contemplate the amount of suffering that went into a meal and the suffering it will cause you later

THERE IS NO UNIVERSAL HUMAN DIET

There is no 'one-menu-fits-all' universal diet for humans.

There is no 'one-menu-fits-all' universal diet for humans. What a person eats depends on lots of factors. People write endless books identifying *the* 'natural diet' of humans, what early humans ate, and what chimpanzees eat. Writers are largely defending what they have chosen as right for themselves. Each person decides what is 'right' for herself in each moment, and what is 'right' changes frequently.

Each person must experiment with her own body. If you make a change to what you think will improve your health and you feel bad in some way, then intuition must be used to figure out why. It might be detoxification symptoms (your body cleaning itself), addiction withdrawal (craving for an effect), or the wrong food choices at the time. (More on addiction in Chapter 9) But if a diet has not been tried for a sufficient period of time (perhaps three months), it cannot be condemned as bad for everyone (or even for yourself at a different time). Also, if a diet does not help you feel wonderful even when adhered to for some time, it cannot be assumed that it is good for no one. Attitude is a huge factor in the body's acceptance of food.

Each person decides what is 'right' for herself in each moment, and what is 'right' changes frequently.

People change, especially when growing spiritually or when physically detoxing. As vibration changes, so do food choices. Humans are complex individuals, following a personal path. Although teachers and role models can help, ultimately each person must find her path alone.

Diet is not the whole key to anything sublime. One cannot become absolutely healthy simply by manipulating the diet. There are lots of other factors, such as emotional wounds, mental attitude, and conscious or subconscious intention. There are lots of activities, such as meditation, that can be incorporated into a lifestyle to enhance spiritual awareness.

Attitude is a huge factor in the body's acceptance of food.

Nevertheless, it does happen that when a person who has been on a degenerative diet adopts a healthful one, she discovers that her entire functional mind is changed. All the mechanisms that feed the brain, that bring blood to the brain, and that transfer nerve energy are purified, intensified, and rejuvenated through fasting and living food. When this secret of happiness is discovered, a way of life is taken up that allows the body-mind to be become more conscious of spiritual truths while still enjoying earthly life. Diet helps one walk more quickly, stabilized on that timeless path, but diet is not *the* path in itself, any more than going to church makes one holy. It is a tool. The diet that most enhances communion with spirit is also quite possibly the most physically healthy and ecologically harmonious. A pure diet seems to makes everything easier.

A pure diet seems to makes everything easier.

REAL FOOD

Real food as it is picked from where it is grown in the soil contains the energy from both the sun and the Earth. This warm, clear vibration reflects the love found at the heart of the universe and conducts it all the way into our cells. Food is a gift of love to us.

Food is the package, but love is our real nourishment—the loving energy found in the ethers. In fact we never feel so close to the cosmos as when we are fasting, eating no food but absorbing the love directly. There are reports of people in the past, and actually living on the Earth today, called breatharians, who eat nothing (imagine their food bills!). They apparently live on divine love and are more vibrant than the rest of us. This phenomenon is rare and is certainly *not* being recommended in this book. The point here is that it is life-force essence (love) that provides people with vital substance, not French fries! The purer the food (closest to the moment it was picked), the more love it contains.

It is up to each person to choose exactly *which* foods they eat on a raw diet as long as they contain living enzymes. Technically, it might include raw meat, but that would involve the violent act of killing so most raw foodists are vegetarian (no animal flesh), and usually vegan (no products from an animal), as well. A raw diet is a compassionate diet which translates to organically produced food from farmers who use methods that are sustainable. Everything on a raw diet is uncooked—not heated above 118°F. Actual diets vary widely in the

The purer the food (closest to the moment it was picked), the more love it contains.

percentage of each food—nuts and seeds, greens, fruit, non-flesh animal products (such as honey), and vegetables. They also vary in the percentage of cooked food tolerated. The focus of a real live-food diet is on eating food in its fresh, raw, living *state*, not on any particular food. Real food still contains love.

VEGETARIANISM

The word vegetable comes from the French word "vegetare," which means "to grow," "to animate," "lively," or "to enliven."[93] It relates to growing like plants (or weeds?). Not at all how society uses the word. Vegetation feeds on minerals and remnants of animals which were deposited in the soil; and then animals in turn feed on the plants. This is the circle of life.

Real food still contains love.

Although vehemently decried by flesh eaters, "it is a well-established fact that the longest-lived people throughout the world, such as the Hunza Kuts, Bulgarians, East Indian Todas, Russian Caucasians, and the Yucatan Indians, are either complete vegetarians or eat meat infrequently."[94] In studies on the physical health of Seventh-Day Adventists (the largest single group of vegetarians in the U.S.), they were found to have about half the colon cancer, coronary disease, and breast cancer than those who ate flesh. The general mortality rate of Seventh Day Adventists was 50-70% of the U.S. population at large.[95] T. Colin Campbell's study of the correlation of diet with the incidence of disease in China in the early 1980s concluded that, "People who ate the most animal-based foods got the most chronic disease such as bone, kidney, vision, heart disease, brain disorders, cancer, stroke, autoimmune disease, diabetes, and obesity." And he

---

93 Merriam-Webster, *Merriam Webster's Collegiate Dictionary, Tenth Edition*, (Springfield, MA: Merriam-Webster, Inc., 1995), 1309.

94 Gabriel Cousens, M.D., *Conscious Eating*, (Berkeley, CA: North Atlantic Books, 2000), 321.

95 "Adventist Health Studies" found at www.llu.edu/health.

says those conditions *can* be reversed largely by eliminating flesh, dairy, and eggs from the diet.[96]

HISTORY OF VEGETARIANISM

The belief persists that our ancestors ate large amounts of meat, but the evidence of hunting has been discredited by some. The very earliest humans were probably foragers, eating a low-fat diet consisting largely of plant-derived foods, with only an occasional bit of meat or fish. Vaughn Bryant, professor of anthropology, who has extensively studied coprolites (preserved human feces), skeletons, and ancient trash pits, writes that the diet of foraging people tended to be mostly high fiber plants, seeds, flowers, nuts, and fruit with occasional low-fat protein such as mice or bird eggs. "Once those groups turned to farming [agriculture and animal herding], however, they became anemic and heavily infected [with internal parasites]."[97]

Their diet surely was much more concentrated in all vitamins and minerals while containing much less fat, protein, salt, sugar, and calories than modern diets. It seems obvious that the animals, who were apparently the forerunners of humans, as well as the first people, ate their food fresh from the bush, tree, or plant. Present day chimpanzees share over 99% of human DNA sequences and their natural diet in the wild is about 50% fruit, 25–50% greens and a small percentage of bark and seeds, and less than 1% insects and other small animals.[98] Before the advent of weapons, aside from slow moving worms and insects, humans could not naturally chase and kill a deer or a rabbit with their hands. They had no human teachers to change the childlike tendencies to play with animals and eat fruit. No one

---

96 T. Colin Campbell, Ph.D., *The China Study,* (Dallas, TX: BenBella Books, 2004), 3-7.

97 Vaughn M. Bryant, Jr., Ph.D., "Eating Right Is an Ancient Rite," *The World & I,* January, 1996, 220.

98 Victoria Boutenko, *Green for Life,* (Ashland, OR: Raw Family Publishing, 2005), 16-17.

knows exactly when humans began to eat flesh, and it doesn't really matter. This is a New Age.

Before Jesus walked the Earth, poets and earnest thinkers were promoting the benefits of vegetarianism. Among these early writers were Siddhartha Gautama Buddha, Plato, and Ovid, beginning with the Greek teacher Pythagoras, who taught vegetarianism on mental and spiritual, rather than on humanitarian grounds. Plato writes that although lesser societies might not be expected to follow a plant-food diet alone, the ideal society, which he was proposing, could and would be confirmed vegetarians.

No one knows exactly when humans began to eat flesh, and it doesn't really matter.

"Alas! What a monstrous crime it is that entrails should be entombed in entrails: That one ravening body should grow fat on others which it crams into it, that one living creature should live by the death of another living creature!" — Ovid

More striking than the *number* of proponents of a non-meat diet, is the variety of their personalities. Such names as Milton, Newton, Voltaire, Swedenborg, Wesley, and Schopenhauer are found among the prophets of reformed dietetics, who, in various degrees of abhorrence, have shrunk from the "*regime* of blood!" Others reputed to be vegetarian are Albert Einstein, Leonardo DaVinci, Gandhi, Dalai Lama, George Bernard Shaw, Shakespeare, Bacon, and Thomas Edison.

A quotation attributed to Plutarch pointed out that man "has no curved beak, no sharp talons or claws, no pointed teeth…on the contrary, by the smoothness of his teeth, the small capacity of his mouth, the softness of his tongue and the sluggishness of his digestive apparatus, Nature sternly forbids him to feed on flesh."[99]

VEGETARIANISM IN THE BIBLE

The first of many passages on dietary law are found in Genesis, the first book of the Christian Bible, which is also part of Jewish

99 Howard Williams, *The Ethics of Diet*, (Urbana, IL and Chicago, IL: University of Illinois Press, 2003), 47-48.

holy scriptures. "And God said, Behold, I have given you every herb yielding seed, which is upon the face of all the Earth, and every tree which bears fruit yielding seed; to you it shall be for food." (1:29) This seems to clearly state what humans should eat and perhaps goes even further to mean that hybrid, seedless varieties are inferior for some reason (no life?). "And to every beast of the Earth, and to every fowl of the air, and to everything that creeps upon the Earth, wherein there is life, I have given every green herb for food; and it was so." (Genesis 1:30) It says that this was "good." (1:12) In Ezekiel 47:12, "all kinds of trees for food and their leaves for healing." There are many vegetarian ideas in the Bible.

There are many vegetarian ideas in the Bible.

The Bible references to killing and meat eating are discussed in a negative way. "You shall not kill." (Exodus 20:13 and Matthew 19:18) It does not say animals or humans or under what circumstances. The book of Isaiah contains a little-quoted passage, "He who slaughters an ox is like him who kills a man." (Isaiah 66:3) In several places the Bible forbids eating fat and blood. (Genesis 9:4 and Leviticus, 7:23) Since it is impossible to eat any flesh without eating fat and blood, this appears to mean we should be vegetarians. "I do not delight in the blood of bullocks, or of lambs, or of he-goats." (Isaiah 1:11)

Genesis says Adam lived a total of 930 years, as did many generations after him. One might wonder why people today rarely live to 100. Some believe that humans were originally made to live forever and that humans were vegetarian from Adam and Eve until Noah, when animals from the ark were eaten. The Bible reports life spans began dropping after the flood from nearly 1,000 years before to 120 years after; it could be that the eating of flesh might be connected to shorter lives.

The Bible also seems to say there will come a time when even carnivores will not kill and eat living animals: "The wolf shall dwell with the lamb and the leopard will lie down with the kid." (Isaiah 11:6-9)

In the story of Daniel (1:8-20), found in the Biblical book of the same name, he and his friends asked for only "vegetables" and water. They became ten times better in "matters of wisdom and understanding" than the rest of the king's "magicians and astrologers." Perhaps that might work today as well.

The Bible also teaches not to use food as a way to judge people or to do them harm. "It is not what enters the mouth which defiles a man; but what comes out of the mouth, that defiles a man." (Matthew 15:11) Philosopher Will Tuttle gives a different perspective on this passage. He writes that uttering a phrase, such as "I'll have a cheeseburger," which will cause an animal agony and terror, is a violent act that "defiles" the speaker.[100]

THE ESSENES

Jesus is thought by some to have been an Essene (a peaceful Jewish tribe). The earliest records of the Essenes were analyzed by Edmond Bordeaux Szekely, who was given permission to study manuscripts written in Aramaic, dating to at least 4,000 years before Christ. From these writings we glimpse the principles which reflect teachings found in Brahmanism, the Vedas, the Upanishads, and the Yoga systems of India. Pythagoreanism, Gnosticism, Kabbalah, and Christianity are all based on these teachings. According to Szekely, these fundamentals were practiced by the Essenes and were known as "The Law." The Law governs all that takes place in the universe, the sum total of life on all the planets in the universe and was called "the cosmic ocean of life." For the Essenes, this 'cosmic ocean of life' and the 'cosmic ocean of thought,' form a dynamic unity of which

---

100 Will Tuttle, Ph.D., *The World Peace Diet,* (New York, NY: Lantern Books, 2005), 211.

man is an inseparable part.[101] Jesus, interpreted these principles in sublime form—the Beatitudes. He said, "You are indeed the light of the world."[102]

For the Essenes, this 'cosmic ocean of life' and the 'cosmic ocean of thought,' form a dynamic unity of which man is an inseparable part.

Szekely describes the Essene diet food principles as divided into four categories:

- Biogenic, or life-generating foods are sprouts and living embryonic vegetables.
- Bioactive foods are fresh unprocessed whole raw fruits, and vegetables.
- Biostatic foods which are cooked and other foods which, although raw, are no longer fresh (losing life force).
- Bioacidic or life-destroying foods, which are flesh foods and foods processed with chemicals.

He says the Essenes recommended twenty-five percent biogenic, fifty percent bioactive, and twenty-five percent biostatic. Under no circumstances are bioacidic foods allowed.

Szekely writes that the topsoil is the focal meeting-point of all terrestrial and cosmic energies. There we find a vital exuberance of biogenic activity, which is continuously creating vegetation full of biogenic energy, particularly in the first few weeks of growth. Since the topsoil of the Earth contains bacteria essential for biogenic energy, the vegetation can then be used for generation of human biogenic energies. This same life-generating force which exists in the few inches of topsoil over the Earth also exists in the biogenic zone of our own human body.

The Essenes encouraged people to expose the skin to the sun, to bathe in water, to breathe fresh air of the forest and fields, and to practice fasting to develop will, thus increasing spiritual power. To them, the young, fast-growing vegetation is a way for the "all-wise

---

101 Edmond Bordeaux Szekely, *The Essene Way—Biogenic Living,* (Nelson, B.C., Canada, International Biogenic Society, 1989), 32–33.

102 George M. Lamsa, *Holy Bible,* Matthew 5:3-14.

super-computer of nature" to impart all the live generating power of the primeval lifestream to the human body and the male and female generative organs.[103]

The Essenes felt that to eat the flesh of slain beasts was to eat of the body of death. "Kill not, neither eat the flesh of your innocent prey…" Interestingly, they wrote that eating meat would poison the blood, cause bad breath and boils, turn bones to chalk, cause the bowels to decay, and scales to form on the eyes (sound familiar?). They tell us to eat the fruits of the trees, the grain and grasses of the field, the fresh milk of beasts, and the honey of bees. Eat all things even as they are found on the table of the Earthly Mother. However, "Cook not, neither mix all things one with another, lest your bowels become as steaming bogs."[104] Food combining was important to the Essenes.

Essene, or biogenic nutrition, emphasized the central, vital principle: foods must be living, and there shall not be a significant time lapse between harvesting the plant and its ingestion in still-living condition into the human organism. Szekely's perfect diet consisted of fresh, organic fruits and vegetables, whole grains, seeds, beans, nuts, yoghurt, clabbered milk, and cottage cheese, made at home from fresh raw milk from healthy, well-nourished goats or cows, and fresh eggs from healthy, well-nourished chickens who have plenty of fresh air and exercise. (I followed this for years and was astounded at the improvement when I eventually gave up dairy products, even raw and organic ones!!)

Essene, or biogenic nutrition, emphasized the central, vital principle: foods must be living, and there shall not be a significant time lapse between harvesting the plant and its ingestion in still-living condition into the human organism.

VIEWS ON JESUS AND VEGETARIANISM

In the beginning, of course, Jesus and all his followers were Jews. Later these 'Jewish Christians' were condemned by what became the contemporary (followers of the writings of Paul), gentile, Christian

---

103 Edmond Bordeaux Szekely, *The Essene Way*, (Nelson, B.C., Canada, International Biogenic Society, 1981) (first published in 1928), 152–158.

104 Edmond Bordeaux Szekely, *The Essene Gospel of Peace*, (Nelson, B.C., Canada, International Biogenic Society, 1981) (first published in 1928), 36–41.

church. Vegetarian writer Keith Akers believes that the church also "lost the core of Jesus' teachings." Most important among these early Jewish Christian groups were the Ebionites, who lived simple, vegetarian, non-violent lives. Akers believes Jesus and these early Christians were influenced by the Essenes. They lived communally, were pacifists, avoided excessive accumulation of wealth, rejected animal sacrifice and slavery, and were vegetarian. So, according to Akers' research, the historical Jesus was almost certainly a vegetarian and a pacifist.

Akers believes that, "cleansing the temple" (when Jesus overturned the tables of the money changers) was not about financial corruption but actually an act of animal liberation, which he knew full-well would anger the priests who greatly benefited financially from selling animals for sacrifice.[105] This was because Jesus was very much against the suffering this practice caused. "Why else," Akers asks, "would Jesus risk his life over an issue if it were not essential to his message?"

Ellen White, founder of the Seventh Day Adventist Church, which advocates vegetarianism, has much to say about diet and health. She also believes eating meat after the flood may have to do with a shortened life span of humans. She writes, "God's original diet for man included grains, nuts, fruits and herbs (vegetables). Flesh food was not included in man's diet until after the flood. When flesh foods became part of man's diet, his life span was greatly shortened!"[106] She believes eating flesh is much more detrimental now, physically and morally because of the conditions in which the animals live.

Since many writers give evidence of Jesus' vegetarian belief, it is supposed that the scriptures were changed when Emperor Constantine decided that his meat-eating edition would be the version everyone would follow (Council of Nicea, 325 CE). Vegetarian scholar Steven

105 Keith Akers, *The Lost Religion of Jesus,* (New York, NY: Lantern Books, 2000), 117.

106 Ellen White, *Finding Peace Within,* (Jemison, AL: Inspiration Books East, 2001), 195.

Rosen writes, "priests and politicians completely altered original Christian documents, through omission and interpolation, in order to make them acceptable to Emperor Constantine, who at the time bitterly opposed the scriptures. Their purpose was to convert Constantine to Christianity and thus make their religion the accepted creed of the Roman Empire."[107] They appointed 'correctores' to 'correct' the text of the scripture to what they considered 'orthodox.' Commenting on this idea in the foreword to his translation of the *Gospel of the Holy Twelve,* Rev. Gideon Jasper Richard Ousley says: "What these correctors did was to cut out of the Gospels, with minute care, certain teachings of our Lord which they did not propose to follow—namely, those against the eating of flesh and the taking of strong drink…"[108] But if the context and tenor of the life of Jesus are taken into account, it becomes difficult to reconcile meat eating with the Christian faith of any era.

Many writers explain the stories of Jesus multiplying the fish to feed the crowd in the New Testament could have been changed in a later translation, since early accounts only mention bread being multiplied and do not include fish. Another explanation is that the word for seaweed (fishweed) may have been translated as "fish." It certainly would have been more appetizing to find seaweed in a basket with bread than a dead fish!

KOSHER KILLING

Jesus may have been a Jew but today Christianity is separate from the Jewish religion, which has its own rules on food (kosher). All fruit and vegetables are considered kosher. The Jewish dietary laws are often thought of as simply primitive health regulations applicable only in ancient times. Many disagree, however, saying these laws are from the Torah and do not specify the reasons. They say the laws are

---

107 Steven Rosen, *Food for the Spirit,* (New York, NY: Bala Books, 1987), 33.

108 Rev. Gideon Jasper Richard Ousley, *The Gospel of the Holy Twelve.* (CA, Health Research, Reprint: 1974, 8. Found in Steven Rosen, *Food for the Spirit),* 34.

to be observed to show obedience and self-control and elevate the simple act of eating into a religious ritual. These laws state generally which parts of which animals may be eaten and how they are to be slaughtered. Kosher foods are commonly available in regular grocery stores and are sometimes considered 'healthier,' or somehow better.

But kosher killing in modern times is a hideous perversion of the original law. The kosher laws in Judaism regarding the slaughter of animals prescribe the reciting of certain prayers and looking the animal in the eyes. Genuine, traditional kosher killing "involves the use of an incredibly sharp, perfectly smooth blade to sever the trachea, esophagus and neck arteries of the animal as quickly and as smoothly as possible, thus ensuring that the animal does not suffer."[109]

Food critic John Robbins says kosher killing *greatly* increases the suffering of an animal. Since the animal must be healthy and moving (conscious) when killed, use of a stunning device is prohibited (not always reliable anyway). The 'Pure Food and Drug Act' requires that animals must not fall into the blood of another animal, so it must be hanging when killed. This means 'kosher' meat animals (already exhausted and terrified) must hang upside down, rupturing their joints, as they twist in agony until the Rabbi is ready to make his cut (two to five minutes or longer). The usually mellow bovine remains conscious, nose clamped for stability, and is provoked into hysteria (though unable to make a sound) until the blood has sufficiently drained from the brain to kill her. Blood vessels cannot be easily removed from some parts of the carcass as required by kosher law, so these parts are sold as non-kosher. All this makes meat-eating more complicated (and expensive) than vegetarian food. A kosher killing adds incalculably to the agony animals suffer.[110]

---

109 Rabbi Zushe Blech, "And You Shall *Schecht*…And You shall Eat, Devarim 27:7," [online article, available from kashrut.com/articles], accessed January 28, 2004.

110 John Robbins, *Diet for a New America*, (Tiburon, CA: H. J. Kramer, 1987), 140-141.

VEGETARIANISM IN OTHER ANCIENT RELIGIONS

In general, the older the religion, the more respect for life. The world's major religious traditions and their earliest adherents were sympathetic toward the meatless way of life and, in many cases, emphasized vegetarianism. Translation and customs change and people tend to accept whatever edition of scripture their church favors. The original intent of the world's major religious scriptures was to encourage a meatless diet.

A kosher killing adds incalculably to the agony animals suffer.

Hinduism, the oldest of the major religions, is a strong supporter of vegetarianism. The ancient Hindus in India always forbade the eating of meat. The *Vedas* (oldest sacred text of Hinduism) state that all life should be revered, for the body is merely an outer shell for the spirit within. The higher castes especially are to observe vegetarianism. Jesus is thought to have traveled extensively and he may have been influenced by the Hindus—the most religiously strict abstainers from eating the flesh of animals—a religion of mercy to all beings, human and nonhuman.

The original intent of the world's major religious scriptures was to encourage a meatless diet.

The term "ahimsa" was originally found in the Vedas, but is now integral to most Eastern religions and means that all life should be revered. For the yogi, all life is sacred; every creature is a living entity, with a heart and emotions, breathing and feeling, so even to contemplate eating meat or fish is quite impossible. Ahimsa means non-injury to living beings and is among the highest laws in moral philosophy for spiritual growth. Many spiritual groups have adopted ahimsa as a lifestyle and advocate a vegetarian diet—sacredness of all life, and the need to live without causing suffering.

While, the majority of Muslims today are not vegetarian, Mohammed's teachings clearly show his ideal was total compassion and abstinence from killing. He said, "Whosoever is kind to the creatures of God is kind to himself." The Holy Book of Islam, the

Koran, prohibits the eating of "dead animals, blood, and flesh." One of the first prophets after Mohammed, (his nephew) advised the higher disciples, "not make your stomachs graves for animals." Muslims discourage overeating in general and Islamic slaughter laws are similar to the Jewish ones.

Other vegetarian groups can be found among religions around the globe. The early Egyptians and Hebrews describe man as a fruit eater. The great civilization of the Inca Indians was based on vegetarian diet. The Taoist saints and sages were also vegetarians. Universal compassion for all of God's creatures is consistent with the highest ideals of many other ancient world religions, such as Zoroastrianism, Jainism, and Sikkism—all of which teach vegetarianism.

The Dalai Lama has publicly declared that he is a vegetarian and suggests vegetarianism to his people. Buddha is believed to have said, "How can a (seeker) who hopes to become a deliverer of others, himself be living on the flesh of other sentient beings?" Buddha, like Jesus, committed nothing to writing and yet his followers would all agree that compassion for all that lives is the foundation of the Buddhist religion. From the Buddhist Canon:

> *There are eleven advantages which attend the man who practices compassion and is tender to all that lives: his body is always in health (happy); he is blessed with peaceful sleep, and when engaged in study he is also composed; he has no evil dreams, he is protected by Heaven (Devas) and loved by men; he is unmolested by poisonous things, and escapes the violence of war; he is unharmed by fire or water; he is successful wherever he lives, and when dead, goes to the Heaven of Brahma.*[111]

---

111 Howard Williams, *The Ethics of Diet*, (Urbana and Chicago: University of Illinois Press, 2003), 295.

TEACHINGS ON DIET IN CONTEMPORARY RELIGION

Most religions have had dietary restrictions at some time in their history, but for various reasons do not currently practice these rules. Some contemporary religions, such as Seventh Day Adventist, Eastern Orthodox, Mormon, and Roman Catholic have dietary observations on meat, caffeine, alcohol, or leavened bread. Some religions have seasonal restrictions or fasting in various forms (during lent, for example) as part of a religious observation, sometimes only during daylight hours and usually as a sort of 'penance' or 'remembering' of a sorrowful event.

While few religions currently teach vegetarianism, some contemporary Christian leaders originally promoted vegetarianism. John Wesley, the founder of Methodism was vegetarian. Bishop Desmond Tutu of South Africa teaches that in God's garden, we are all vegetarians, since that was God's original plan. Many Seventh Day Adventists follow Ellen White's teachings to eat a moderate, simple vegetarian diet with no stimulants like coffee or drugs in order to lead a spiritually sensitive, moral and physically healthy life, which enables one to serve God to one's highest ability. Her teachings make a clear connection between the diet one eats and the spiritual sensitivity, clarity of mind, and strength of character needed to follow an enduring spiritual life.

Other modern denominations that have a meatless contingent include Quakers, Mormons, and members of the Baha'i Faith. The list goes on: the Magis, Theosophists, Salvation Army, Sufis, and many others have advocated the vegetarian diet for those seeking spiritual advancement. Although the Unity church is not considered vegetarian, its founders, Charles and Myrtle Fillmore, strongly advocated the vegan ethic of kindness. Vegetarianism is compatible with the teachings of all religions, but there is little evidence that today's religions are attentive to any connection between nutrition and spiritual health.

PHYSICAL TOXICITY OF COOKED FOOD

If asked, most people would agree that chemicals sprayed on food as it grows and those added later for preserving and flavoring make food toxic to some degree. Spoiled food and food that is dirty or otherwise polluted would also be considered unfit to eat by most people. But to a raw fooder, even ways of preparing food that are common to people on a SAD, like heating with a stove or microwave, renders food toxic. Cooking (even organically grown vegetables) distorts the molecular bonds, denatures the protein, and disrupts the patterns of nature. Heating conventionally grown food to extreme temperatures is even worse, as heating distorts and intensifies the toxins from pesticides applied to the crop as it grew in the field.

There are some researchable studies that show the physical toxicity of cooked food. The Paul Kouchakoff study showed that the phenomenon, known to medical professionals as "post-parandial leucocytosis" (increase of white blood cells after eating), does not occur if the meal is raw.[112] Another study done on cats by Francis Pottenger, a friend of Weston Price, showed that animals who received an all raw food diet bred normal litters generation after generation, but cats who were fed mostly cooked food became progressively degenerate.[113] These studies need to be repeated.

Cooking food turns many components of natural food into foreign toxic substances. According to Gabriel Cousens it coagulates the bioactive mineral and protein complexes and therefore disrupts mineral absorption, including calcium. It creates carcinogenic structures in fats and produces free radicals. Heating carbohydrate-

---

112 Paul Kouchakoff, "The Influence of Food Cooking on the Blood Formula of Man," (seleneriverpress, 1930) pdf article found online August 13, 2013.

113 Francis M. Pottenger, Jr., *Pottenger's Cats,* (Lemon Grove, CA: Price-Pottenger Nutrition Foundation, 1983), 11.

rich foods, such as potatoes, rice, and cereals, creates acrylamide, a probable human carcinogen that also causes damage to the central and peripheral nervous systems. Cousens also believes cooking transforms pesticides, herbicides, and food additives into different compounds that are even more carcinogenic.[114]

Raw food proponent T.C. Fry writes, "Cooking disorganizes, oxidizes, and makes nonusable a food's mineral content. It deaminates [changes the amino acids] the food's protein content, thus rendering it worthless in human nutrition. To the extent that a food has been cooked—reduced to inorganic minerals, caramelized sugars and starches, coagulated and deaminated proteins, poisonous acrolein-laden fats, devitalized vitamins…it is not only worthless, but the ash becomes toxic debris in the body."[115]

As discussed earlier in Chapter 7, these toxins are stashed and accumulate in non-essential parts of the body in order to keep the person alive. But as the 'toxic load' builds up over a lifetime, the body's ability to eliminate them is progressively diminished. Eventually, the natural defenses of the body are overwhelmed, leading to such conditions as cancer, dementia, cirrhosis, gout, and kidney stones. The kind of toxin, together with the parts of the body most often bombarded by negative thoughts, determine which areas will break down first leading to a diagnosis.

Toxicity of food has a threshold like other poisons and medications. At one dose there will be no symptoms and with one more bite it might be overwhelming. According to the Law of Vital Adaptation (see Chapter 6), the more polluted the body, the more pollutants it will tolerate—to a point! Toxic substances are not often considered when diagnoses are made. Many diagnoses such as fibromyalgia and colitis might simply be the result of pollution on a physical level. These

---

114 Gabriel Cousens, M.D., *Rainbow Green Live-Food Cuisine,* (Berkeley, CA: North Atlantic Books, 2003), 109.

115 T. C. Fry, "Criteria for Selecting the Highest-Quality Foods," found in Dr. Douglas N. Graham, *80/10/10,* (Key Largo, FL: FoodnSport Press, 2006), 65.

and other diseases often clear up quickly when the person shifts to the raw organic vegan diet. It often remains a mystery to health providers why a particular person will contract a particular disease. If toxins were considered, it might be discovered that the affected person is 'cleaner' and therefore more susceptible. Or conversely, they might be very toxic and at the tipping point.

Stimulants like 'power-drinks' appear to give an energy buzz, but this too is misleading because the excited feeling is created by the tremendous energy needed to clear them from the body. The desired rush comes from the energy system going into emergency protective overdrive, depleting stores of energy and resulting in a later 'crash.' This is commonly referred to as 'rebound.' Victoria BidWell, a student of the effects of the live food diet, calls this phenomenon "The Law of Stimulation or Dual Effect." She writes, "Coffee is a drug. Coffee does not give [the] body energy. It causes the release of stored energy, thereby further depleting the body. Whenever a toxic or irritation agent is [ingested], the increased action is caused by the extra expenditure of vital power called out [to detoxify the body of that substance], not supplied, by the stimulatory process."[116] The result is an overall diminishment of vital energy.

Cooked food contains more simple sugars, which produce the 'numbing' feeling after eating that is thought to contribute to the addictive effect. People literally use cooked food to self-medicate much the same as alcohol, prescription, over-the-counter, and illegal drugs. Highly processed food creates a foggy, sluggish, 'I-don't-care' effect. Raw foodists do not report that bloated, lethargic, sleepy feeling after eating, just the gratification of their healthy hunger. In fact that might be the major reason people slip back to cooked food even though they have strong evidence that it was the food that created their

116 Victoria BidWell, *The Health Seekers' Yearbook,* (Mt. Vernon, WA: GetWell StayWell, America!, 1990), 8, 15.

problem. Whether it is the sugar, or the chemicals, or the changed food molecules that people crave, it sure sounds like addiction.

COOKING DEPLETES NUTRIENTS

Cooking does more than rearrange molecules into new toxic foreign chemicals. Viktoras Kulvinskas, a raw diet researcher who worked with Ann Wigmore, estimates that heating food above 118° F depletes around 85% of its nutrient value.[117] He quotes a USDA study on meat protein cooked at 400°F, which found this "caused a very marked decrease (4 to 30 fold) in the soluble protein nitrogen of the steaks." Non-soluble nutrients cannot be effectively utilized by the body. Kulvinskas writes that cooking meat with sugar destroys 50% of the amino acids lysine, argine, tryptophane, and histidine content. Heat denatures proteins and denatured protein cannot sustain life. A cooked seed is dead and will not grow.

Raw foodists do not report that bloated, lethargic, sleepy feeling after eating, just the gratification of their healthy hunger.

> For an example of denatured protein, try breaking an egg into a dish and mix in a small amount of water; it absorbs right in (like when making an omelet). BUT if you cook the egg first and try to get it to absorb water, it will not. The protein is no longer water soluble.

Gabriel Cousens writes that cooking destroys over 50% of B vitamins and 70–80% of vitamin C.[118] Many sources show cooking destroys at least 50% of protein and about 70% to 80% of vitamins and minerals, including almost all vitamin B-12. The fat soluble vitamins A, D, E, and K are less vulnerable and can remain stable up to the boiling point of water, but about 50% of them are destroyed in frying and baking at higher temperatures.[119] Half as much live food is needed

A cooked seed is dead and will not grow.

---

117 Viktoras H. Kulvinskas, *Survival in the 21st Century*, (Mt Ida, AR: 21st Century Publishers, 2002), 46.

118 Gabriel Cousens, M.D., *Conscious Eating*, (Berkeley, CA: North Atlantic Books, 2000), 563.

119 Ann Wigmore, *Scientific Appraisal of Dr. Ann Wigmore's Living Foods Lifestyle*, (Boston, MA: Ann Wigmore Press, 1993), 21.

to get the same nutrition as from cooked food and requires less stress on the digestive system and the energy stores of the body.

Question: When food is cooked, in the name of 'improving' it, does the cook believe that nature has made a mistake? Can nature be improved? Not only is cooked food destroyed on the molecular level and measurable nutrients (the ones we know about) reduced, but also the unknown essential natural substances (that future generations will isolate and name) are probably destroyed as well. It is impossible to believe that taking a tablet containing a manufactured facsimile of vitamin C can be better for the body or the connection with spirit than a bright-colored orange eaten with juice dripping. Aside from nutrients, the pill lacks joy, while the fruit stimulates our connection to universal love by vision, smell, tactile, and gustatory pleasure.

COOKING DESTROYS ENZYMES

Half as much live food is needed to get the same nutrition as from cooked food and requires less stress on the digestive system and the energy stores of the body.

While enzymes are not exactly nutrients, they are essential for digestion and absorption of nutrients, cooking destroys the self-digestive enzymes found naturally in all foods. Enzymes are living proteins that act as catalysts, directing the life force in basic biochemical and metabolic processes. They regulate all body functions, but are not themselves changed in the process. It is unknown how enzymes work, but they break molecular bonds, changing one substance into another (or several others). There are thousands of kinds of enzymes, because mostly they only work on one type of substance. They are often named for the type of substances they work on, adding the ending "ase". For example, an enzyme that breaks down protein is called a 'protease' and fat-digesting enzymes are called 'lipases.'

Enzymes are essentially unchanged in the process of their work, but they do wear out and need to be replaced—some after 20 minutes, while others work for several weeks.[120] The body makes some

120 Anthony J. Cichoke, *The Complete Book of Enzyme Therapy,* New York, NY: Avery, 1999), 5.

enzymes, but the ideal specific digestion enzyme for each food is found inherently in all living, uncooked food. Vitamins work with enzymes as coenzymes. Opinions vary, but enzymes are considered destroyed when the food is held above 118° for a half hour. So pasteurization as well as cooking destroys enzymes. Freezing, however, does not seem to harm them, for they are no less alive at temperatures of fifty to sixty degrees below zero. Many seeds will grow after being frozen. Since 'life' can ordinarily only be detected in food by observable signs such as a seed sprouting or green leaves appearing on a tree, food is considered living when the enzymes are alive. Whatever is alive has enzymes in it.

This enzyme-killing temperature will redden human skin and prevent germination of most formerly viable seeds. Food can be warmed and eaten just below this temperature and still be considered raw. Even food that has been cooked is eaten at about this same temperature, because it would burn the mouth if it were not cooled from the scalding temperature at which it was cooked. If a finger can be held in the soup comfortably, it will be the perfect eating temperature and still retain its life force energy. No need for a thermometer.

Whatever is alive has enzymes in it.

> Try making a batch of gelatin dessert with canned and one with fresh pineapple in it. The batch made with fresh pineapple will not jell because the enzymes in the fresh pineapple digest the protein in the gelatin, thus showing that canning fruit destroys its enzymes.

Biochemist Edward Howell believes that the upper peristalsis-free portion of the stomach (cardiac) which secretes no enzymes or acid was intended to allow the enzymes in raw food as well as the salivary enzymes added in the mouth to begin digestion. The food then moves to the pyloric portion of the stomach which secretes peptic enzymes and hydrochloric acid for the next step in digestion. If the natural enzymes are destroyed by cooking, this first step does not take place.[121]

KILLING BACTERIA

Another problem with cooking is that it destroys bacteria found naturally on raw food. That is the major reason given for cooking—to sterilize it so it keeps longer (such as in canning food at high temperatures). These naturally-occurring bacteria were intended to end up in our intestines. Recently, in an attempt to help patients overcome digestive disturbances such as colitis, irritable bowel syndrome, and constipation, stool (with living microbes) from healthy patients was infused into the digestive tracts (usually with a tube) of suffering patients. Called "fecal microbiota transplantation" (FMT), it is the only non-surgical therapy for ulcerative colitis that has demonstrably induced persistent medication-free relief. "Symptom-free remission with no histological signs of inflammation has been documented during follow-up as long as 13 years."[122] Perhaps the reason one person would have colonies of healthy bacteria in their digestive tract while others do not has to do with sterilization of food or maybe the use of antibiotics or disinfectants? Health begins at the gut level.

These naturally-occurring bacteria were intended to end up in our intestines.

OTHER DISTORTIONS OF FOOD

Other molestations of food (besides cooking) include radiation, genetic modification, microwaving, and the use of chemicals to preserve and 'enhance' flavor or appearance. Scientists, declaring them safe, often distort 'scientific findings' and are not considering energy as

121 Edward Howell, *Enzyme Nutrition,* (Wayne, NJ: Avery Publishing, 1985).

122 Borody T.J., Warren E.F., Leis S., Surace R., Ashman O., "Treatment of Ulcerative Colitis Using Fecal Bacteriotherapy", *J. Clin. Gastroenterol.* 2003;3 (1);43-47. Found in article "Fecal Microbiota Transplantation for Ulcerative Colitis" posted January 24, 2012 by Mark Davis, N.D.

a factor. Containers, like plastic made of chemicals, also leach toxins into the food, especially if exposed to sunlight or microwaves. While not actually a 'food,' 80% of Americans take at least one drug every week, sometimes by the handful, and carry them along like a 'snack.' All drugs are toxic. Many people believe taking medications will keep them healthy, but adding more toxins in the form of medication, alcohol, caffeine, or junk food will not heal symptoms most often already caused by toxicity!

FOOD AFFECTS THOUGHT

'Intoxication' is a familiar term because the effects of alcohol on the mind and body are almost instantly noticeable. It is also clear that thoughts have an effect on the body, too (as evidenced by the 'electric' feeling when realizing you forgot your purse). What is not commonly known is that what we eat has nearly as great an effect upon the mind, body and affairs as what we think. We know that alcohol is composed of carbon, hydrogen and oxygen (C.H.O.) and so are many foods such as sugar and starch (which is converted to sugar by cooking). The consumption of refined carbohydrate food is slower than alcohol and usually mixed with other substances, which delays effect. The meal, therefore, is not suspected of changing us mentally. Over time, as much alcohol will get into the brain from cooked, sugary food as from drinking gin. This slowly results in physical deterioration, chronic 'brain fog,' and addiction—just like with alcohol.

Many people believe taking medications will keep them healthy, but adding more toxins in the form of medication, alcohol, caffeine, or junk food will not heal symptoms most often already caused by toxicity!

BRIEF HISTORY OF EATING FOOD IN ITS NATURAL STATE

The point in human history when cooking began is disputed. Vaughn Bryant says, "I believe the deterioration of health found in modern humans is due not so much from the kinds of food that we eat, but that in ancient times the food was eaten in its natural,

Over time, as much alcohol will get into the brain from cooked, sugary food as from drinking gin.

unprocessed, and often uncooked form, which was not contaminated with chemical sprays, preservatives, and additives."[123] He says humans began using fire about 750,000 years ago but do not appear to have begun cooking foods on a regular basis until perhaps 150,000-200,000 years ago. He also says that "Cooking created major changes. Jaws and teeth got smaller in humans."

Hippocrates

Hippocrates, who was known as the Father of Medicine, said, "Your food shall be your medicine and your medicine shall be your food" some 400 years before the birth of Jesus.[124] Hippocrates also maintained that food must be taken in the condition in which it is found in nature—uncooked. He taught people how to help themselves be well and that the body cannot act as its own physician when nourishment is destroyed through the process of cooking. His family claimed to be descended from the mythical Asclepius, Greek god of medicine. Hippocratic medicine was humble, passive, and based on "the healing power of nature." According to this doctrine, the body contains within itself the power to re-balance and heal itself. His therapy focused on simply easing this natural process. He was reluctant to administer drugs and give treatment that might prove to be wrongly chosen, and he thought patients in good spirits (happy) would heal faster.

Natural Hygiene

Natural Hygiene, a field filled today with practitioners holding very conflicting views on a lot of topics, is founded on the principle that the body is self-cleansing, self-healing, and self-maintaining and that we only experience illness when we break the natural laws of

---

123 Vaughn Bryant, Ph.D., Professor Department of Anthropology, Texas A&M University, College Station, TX, personal communication, August 9, 2013.

124 Ann Wigmore, D.D., N.D., *Naturama Living Textbook,* (Boston, MA: Hippocrates Health Institute, around 1978), 5.

life.[125] The Natural Hygiene movement was started in 1830 by Sylvester Graham (think graham crackers), William Alcott, Mary Gove, and Isaac Jennings, all medical doctors. They were followed by Russell Trall, Herbert M. Shelton, St. Louis Estes and many others. T. C. Fry seems to have been a bridge between Natural Hygiene and the raw food philosophy. His famous quote is, "It's better to be ignorant than to have learned so much that isn't so." He founded the Life Science Institute in Texas, which has over 4000 graduates, including Harvey and Marilyn Diamond.[126] Fry wrote extensively of the benefits of raw living food.

Well-Known Raw Food Enthusiasts

Typical of the early pioneers of raw foodism, many of whom were doctors who defied the medical establishment's practice of giving medicine, was John Tilden, a medical doctor who used no medicine but "practiced cleaning the body of toxic matters and then allowing inherent healing powers to restore health."[127] Dr. Max Bircher-Benner, who was excommunicated from the Medical Society of Zurich, advocated raw fruit and vegetables, "at a time when the accepted wisdom attributed all strength and nourishment to meat."[128] There are many other advocates who spoke up about the benefits of the live food diet and called for the cessation of cooking. Some of the louder or more eloquent were: Hilton Hotema, Arnold Ehret, Morris Krok, A. T. Hovannessian, Viktoras Kulvinskas, Harvey Lisle, N. W. Walker, Paavo Airola, John Tobe, and Ann Wigmore. Each of these blazed a trail for all to follow in solving the mysteries of wellness. The list keeps growing.

---

125 Harvey and Marilyn Diamond, *Fit For Life,* (New York, NY, Warner Books: 1985), 19.

126 David Klein, Article published in *Living Nutrition* magazine, "In Memoriam T. C. Fry" (1926-1996) from website livingnutrition.com, June 2, 2007.

127 John Tilden, M.D., (1851–1940), *Toxemia Explained,* (No publisher listed), v.

128 Ruth Kunz-Bircher, *The Bircher-Benner Health Guide,* (Santa Barbara, CA: Woodbridge Press, 1980), 16.

PATTERNS OF NATURE

In quantum physics we see scientific evidence that everything in the universe is vibrating and connected and that each part of the universe includes the whole—like the pattern of a leaf resembles a miniature tree. When one part of the universe is ill, it affects all the parts. So when one person takes a step toward enlightenment—everyone benefits. As above so below—macrocosms and microcosms, the patterns of nature are endless. There is symmetry between the tree and its roots.

> Cut open a fresh ripe tomato in late August and meditate upon its beautiful pattern.

Nature created delicious food in elegant abundance with fragrance, nutrients, enzymes, and intricate molecular patterns undamaged by heat or microwaves. Medical science has come a long way from the first discoveries of scurvy in sailors and yet, nature is older than science and has held things together despite man's efforts to the contrary with pesticides and logging, for example. Consider the possibility of a myriad of unseen factors, nutrients, and energies around and in the tomato as yet unidentified by science.

As above so below—macrocosms and microcosms, the patterns of nature are endless.

Animals cannot absorb minerals and other nutrients directly from soil. We must get them pre-digested through the system of a plant. Necessary minerals like sodium and calcium are found in just the right balance in plants such as green leafy vegetables relished by herbivores. Fruit and green leafies contain protein, fat and carbohydrate that are in perfect combination for humans. Human cells, especially brain cells, run on natural raw carbohydrates, not protein. Eating food the way it is delivered from the breast of mother earth (as wild herbivores do) is more likely to insure that needed nutrients, even those not yet named, are included.

Consider the possibility of a myriad of unseen factors, nutrients, and energies around and in the tomato as yet unidentified by science.

Plants and animals were intended by nature to be mutually beneficial. Animals eat various parts of plants, process them with natural enzymes, infuse them with animal energy, and expel the fiber and nutrients back to the soil in exactly the form the plants need. Bacteria and enzymes assist every part of this process. Animals also cart away the seeds and conveniently deposit them in distant locations on the ground, surrounded by a nourishing ball of plant-food (manure). Animals are breathing creatures whose life is sustained by the oxygen part of the air molecule and they eliminate carbon dioxide, while plants breathe in the carbon dioxide and give off oxygen. The animals' hooves and claws scratch the soil, letting the seed enter the Earth's skin where it can grow into food for other animals. Plants feed, nourish and shelter animals—animals make compost which nourishes plants—a symbiotic relationship made in heaven!

Plants and animals were intended by nature to be mutually beneficial.

SPIRITUAL VIBRATION OF FOOD

Beyond the physical problems that are obvious when a person changes to a raw food diet, cooked food deadens the spirit. Lifeless food depletes the energy system of the body and impairs the flow of life-force in the cells, the circulatory, skeletal, muscular, lymphatic, endocrine, nervous, urinary, immune, skin, respiratory, reproductive, and especially digestive systems. When energy systems of the body are blocked, thoughts are more likely to be dark, adversely affecting the vitality of the body. Cooked food impairs both the physical vehicle and the mind as a direct result of the lack of energy in the food moving through the center of the body in what is known as the gastrointestinal tract leading from the lips to the anus.

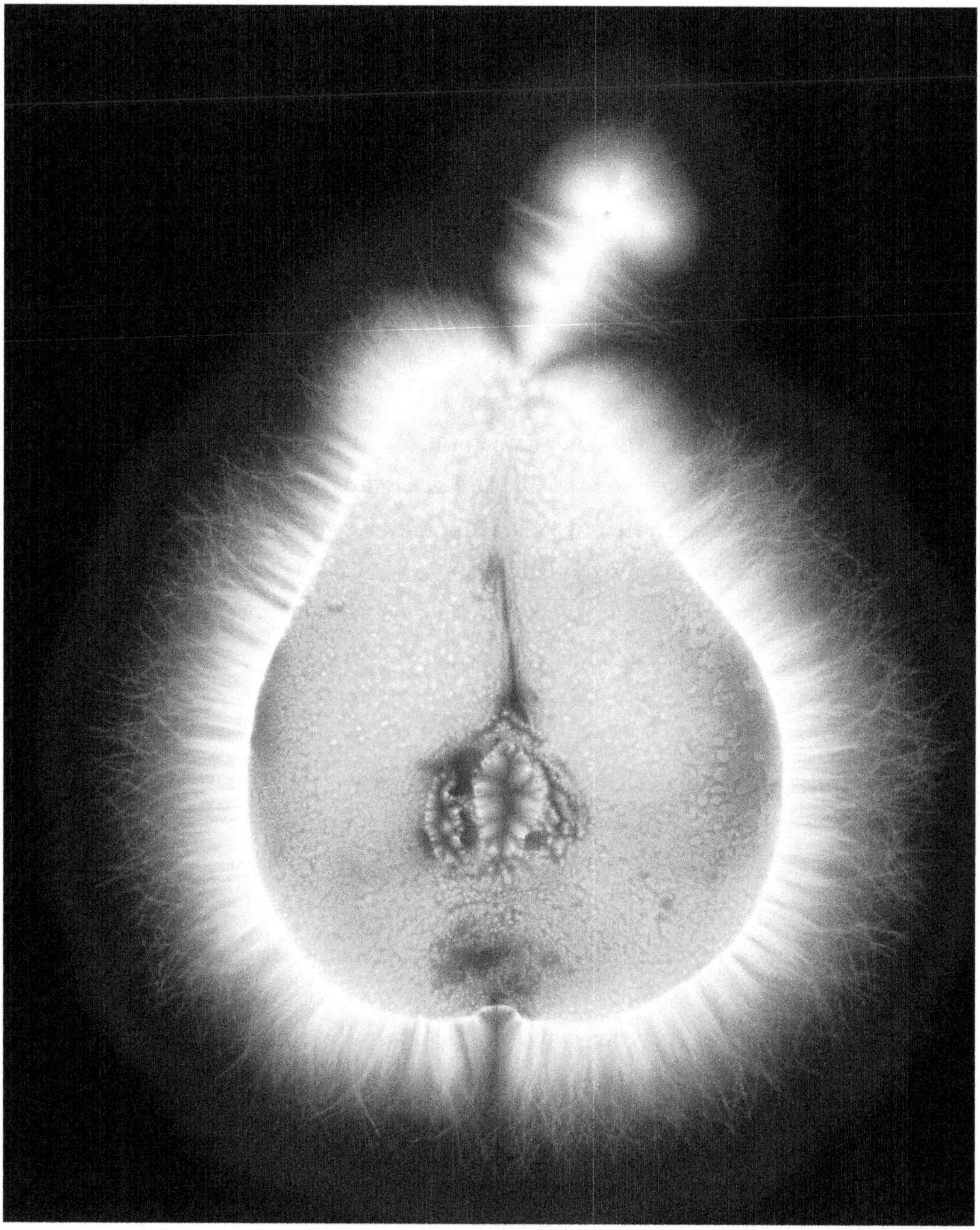

Photo credit Science Source.

Kirlian photograph of pear half showing energy.

Gabriel Cousens calls the energy that surrounds living bodies Subtle Organizing Energy Fields (SOEFs) and writes that they exist prior to the existence of the physical forms and are blueprints or templates *for* the biological forms and structures. He states that one way humans get SOEFs is from food. "Whenever food is cooked or processed in any way, it loses the strength of its SOEFs. Cooked and processed foods actually take energy from our bodies in order to properly assimilate them and theoretically at the SOEF level, this same type of depletion of energy also happens." Cousens observes that people who change to a raw-food diet energize their SOEFs, reverse the entropic process of aging, and seem to get younger.[129]

Karma affects the energy of everything involved, including food.

Artistic painter Joe Alexander writes, "Cooking food kills the life-force in it." He believes that when he ate cooked food his paintings were "bleak, grotesque surrealist-type pictures with drab and dull, muddy colors; I was a creator of deserts in my art. But when I became a raw food eater, all of a sudden I began to paint instead, vibrantly alive pictures with lush abundance of healthy shapes and brilliantly beautiful colors."[130]

KARMA

Karma is the ever-just inevitable order of cause and effect (both positive and negative) that governs all existence. Each thought and action brings about future situations on both large and small scale until a new intention intervenes. It is also known as *reaping what we sow*, self-fulfilling prophecy, and the Law of Attraction. It all means the same. Karma is not a hard and fast rule. It is changeable by changing attitude and intentions, and by learning from experience.

Karma affects the energy of everything involved, including food. One could say all thoughts and actions are prayers, so pausing to

---

129 Gabriel Cousens, M.D., *Conscious Eating*, (Berkeley, CA: North Atlantic Books, 2000), 279–281.

130 Joe Alexander, *Blatant Raw Foodist Propaganda!*, (Grass Valley, CA: Blue Dolphin Press, 1990), 75.

express gratitude before eating increases the vibration (karma) of the food. Victoras Kulvinskas, believes that all of us are on the journey of enlightenment together and the right food can be an aid. He writes that fruit is the only food that is 'karma-less.' All other food involves killing, whether it be animals, plants, or seed. Fruit is offered from the plant by nature. When ripened to perfection by the sun, the taste is perfect and it is the easiest food to digest.[131]

Fruit, it seems, wants to be eaten. It comes in bright colors which attract our attention and when fragrantly ripe and succulent is the most tempting and delicious food it is possible to savor in the mouth. It is usually pleasantly sweet and often tart at the same time and appeals to the natural choices of humans, who have hands shaped to pick it. How can anything be better than a ripe peach or cantaloupe? Eating fruit does not destroy the plant. By eating the fruit we are completing and repeating the life cycle of the plant or tree when we save, dry, and put its seeds back into mother earth the next year.

Cooked food has no life force energy.

Food has a spectrum or scale of karma, its spiritual vibration. Raw vegan food is of a higher vibration than cooked, and some living foods are even higher than others. Eating that which does not destroy the plant (lettuce harvested by the individual leaf) is of a higher vibration than eating the entire plant (say a carrot). The choices range from slow deadening energy of cooked animal flesh to the happiest of food—the milk from a happy mother who wants and loves her child. Somewhere near mother's milk is fruit—apples, cucumbers, oranges, tomatoes, raspberries, kiwi etc. These contain the seeds which (not hybridized) will bring forth more fruit similar to the one in which the seed is found. There are other ways for plants to be propagated, of course, but this is the general plan. The spiritual vibration spectrum runs from fruit to vegetables and root crops. And finally, to eggs, milk, and the flesh of animals, containing fat and blood.

Foods affect us spiritually by the level of energy or karma it contains.

131 Viktoras Kulvinskas, *Survival in the 21st Century*, (Mt Ida, AR: 21st Century Publishers, 2002), 21.

The ultimate evidence that a food is alive is whether it will reproduce itself (if it is a part of the plant that *will* grow and it remains intact). A cooked seed is dead and will not grow. Chemically, they are the same, but if a roasted almond and a really raw almond are planted, the cooked seed will rot and the raw one will grow and replicate itself many times. Cooked food has no life force energy. Fire is a destroyer; when food is cooked it always becomes less than it was before, never more. It makes no sense to destroy food before eating it.

Rudolf Steiner taught that enzymes are the bridge between the physical and the spiritual worlds.

The eating of food grown with compassion, prepared preserving the sun's prana, and eaten with gratitude is a powerful enhancement to efforts of the incoming spiritual energies. It appears to increase the flow of life force energy in and around the body of an aspirant. Even people without a professed interest in things of a spiritual nature remark on the 'glowing' appearance of raw foodists.

Some say enzymes are life itself, prana made physical.

The raw vegan diet enhances physical healing and mental clarity, which removes major stumbling blocks to meditation and connection with our true selves. When energy is enhanced, it seems to take less effort to connect with 'all-that-is' and receive intuitional information needed to make decisions, escape peril, enhance relationships, express opinions, or see the good in others. With the challenges of physical pain and mental fogginess gone—there is a clear view through a break in the clouds. Blessing your food before eating it enhances your own body cells. Foods affect us spiritually by the level of energy or karma it contains.

Howell believes that the length of life is inversely proportional to the rate of exhaustion of the enzyme potential of an organism.

SPIRITUAL ASPECTS OF ENZYMES

Rudolf Steiner taught that enzymes are the bridge between the physical and the spiritual worlds. Enzymes carry a unique energy, a spark upon which all life depends. They seem to have the intelligence to act in highly specific ways in response to the needs of the body. Mysteriously, they represent a life element which is biologically recognized but can be measured only in terms of activity. The true nature of enzymes cannot be explained, either by biology or chemistry at this time. It seems that at a certain point in their research, scientists are faced with an 'unknown factor' in the life process. Modern scientists generally are not yet able to test the spiritual qualities of enzymes. Some say enzymes are life itself, prana made physical.

The water-loving cells of the body love raw food because it is full of the nature's life juice.

Dr. Edward Howell, an American medical doctor, believes there is a fixed 'enzyme potential' in all living creatures. This potential diminishes over time, subject to the conditions and pace of life. He believes enzymes are 'protein carriers,' charged with vital energy factors, and not merely catalysts. Howell even goes so far as to say there is evidence that might indicate an intimate connection between metabolic enzymes and the phenomenon we call *life*. When dead food is eaten, the body, searching for the natural enzymes and nutrients that should accompany the calories, remains hungry, which leads to overeating. Howell believes that the length of life is inversely proportional to the rate of exhaustion of the enzyme potential of an organism.[132]

WATER IS SPIRIT

Digestion depends upon food's ability to be turned into a liquid and dissolve in water.

The steam leaving a pan of frying vegetables is the natural pure water—life force energy from nature *escaping*. The water-loving cells of the body love raw food because it is full of the nature's life juice. Cooking removes natural water and destroys much of the life force energy, which leaves the body of the eater starving for what it really wants—prana. The person, still hungry, often craves more food, leading to a starved, obese body.

Water, a major portion of the body, is a mysterious substance. It literally regulates all functions in the body and on the Earth. It

132 Dr. Edward Howell, *Enzyme Nutrition,* (East Rutherford, NJ: Avery, 1985), 29, 49, 73, 85.

has a high specific heat value (amount of heat required to change its temperature) which helps our body withstand wide variations of ambient temperature. Without the ionization of water (the exchange of positive or negative electrical charge of molecules), bodies would cease chemically reacting—meaning they would be dead.

Oxygen, the 'breath of life' enlivens physical matter, the temples of living souls.

Live vegan food contains an abundance of the very highest quality water, because the plant has filtered it through its root system from the Earth into itself. Cooked food, even if boiled in water, ultimately contains less water than the food in its natural raw state (note the moisture in raw potato versus cooked). Digestion depends upon food's ability to be turned into a liquid and dissolve in water. When the previously mentioned cooked egg will not absorb water, it cannot be utilized as effectively by the cells of the body.

And if water is alive, it is possible that the nature of the water itself is affected by heating it (as with other living things). Eaten in its natural form, food contains the full measure of cosmic energy sent from the sun and is the natural pure form of living sacred water. Water contains spirit energy, and people can partake of life force energy simply by feasting on living food.

Water contains oxygen, the primary nutrient of all living things. Cooking decreases the oxygen in food. It is no coincidence that the word 'inspiration' means both the physical act of breathing oxygen into the lungs *and* the spiritual phenomenon of intuitive illumination. Oxygen is spiritual energy made physical—spirit being absorbed into matter. Oxygen, the 'breath of life' enlivens physical matter, the temples of living souls.

If there is anything that cures and heals everything, it might be pure water.

Masaru Emoto photographed ice crystals after the water had been exposed to various human emotions. In his words, water is "like the portal into another dimension."[133] Emoto's photographs of frozen

133 Massaru Emoto, *The Hidden Messages in Water*, (Hillsboro, OR: Beyond Words Publishing, 2004), xxv.

water crystals show grotesquely distorted crystals when the water was exposed to negative emotions such as the word "hate." The crystals from water that was blessed or exposed to positive words like "gratitude" or "love" were symmetrical and beautiful. He believes that water may be the carrier of souls and that water is the same as the soul.

The universe is of a mental nature and thoughts matter very much.

Water is life-force and when the life-force of the body is enhanced, health is improved. Rain is truly a divine gift eaten in living food! Just as Emoto's water absorbed the energy of the words and attitudes around it, the water contained in food will pick up the attitude of people it encounters and carry it into the body of the eater. Live food contains exponentially more water than cooked food and therefore is capable of more energy transport. If seeds are planted, watered, tended, and harvested with loving attitude and the food is prepared with loving hands, the water it contains will be greatly enhanced. So sing in the kitchen, bless your food before eating, and dine with gratitude and laughter. If there is anything that cures and heals everything, it might be pure water.

As with addictions other than food such as smoking, alcohol, violent movies, or rage—in order to avoid the addiction, a person needs to control the thoughts about it.

WHICH CAME FIRST?

So which comes first: spiritual enlightenment or love for the physical body? Do people first become conscious of the impact of food choices and then choose fresh vegetables? Or do they wait for the live organic vegan diet to become popular and then discover the spiritual benefits? Is it a willful decision to be healthy, peaceful, and conscious that causes a seeker to change her diet? How will she learn of the benefits of a diet without sugar, white flour, and animal parts?

The universe is of a mental nature and thoughts matter very much. A thinker has full control over her thoughts, and if she chooses to change her thoughts, she possesses the will to do so. A conscious decision to be healthy is a loud and clear message to the subconscious mind to make healthy choices on all matters. As with addictions other than food such as smoking, alcohol, violent movies, or rage—in order to avoid the addiction, a person needs to control the thoughts about it. Constant thoughts of revenge lead to violence; better a peaceful thought on the matter. In other words, thinking about hamburgers and french fries will lead to eating them. So ponder fresh salad ingredients, instead.

It is difficult to distinguish whether a desire for a food is the imagination of the diner or the content of the dinner. Disregard for the holiness of food changes its energy. Food faces other negative effects, too. Americans worry about food. They anguish over what kind, its safety, or what type causes which diseases, often turning to experts or the news media for information. Usually this worry is centered on fat and bacteria content. Nutrition experts are often confused and confusing. Food also invokes guilt for destroyed rainforests and whether it is 'fattening.' We joke about moral values, calling our favorite dessert 'sinful.' Food is thus imbued with negative attitudes, changing both the vibration of the food and the thoughts of the eater.

Pay attention to your health before it demands all your attention.

Each of us can take conscious control of our thoughts and choose the best nutrition for ourselves—food 'to live for.' Eating sugar ultimately causes depression (after the high is gone), but fruit and leafy greens vegetables create a predominantly positive mood. Most people begin their spiritual journey at the physical level, so that is a place to begin change. The same 'sinful' desserts *can* be made 'soulful' by using organic living ingredients (and they taste even better)! Pay attention to your health before it demands *all* your attention.

READINESS

Some people feel that the majority of the population is not able and will not benefit if they start on the spiritual path by changing their diet first. Dr. Norman Walker, famous health writer, says that not all people are ready for a raw food vegetarian diet. People choose their diet, friends, and pastimes according to their state of consciousness in each moment. When we are upset, depressed, or fearful we tend to choose food with a lower vibration. We choose the easier path—drive-through restaurant, microwaved supper, frozen pizza. Often we don't consider how we will feel in the morning when we order the next meal or drink, even if we know better. When a person has changed her own vibration, whether by accident or design, she will often naturally move toward food of a higher vibration. Walker writes, "In the lower state of physical and material consciousness, it would seem, most people would rather take something to give them instant relief and let the future, including the undertaker, take care of them."[134]

Like a tulip in spring, raw vegans will awaken in the New Age.

Da Free John, a controversial spiritual leader, writes in his book *Raw Gorilla* that the disciplines of eating raw food and fasting are not for beginners. "They [diet disciplines] assume a level of maturity wherein we are stabilized and in a problem-free disposition." In other words, he is saying that awareness comes before diet changes. Da Free John writes, "It is a simple and natural development of a life already healthy and founded in the spiritual secret of happiness."[135]

Changing to a live diet might be a good first step for many people. It is helpful to be aware that physical cleansing leads to emotional, mental, and spiritual changes, though. In fact, health concerns are often a major motivator to seeking a spiritual path searching for truth.

WE ARE WHAT WE EAT

Others feel that the spiritual path can be accessed from any point. It is reasonable that by changing your diet you can enhance spiritual consciousness. If people really are what they eat, perhaps while eating

---

134 N. W. Walker, *Become Younger,* (Prescott, AZ: Norwalk Press, 1949 revised 1978), 62.

135 Da Free John, *Raw Gorilla,* (Clear Lake, CA: Dawn Horse Press, 1982), 17.

vegetation, they too will turn toward the light, as plants do. Like a tulip in spring, raw vegans will awaken in the New Age.

People are unaware of these truths and their ignorance subjects them to greater pain. Many doctors are simply unaware of the amazing power of the live vegan diet to reverse physical diseases currently considered incurable. Diabetes is one example. Gabriel Cousens invited a group of severe diabetics to his healing center in Arizona and fed them a raw vegan diet. The results were miraculous to a medical person who has observed the chronic and usually progressive nature of diabetes. All but two of the eight subjects were off insulin in 30 days. One had a greatly reduced dose of insulin and one gave up and went home. The majority of the subjects had type-two diabetes and two were type-one. Of the type-one diabetics, one had his insulin requirements drastically reduced and the other was able to come off the insulin altogether."[136] This is considered impossible by most doctors.

Mental health workers, teachers, and parents are not aware of the power of diet to manage behavior and learning problems. The resources of the 'sick care system' cannot keep up with the children and adults with these issues. Healing begins, as with all revolutions, at the grass roots. But everyday people are not aware, either, that there is something doable, affordable, and controllable that heals many conditions. It is simple, *but not easy* to overcome addiction and endure detoxification withdrawal symptoms to get to gleaming health on the other side. Spiritual teachers and leaders, although aware of the possibility that meat is not a good thing, are hesitant to practice and teach vegetarianism—churches, too, must please the masses or risk financial ruin.

Health (physical, mental and spiritual) can buy wealth or anything else that can be imagined because success becomes more likely when you are physically healthy, mentally alert and spiritually peaceful.

136 "Simply Raw: Reversing Diabetes in 30 days", DVD, website www.rawfor30days.com, Raw for Thirty Days, LLC, and from personal communication with April Davis of the Customer Happiness Team at Raw for Thirty Days.

It is up to you, the reader. While there are no guarantees, you have nothing to lose but fat tissue, depression, cancer, arthritis, and whatever else is beginning to develop as yet undetected. There is everything to gain—freedom, flexibility, comfort, natural color hair, bright eyes, and easy bowel movements. The broader results could be an end to war, world hunger, and greed. Wealth does *not* bring health nor does it buy one more minute of life. Health (physical, mental and spiritual) *can* buy wealth or anything else that can be imagined because success becomes more likely when you are physically healthy, mentally alert and spiritually peaceful.

When an aspirant adopts a living food diet she becomes, to a great extent, a different person. Not only will the body become 'younger,' and healthier, but the mind opens, new interests are explored, new goals and philosophies are attracted. Some refer to this as "youthing" (as opposed to aging). There is a glimpse of how much better life can and should be than most humans on the Standard American Diet can even wildly imagine. There is a glow about the face and sereneness in the eyes. There is a peacefulness of actions that tends to ripple out to those around. A person has to test for herself the truth or fallacy of any written or spoken declaration, for it is impossible to imagine how much diet affects life unless a change is actually made. Try it. What if it works?

Although illnesses can be turned into an important opportunity for spiritual growth, people with low physical vitality have less energy available for their spiritual focus. The electrical potential in our tissues and cells is a direct result of the liveliness of our cells, and live food enhances this. Electron-rich live foods have an abundance of life force energy which brings prana not only into the body, but also into the mind, helping to purify and expand the energy centers and channels, thereby enhancing consciousness. Natural energy acts as the most powerful fuel, and we become 'superconductors' of prana. As the prana in our body flows, we are allowed deeper perception of truth and reality as 'Oneness.' Kirlian photography clearly shows that live foods have a much stronger aura. Choosing live food is a way of deliberately and consciously choosing to cooperate with the patterns of evolution.

Physical illness depresses the ability to feel joy and to allow joyful thoughts—illness is the 'ill-usion' of a lack of love.

S.E.L.F. STUDY SPIRITUAL RESULTS

Spiritual 'problems' are difficult to quantify and put into language, and therefore not usually studied. On the S.E.L.F. study questionnaire, students were presented with statements like: "I am afraid to die," "I am a divine being," "My life has bigger meaning," and "I can trust my "inner guide in choosing food." They were asked to determine "To what extent are they true for you?" The study found that of the 183 spiritual 'problems' the students reported at the beginning of their two weeks on exclusively raw vegan food, 42.6% of them were reported resolved before the students went home and 25.1% were improved. Overall the 12 students believed that they were 67.7% more spiritually content than they were before changing their diet. Other factors (like two weeks away from home) were not controlled for, but the results are still impressive.

Change on one level automatically affects all the other aspects of our 'self.'

PHYSICAL DETOXIFICATION IS SPIRITUAL

Physical illness depresses the ability to feel joy and to allow joyful thoughts—illness is the 'ill-usion' of a lack of love. Diseases are a result of a block in the flow of energy, either physical or mental or both. People don't realize they are half-sick and mentally foggy. Symptoms are actually the body trying to rid itself of toxins and heal. The liver, pancreas and the lymph/blood system work on the inside to pull toxins out of the cells and dump them into urine, skin, and feces for elimination—a most marvelous and divine system! When the body is purified and returned to a state of harmony and health, energy is freed up to ponder emotional and mental errors, SINs that have blocked access to the spiritual 'river of love.'

The process can be trusted because it is guided by the older, wiser part of the soul.

Change on one level automatically affects all the other aspects of our 'self.' The physical symptoms of detoxification are discussed in Chapter 7. While a toxic attitude and lifestyle are often unconscious, change is a *conscious* choice. The purification of the body/mind can begin at any level, but all levels are controlled by the mind, so major detoxification cannot happen without a mental choice. The decision to be healthy comes first, followed by actions such as diet changes and exercise that allow the body to detoxify. On the physical level it is simply called detoxification, similar to the 'withdrawal' experiences of people overcoming a drug or alcohol addiction. When decisions and actions have convinced the subconscious mind of the intent to be well, there follows a change of energy, a cleansing called a 'healing crisis.'

The length of time each of these stages takes is very individualized.

The changes often lead to discovery of unprocessed and suppressed emotions, thereby allowing them to be released. This begins the awareness of the fallacy of previously held beliefs, triggering enhanced spiritual awareness and sometimes a 'spiritual emergency.' It is a process that can be gentle or shocking and can lead to the spiritual 'dark night of the soul' (see Chapter 12). There is an *ongoing* 'scrubbing' of the self-cleaning physical body that removes accumulated 'trash' and 'poison.' This 'scrubbing' process clears emotional and mental baggage as well. The process can be trusted because it is guided by the older, wiser part of the soul. Supportive people can be also helpful.

The length of time each of these stages takes is very individualized. Some say detoxification of the physical body after changing to a raw vegan diet takes one month for every year the SAD was eaten, so a

30-year-old would take about 2½ years. It is ALWAYS an ongoing process. Who knows if anyone is ever cleared on all levels? Spiritual awareness is ever unfolding.

Brian Clement of the Hippocrates Institute in Florida tells of three phases of growth with live food, each lasting seven years. Phase one is rebuilding and revitalizing the physical body by nurturing the cells with pure water, living foods, and exercise. Phase two develops emotional health, which must wait until the needs of the body are met so there is enough strength and openness to look in the heart, focus, and create goals. In the spiritual phase three, the question is asked, "Why am I here?" Clement sees 21 years to complete the journey using live food to restore physical, mental/emotional, and spiritual health.[137]

Embarking on a path of spiritual growth using live foods is indeed a journey, different for each individual. The decision to improve one's life begins the journey, and physical purification aids the process. It is exciting and ever-changing, even from meal to meal. It is a gift no one can give you but yourSELF.

MENTAL/EMOTIONAL HEALING CRISES

At the mental/emotional level, detoxification is called a 'healing crisis'—a time of facing distortions in thought and the emotions that have resulted from those errors. Healing crises also often happen after a massage, an energy healing session, or a good session with a psychotherapist. These assist in moving etheric 'log jams' by moving energy and fluids with magic hands, positive intentions, and probing questions. Healing crises cause a person to feel unsure of themselves, even ill for a time. Healers advise drinking water to wash out freed toxins. Release is always on all levels.

137 Brian Clement with Theresa Foy DeGeronimo, *Living Foods for Optimal Health,* (Rocklin, CA: Prima Health Publishing, 1998), 119–122.

People who adopt a raw vegan diet can uncover rage or fear that was covered with guilt, shame, or regret. For example, people who are reaching spiritual maturity might discover that they still hate their first spouse and have to forgive again for the hundredth time. But emotional 'pus' (pockets of unconscious shame) left inside, will fester and eventually erupt into a 'boil,' perhaps in violence against self or another. It might also result in cancer or account for the occurrence of an accident to the affected part of a healing person.

The mental symptoms that occur with the withdrawal from SAD are similar to what is experienced by anyone who has rapid increase of consciousness. There will usually be a period of transition (feeling worse) as the body, mind, and emotions are purified. A sluggishness of mind or body may be a clue that change is taking place. There may be unusual reactions or feelings of low self-worth. When changing to a lighter diet, one may experience this release of energies in the form of heightened emotions, insecure feelings, aggressive tendencies, depression, or anxiety, which may alternate with feelings of elation and expansion (hence the term "flipped-out vegan"). Many people have told me they needed meat to feel "grounded," but actually they were having withdrawal symptoms and may have started to encounter previously buried emotions. Unaware that they were addicts, they needed a 'fix.'

But each person finds consciousness in their own way and in their own time.

The process usually follows a pattern. At first a person feels better physically, mentally and emotionally. But if not prepared for detoxification withdrawal symptoms and healing crises, it can seem like something is wrong or the diet is not good for them. These symptoms are temporary and depend upon a person's stage of cleansing. If they seem intense, however, a more gradual transition to all raw might help moderate them, like adding some organic steamed vegetable or grain, until they subside. Eventually the crises pass, the detoxification symptoms of fatigue and body aches subside, and moods settle into a mostly peaceful space. If the diet is continued, the light will dawn and energy will soar—this time for good. By eating food that enhances the flow of cosmic energy, the ability to sustain meditation will eventually be enhanced and one experiences greater harmony with nature. But each person finds consciousness in their own way and in their own time. Aspirants should go to 'all raw' when it feels wonderful—when finally the annoying 'hangover' seems worse than the craving for junk. This is an ongoing process and there are no contests!

Food acts as an energetic bridge through which the soul maintains the physical body that interacts with the physical world. When heavier foods are consumed (such as meat and cooked foods), there is a dampening in the energetic field, which tends to keep energy from moving through the person's subtle bodies. When lighter foods are consumed, the energetic field is lightened, which allows energies which have been stuck to be released. This explains why so many find it difficult to maintain a lighter diet—it requires learning to process our suppressed emotions, insecurities, pain, anger, and fear. It is not easy to face responsibility for creating past (or future) situations. It is easier to blame genes, gods, germs, and Henry (the first husband).

But each person finds consciousness in their own way and in their own time.

When the physical (body) is cleared of toxins, emotional pain exposes flaws in thought so they may be examined and corrected. Physical habits are then easier to change. For example, when feelings of inferiority or guilt are gone, it becomes easier to stop punishing the body with cigarettes and sugar.

COMPASSION

John Robbins was heir to the Baskin-Robbins fortune when he turned vegan activist. He tells many stories of animals' devotion and heroic efforts to assist humans. In writing about the deplorable conditions and the suffering lives of animals raised for human food, he says, "There is a relationship between the capacity of a being to love, and its capacity to suffer, regardless of its species."[138] We humans like to pretend we are merely eating food and not the dead carcass of an affectionate, gentle animal (we don't eat the dangerous carnivores). Robbins observes, "It has often been said that if we had to kill the animals we eat, the number of vegetarians would rise astronomically." The physical and emotional toll on the slaughterhouse workers is enormous. He says, "The industry chooses the cheapest possible methods of killing. They do not purposefully choose to be brutal and sadistic; it just often works out that way."

Mystic healer David Cousins explains that "Although we did have a peaceful contract with animals whereby they were willing to be eaten by us, they did not agree to die fearfully." This part of the contract was broken a long time ago. The result is a lot of meat impregnated with the slow frequency energy of fear which animals experience at slaughterhouses. When people eat meat, they absorb that fear vibration. Cousins says this energy attracts other fear vibrations to it and will create a band of fear around the lower chakras. He advises when selecting which foods to eat to begin looking beyond the normal awareness and look at the magnetic imprints which have gone into the food.[139]

Meat-eaters do not ponder the anguish and terror of an animal being taken to slaughter.

There is nothing spiritual about torturing and killing animals, just as there is nothing spiritual about killing at all. Even if one is in the position of having to kill in self-defense, the argument could be made that the person has called in the violent energy before the event. Eating a hamburger is premeditated. The human knows it and undoubtedly, the cow knows it, too. A decision to stop causing the torture and murder of gentle sentient beings is a clear step on the path to enlightenment.

---

138 John Robbins, *Diet for a New America*, (Tiburon, CA: H.J. Kramer, 1987), 37.

139 David Cousins, *A Handbook for Light Workers*, (Dartmouth, UK: Barton House, 1993), 151–152.

Eating flesh, which has had the killing covered up by attractive packaging, roasting pans, and garlic, is a product of mass hypnosis and brain washing. This is the same phenomenon that has occurred in war and slavery. If you do not think about it, the suffering of animals, enemies, and slaves is OK. Meat-eaters do not ponder the anguish and terror of an animal being taken to slaughter.

Cheap animal products are produced now in CAFOs (Concentrated Animal Feeding Operations), where animals are kept in close confinement and food is brought to them instead of them walking to graze for themselves. In fact, these factories are so concentrated that there is no vegetation in sight. Chickens, cows, and pigs are especially kept this way for the production of meat, eggs, and milk. While the males of these species are of course killed for meat, the female is further exploited by arranging for her to bear young for the production of milk (after removing her baby to be raised on artificial food) and eggs.

Will Tuttle wrote, "One would almost hope that for their enormous sacrifice, the cows would at least be supplying humans with something beneficial. And yet the deeper justice is inescapable; by killing them, we kill ourselves; by enslaving them, we enslave ourselves; by sickening them, we sicken ourselves."[140]

Eating live food can be made into a sacrament.

When encountering animals, young children understand that these creatures are in tune with the universal source of love. A child can see the mother cow and hen love their calf and chicks. We will all be healthier and lifted in consciousness when we adults take an honest look at those truths, too.

DIET FOR A NEW AGE

In writing about humans making preparations for the New Age energies, spiritual teacher Vera Stanley Alder says to make eating a

140 Will Tuttle, *The World Peace Diet,* (New York, NY: Lantern Books, 2005), 122.

'sacrament.'[141] She believes that living food has nutrients which are not assimilated as material substance, the benefits being derived entirely from the spirit and life in them. The act of eating is performing a miracle, but the miracle is only as complete as the enthusiasm applied; therefore, we must always eat when we are calm. She explains that a large part of the digestive process should take place before the meal is swallowed, so slow and thorough chewing is important. She says that the "vital *living* forces" of the food are abstracted through the walls of the mouth and that part of this energy is lost once it reaches the acid of the stomach. People who bolt their food do not obtain the stimulation to the brain and nerves which is the reward of eating slowly. Eating live food can be made into a sacrament. Communion and baptism are thought to infuse divine energy into the body. The same can be said of blessing our salad, filled with the sun's love and then taking that divine energy directly into the 'chalice' of our body. It raises the vibration of body and mind, which reflects in the skin, posture, and the sacred eyes. Alder declares that food eaten in its raw state is more than twice as strengthening as cooked food.

Annie and David Jubb, healers and live food advocates, write, "Life-force is the electric energy a living animal has between its nerves and blood. When the animal is dead, this force is no longer present. Yet, in vegetation, the sun's light (life force) remains within it for some time after it has been harvested. Each cell of the plant stores the energy of the sun within it."[142]

Gabriel Cousens suggests people with eating disorders and addictions do best when they begin a live-food diet which he calls the Lover's Electron Diet, a high electron diet which creates an endorphin-high feeling all day and increases the experience of the flow of cosmic energy in our lives. He writes, "We are human photocells whose

141 Vera Stanley Alder, *The Finding of the Third Eye,* (York Beach, ME: Samuel Weiser, Inc, 1970), 118-119.

142 Annie Padden Jubb and David Jubb, *LifeFood Recipe Book,* (Berkeley, CA: North Atlantic Books, 2003), 8.

ultimate biological nutrient is sunlight."[143] Cooked dead food and even highly hybridized raw food uses up electrons, creating destructive free radicals. Live food contains antioxidants, which give up spare electrons to their 'hosts,' stabilizing the electron-seeking free-radicals which are believed to 'cause aging.' Cousens quotes Johanna Budwig as saying "electron-rich foods act as solar resonance fields in the body to attract, store, and conduct the sun's energy in our bodies."[144] He also quotes Rudolf Steiner as saying, "The more we increase our ability to absorb and assimilate light, the more conscious we become."[145]

Taking life-force into the body is the very definition of a sacrament, Joe Alexander declares the greatest value of the raw food diet is in its 'transformative value.'[146] When one begins the raw food diet, a new and better person emerges. There is more of the true essence, the natural self, becoming more a part of the 'One-Great-Life-of-Nature.' Raw foodists get new insights into how much better life can and should be—how Nature intended it to be. Alexander believes the discipline of eating raw makes a person freer to be more creative, work harder, and think more clearly to enjoy the beauties and wonders of the natural world.

The coming new enhanced energies will be conducted through purified energy channels in the body.

The New Age represents an era of changes. In this time, each member of the human family will link with all creation. There is a need to reconstruct human bodies through living foods not only to become healthier, but to develop advanced communication skills with each other and with the wiser, older Self within. The physical body is a holy temple, and only through healing the body is spiritual evolution possible. The coming new enhanced energies will be conducted

---

143 Gabriel Cousens, M.D., *Conscious Eating,* (Berkeley, CA: North Atlantic Books, 2000), 224-225, 578.

144 Gabriel Cousens, M.D., *Conscious Eating,* (Berkeley, CA: North Atlantic Books, 2000), 579.

145 Gabriel Cousens, M.D., *Conscious Eating,* (Berkeley, CA: North Atlantic Books, 2000), 581.

146 Joe Alexander, *Blatant Raw Foodist Propaganda!,* (Grass Valley, CA: Blue Dolphin Press, 1990), 75–76.

through purified energy channels in the body. A diet of living foods and a lifestyle which increases a healing energy flow will release the power and guidance from within.

To prepare the sacred meal, spiritualize food by preparing it consciously, visualizing the pleasure of eating and the pleasure of cells receiving the light from the sunshine. It is good to prepare one's own food or when possible, do it together as a family or community. Always, before beginning the meal, hesitate and think about the food, its journey through the body, and the hands that have touched it, asking a blessing for the gardeners, cooks, and laborers. Before the first bite, bless it and balance it to the energy of your body, as if for communion, instilling spiritual love. Enjoy each bite!

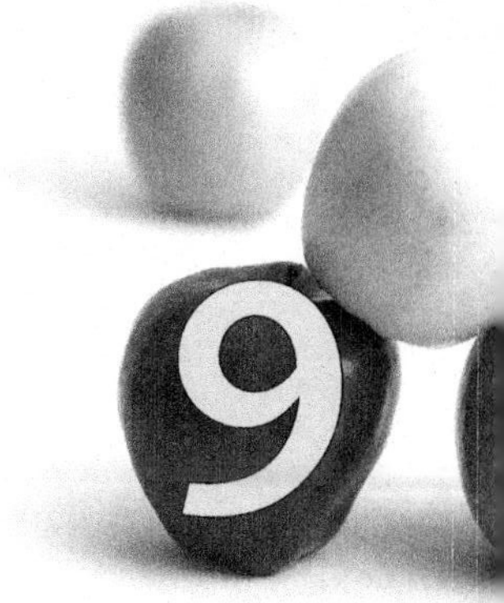

The Live Vegan Diet

Living food is rejuvenating, enzyme-rich food that is ideally assimilated by the body.

— Ann Wigmore

Food fresh from the garden contains living enzymes which help it easily assimilate into the bodies of sentient breathing animals. *It is a diet of pure love.* What better cuisine in summer than to lunch, sitting on the Earth in the garden—a bowl of lettuce, a ripe tomato, an ear of sweet corn, a whole cucumber, and a handful of crisp green beans. No need to wash, cut, dress, or cook—just bless it. When the snows of January blow bitter, dried sun-ripened tomato and a handful of almonds—life force energy intact, blended into a warm creamy tomato soup soothes the soul. Unbeknownst to the uninitiated, live food tastes better than any cooked version.

Real food enlivens everything from the gardener to the compost at the next cycle of life—always in the rhythm of the heartbeat of nature, the physical evidence of the intelligence of the universe. Living food contains the life-energy that allows a seed to sprout (in the presence of life-giving water) and grow into a new plant to produce more food. It is not pie in the sky to wish to be well; it is the sky *in* the pie diet.

Unbeknownst to the uninitiated, live food tastes better than any cooked version.

The diet described in this book would appear to be quite specific and defined. But in practical application, there are as many definitions as there are people pursuing youth, health, beauty, or spiritual wisdom by eating this way. What is described here is the array of versions of the fresh living diet. The reader is encouraged to experiment, observing herself physically, mentally, emotionally, and spiritually for clues leading to her perfect combination. Each food selection (or choice to fast) must be made using inner guidance and not the opinion of others.

C.L.O.V.E.R.

Living food is straight from nature. Basically, don't eat anything that is advertised anywhere! An easy way to remember the spiritual diet in this book is the acronym "CLOVER." This stands for complete, local, organic, vegan, exquisite, and raw. CLOVER is a guideline, subject to what is available. There is probably no perfectly pure air, soil or water left on the planet, and attempting to avoid all traces of modern toxins would be not only futile but would drive a person crazy. Nature is forgiving, however, and self-healing as well. The road to heaven and health really *is* paved with good intentions. Live in the 'clover'!

The road to heaven and health really is paved with good intentions.

"C"—Complete

Complete means including the edible skins of fruits and vegetables, hulls of seeds, and stems and other fibrous parts when possible. Complete food means no juicing (which discards vital fiber). It is eating all parts of the food that can be eaten, such as the white part under the skin of an orange, the apple peel, and whole kale or chard leaf (in a smoothie, for example). The green part of a green onion is the best part. Fiber is very good for cleaning the colon. When making seed 'milk' (often spelled mylk), the whole nut or seed can be blended until creamy with a small amount of water; then add more water, utilizing the whole seed. Eat the section dividers in the grapefruit and orange. Scrub the carrot and leave the peel if possible.

Complete means including the edible skins of fruits and vegetables, hulls of seeds, and stems and other fibrous parts when possible.

But don't throw away the seeds, skins, roots, and stems—worms love them! Keep a kitchen bucket and carry the precious living material to the compost pile. Layer the still-live kitchen 'scraps' with weeds/grass clippings, dry leaves/hay, and a layer of soil or animal manure and the pits and peels will live again—continuing to feed the planet.

"L"—Local

Local food is raised within 100 miles, or better yet, just outside the door. Most food in the grocery travels 1000 miles or more. The number of miles is not as important as being conscious of the long term *cost* of shipping. It is not just the freight bill but the cost in terms of depletion of fossil fuels, pollution of air, and loss of nutrients in transit. It is almost always possible to grow some of your own food, even if you live in a motel room. Sprouting in jars is within the reach of anyone with a water supply and access to seeds (more on this later).

Local food is raised within 100 miles, or better yet, just outside the door

Food grown nearby contains the energy of the area and is more healing. It has grown in harmony with local animals. Seeds pick up the energy of the gardener as she tills, plants, weeds, and waters. Local weeds are particularly healthy to eat. Locally produced honey is said to have special healing qualities. Eating tropical foods in cold climates might cause an arctic dweller to be less tolerant of the cold; conversely, eating fruit grown nearer the poles might make equatorial heat oppressive. There are no laws or rules. Select from available food with wisdom and thrift.

"O"—Organic

The term 'organic' literally means it contains carbon because it is or was once alive and either has or will decay. For this book organic refers to food grown according to standards set by governments and international organizations—Certified Organic. Organic certification emerged only in the 20th century because of the assault of new chemicals introduced into the food supply when agriculture became industrialized. You vote to maintain high standards when you buy organic food, and eventually it should become cheaper because the farmer has no chemical bill to pay.

In general, the label "organic" means the food was grown naturally, with no chemical fertilizers or synthetic pesticides. It cannot be processed with irradiation, industrial solvents, or chemical food additives or preservatives nor can it be genetically modified. Organic food means it has been grown as much as possible the way food was grown before chemical corporations took over the food system—in deep rich composted topsoil not corrupted by deadly poisons. Only natural fertilizers are used, like animal manure. Sea water, rocks and shells that have been dried and ground into powder, sea weed, compost, and wood ashes are also used for fertilizer, depending on what nutrient is lacking. Organic certification means the farm is inspected for use of prohibited chemicals and other unsafe substances. Genetic modification (GMO), which uses genes from another species of organism (like bacteria) to change a plant—an event never found in nature—is also prohibited under organic standards.

In general, the label "organic" means the food was grown naturally, with no chemical fertilizers or synthetic pesticides.

Conventionally grown food can be living, but the chemicals make it toxic. If a 'space suit' is required to apply the stuff, better not to eat it. Insects and microorganisms will, by nature, attack only a plant or animal that is weak or lacks vital energy; it is natural selection in operation. Chemical fertilizers and pesticides weaken plants because they are toxic. And then more chemicals are needed to kill the bugs that naturally attack the weak plant. It is a vicious cycle; using chemicals increases the amount of chemicals needed. If insects are eating a plant, the farmer should check to see what is wrong with the soil or environment. The term "cide" means "kill" no matter what pretty name is on the label. These toxins are drawn into the whole plant and cannot be washed, cooked, or peeled away. All of these practices decrease the life force energy in the food.

Artificial hybridization (which is allowed in certified organic food production) also is to be avoided. A 'hybrid' plant is simply the result when one variety of a species has been pollinated with another (usually by hand). Growing striped watermelon near spotted ones will render seed that will produce a melon with both spots and stripes, for example. While plants have hybridized themselves for ever, modern hybridization renders seed that is sterile or will not grow fruit like the one from which it was saved. Some plants are bred to eliminate seeds altogether. Better to go for the open-pollinated or heirloom kinds and then the seeds can be saved, too.

Artificial growing yields food of inferior quality. This would include plants grown in a soil-less chemical solution or under artificial lights. The plants do not have a chance to absorb energy from the sun, rain, and live organisms in real soil. It is like living in the dark—on vitamin pills, coffee, beer, antibiotics, and laxatives. It is out of harmony with nature.

"V"—Vegan

'Vegetarian' refers to a person who eats neither flesh nor any part taken from the carcass of a previously living animal. That means any animal that lives on the Earth, in the sea, or in small cages. 'Animals' include ones with four legs, two legs or no legs at all. Yes, fish, shellfish, birds, all bovine animals, insects, worms, snakes, sheep, goats, rabbits, and game animals, as well as chickens and pigs, are included (even human flesh for that matter). This would even mean carnivores, but flesh eating humans shun the meat from animals that eat flesh. There is no such thing as a vegetarian who eats "a little chicken or fish." A person who calls herself vegetarian might, however eat dairy, honey, or eggs (no killing). A raw vegetarian would eat these foods in their live state.

The term 'vegan' strictly means a menu without any foods taken in any way from any animal.

The term 'vegan' strictly means a menu without any foods taken in any way from any animal. This would mean no flesh, bee products, anything made from the milk of any animal, or any animal's eggs, including those of fish and ducks. There would be no meat, cheese, yogurt, butter, or caviar, even mixed into a product, such as cake. Vegan food is made with ingredients taken strictly from some part of a plant—roots (carrot), stem (rhubarb), leaf (spinach), flower (broccoli), sprout, or seed (nuts). It is not only possible to be a junk food vegan (think potato chips) but very easy. That is why preparation of the food is so important. A new term, "beegan," has recently been coined which means no animal products except honey.

"E"—Exquisite

The term exquisite means the food looks, smells, and tastes amazingly delicious and is naturally fragrant.

The term exquisite means the food looks, smells, and tastes amazingly delicious and is naturally fragrant. It must be fresh and appeal to the very soul of the diner. Using spices and seasonings from nature, the food is in harmony with both the taste buds and the digestive tract. It makes the eater feel delighted while eating it, an hour, and a week after the meal (and for years to come). The flavor and life burst into her cells right through the oral membranes to the brain next door and feel "right!" In the stomach it must feel divine, completely comfortable and fulfilling, producing no gas as it progresses through the body (except as the colon is cleared initially). It will fill the cells of the diner with a joyful singing and bring an unbidden satisfied sigh. It must be a feast for sight, smell, and taste. It can be a plain salad or a fancy warm casserole but it must be luscious.

The eater feels wonderful after the meal partly because it is harder to over-eat raw food. The body says "stop."

"R"—Raw

Although often considered interchangeable, raw, fresh, and live are not identical. Raw means 'uncooked' but sometimes gets distorted to mean things that have been pasteurized (like almonds) or steamed (like cashews), so in these cases it means 'not roasted' (it is still probably dead). Live food means not killed by any means, cooking, pasteurizing or over-long storage. It means not heated above 118°F—by microwaving, boiling, canning, irradiating, frying, baking, steaming, roasting or any other means. Pasteurization simply means the heating of any substance to a certain temperature for a specified period of time. This kills flavor and valuable nutrients (known and as yet unknown), like vitamins (especially the water soluble ones), and over 90% of the enzymes. Pasteurized food is *not* live.

'Living' means much more than that; it implies that the delicate enzymes and the 'spark of life' are still alive. Live food embodies the elusive life force energy from nature that leaves at death. Since our bodies are alive, if our fingers find it too hot to touch, the food is dead. You don't need a thermometer. A living sprout may be blended, and even though it would not be able to grow again in that form, is still considered live if eaten very soon—before the enzymes die.

'Living' means much more than that; it implies that the delicate enzymes and the 'spark of life' are still alive.

> Try roasting a handful of lentils or buckwheat groats in a 350° hot oven for half an hour. Then put the roasted seeds in a jar and soak in water for 8 hours. Soak some raw seeds in another jar. Cover with a mesh and sit the jars at an angle, rinsing twice a day. Within a few days you should see the real difference in live and dead food—life!

'Fresh' can mean raw but it might also refer to whether food is spoiled or not. The presence of life might not be apparent by simply looking at a seed or plant—a deciduous tree in winter looks dead but will bloom again in spring. To see if a seed is alive it must be exposed to the right conditions of moisture, temperature, and light. There are levels of 'aliveness.' A dried lentil is alive; but when it is soaked and sprouted, it is actively growing and considered more alive—biogenic or 'life-generating.' White flour, dry pasta, and irradiated potatoes, while 'uncooked' or 'raw' are considered dead because the processing is intended to kill enzymes in order to prolong shelf life. Live food, if intact, would grow. Live food is always raw; not all 'raw' food is alive.

People often lament they 'need' hot food in the winter to 'warm' them. But, no one can eat cooked food right off the stove—it must be cooled to a comfortable temperature so it will not burn the tongue. Raw dishes are served at about the same 'mouth temperature.' Raw soups are heated up to approximately the same temperature of cooked soups (after blowing on it). Unlike in the commercials where the food 'fights back,' live food loves to be eaten and feels good in your body.

Live food is always raw; not all 'raw' food is alive.

The "R" in CLOVER also stands for ripe. Food that is not mature is not digestible and not nearly as sweet as ripe food. Peppers, for example should not be eaten green. Most of the varieties that are sold green would turn red or another color if left on the plant a little longer. That is why red bell peppers are more expensive than green ones. Jalapenos will also turn red and are much better for you after they mature. Bananas should be left until they have at least a few brown 'freckles,' little or no green at the tips, and will peel easily. Let them ripen and then refrigerate. The skin will darken but the insides will be sweet and delicious for about a week. Avocados will keep better if you refrigerate them when hard and green. Bring them out into the fruit bowl a couple of days before you eat them soft, ripe, and buttery.

The diet discussed in this book is any version of fresh vegan, organic food that may be prepared by blending, chopping, fermenting, freezing, or dehydrating. It is not, however, heated above 118° F, irradiated, or preserved with chemicals other than pure sea salt (and that used sparingly). Delicious and simple recipes are to be found in over a hundred published books on the subject. A living diet is a whole new experience of creating living dishes—food the whole world can feel good about.

ISN'T THAT KILLING THE PLANTS?

Why (one might ask), is it okay to kill a plant and not an animal? That does cause a problem for some, and that is why some strict religions declare fruitarian as the best diet, which only includes fruit, seeds, and leaves that when removed or harvested do not harm the plant itself. Tomatoes, squash, eggplant, peas, avocados, cucumbers, and many other vegetables are really the fruit of the plant. Berries and seeds are also dropped by the plant. All nuts, legumes, and grains are seeds.

In nature, wild animals browse and under ordinary circumstances almost never destroy all of a particular species. They leave some to go to seed for the next year's crops. That is the way of nature and humans are part of nature. Most of a harvest may be eaten, but leaving some plants (like parsnips) or fruits (like tomatillos) in the garden to reseed is in harmony with natural cycles. Some biennial crops must be stored and replanted in spring (like carrots and cabbage) in order to form seeds. Lettuce, broccoli, kale, and many other plants will naturally bolt if allowed and produce abundant seeds. Other crops, like garlic or raspberries, do better if a few plants or roots are dug and moved elsewhere each year or every few years.

Plants have beautiful auras when viewed with Kirlian photography (or give it a try with the naked eye). It is known that spending time focusing loving attention on a plant helps it thrive. Humans have a connection with plants. They are also living, intelligent creatures, and it has been suggested that plants and fruits might wish to be eaten if in loving, grateful communion. And if you are really concerned about killing plants consider the number of plants it takes to feed animals for meat as opposed to the vegan way. (See Chapter 11.)

Plants might be part of a loving plan to support humans as they evolve, much the same as pets agree to love and heal their owners and be fed in exchange. Plants fill the human body with Divine Light as mankind struggles to become aware of that light. Fruits depend upon animals eating the pulp from around the seed, in order to propagate themselves. The seed is then deposited in nature, surrounded by a 'nugget' of the animal's nourishing manure to grow and fruit again. Perhaps 'humanure' (human manure) might be used to feed plants (instead of building costly sewer treatment plants) if human bodies were chemical-free and had healthy flowing energy systems. Eventually plants eat animals.

Eventually plants eat animals.

TYPES OF RAW DIETS

There are about as many raw diets as there are raw foodists and the discussions (not the food) can get heated over which is best. The topic of diet can be touchier than politics, religion, or sex. Most raw foodists aspire to a 100% raw diet as an ideal, and those who reach that goal are very enthusiastic about the benefits. But there are very few who maintain this stringent rule. Even strong advocates allow that being 100% anything is mentally unhealthy. Even 'all raw' people will have to concede to 95%, because it is impossible to be certain what temperature was used when foods are prepared by others—almond

Most raw foodists aspire to a 100% raw diet as an ideal, and those who reach that goal are very enthusiastic about the benefits.

butter or raisins from a store, for instance. All would agree only on the importance of eating most food in its natural state—live—and the only food item usually excluded is flesh. Some raw food diets are high carbohydrate and low fat and some are the other way around. Each person is looking for a personalized result.

Some say since we are closely related to chimpanzees, we should eat what they naturally eat. Most agree these relatives are strictly vegan, but people are not chimpanzees. They are unique and each person walks a different path, changing as she heals, learns, and becomes conscious. What is needed at one stage feels wrong at another time, climate, age, detoxification, or initiation level.

Most agree that fresh deep, green leafy vegetables are excellent for human food, and all raw foodists allow at least some fresh fruit. Many say greens and fruit are ideal food for humans; but some restrict them, especially sweet ones, maybe until a health condition reverses. Sprouted seeds like alfalfa and clover are usually acceptable and some eat legumes like lentils and mung beans this way. Most also would eat micro-greens like buckwheat shoots, especially in winter. Fresh raw lemon juice is usually an acceptable dressing ingredient, but vinegar sometimes is not. Locally grown food is really important to some, and in northern climates, vinegar could be local while lemons would not.

Honey and maple syrup also are cold climate food, while agave is from warm areas. Dried fruit is often used for sweeteners and some (like dates) are tropical, while others (like raisins) can be grown in lots of areas. Honey is an animal product and maple syrup is cooked. Probably everyone would agree that honey, maple syrup, dried fruit, and agave are all better than sugar and high-fructose corn syrup. All of these are available organically grown.

Labels can be very misleading. Almonds, for example, are required to be pasteurized if they are to be sold retail in the United

States (even though labeled raw). Cashews found labeled raw in stores are not, either. They have been steamed to remove the shells. It is possible, however, to obtain both of them unpasteurized—truly raw. Rolled oats and wheat bulgur are both steam processed, and are not raw. All commercially frozen vegetables have been blanched (plunged into very hot water) before freezing, but frozen fruits are generally frozen raw. Anything that is canned is cooked. Commercially ground nut and seed butters like tahini have been ground at very high speed and probably have been 'cooked' in the process. The labels on some sprouted grain frozen bread labels say they were baked at low heat but if above the 118°F limit, are not raw. Look at labels, contact the company, and ask your body and inner guide if this food is good for eating right now and *listen* to the answer.

Raw foodists often start eating later in the day and stop earlier than the majority of Americans. They will often start the day with fruit or fruit blended with greens and most will have at least one meal a day of a large green salad, plain or fancy. Live cuisine can get as elegant as any SAD meal, and dinners of several courses from appetizers and dips, entrees of vegetables marinated, shredded, sauced and seasoned can be created. Raw desserts are to live for!

RAW CONTROVERSIES

Live food vegans are conscious of each food in their diet. The same food might be indispensable to one or abhorrent to another. Some say only birds should eat grains because only they have a 'crop' to grind it. Sea vegetables and algae might be considered an important food or a supplement. Salt is a hot topic—it can be used liberally or sparingly in various forms, like different sea salts or nama shoyu (a raw soy sauce). Each salt imparts a different flavor. Often oil is limited or eliminated but lots of 'rawbies' eat organic, cold pressed oils like olive and coconut,

Raw desserts are to live for!

as desired. Many raw foodists find legumes difficult to digest and will substitute nuts in bean recipes like hummus. Lentils can be sprouted for salad, used as 'chunks' in soup, or made into 'burgers.'

Supplements, especially Vitamins B12 and D, are arguably problems with the live vegan diet. Some raw lovers allow them but many are vehemently against any pills (as was Ann Wigmore). Nutritional studies are rarely done on raw foodists. Nutritional yeast is controversial, depending on beliefs about vitamin B12, cooked food, and taste. B12 is made only by bacteria found in animals and soil. Both the bacteria and B12 is destroyed when food is sterilized by cooking. Of course, supplements are made by corporations and it is hard to know what is actually in the little capsule. (More on micronutrients later.)

Food combining is important at first; others say it is less so with raw food. Food combining rules say to eat food that digests quickly first. Fruit, especially melons, should always be eaten first and alone because they digest so much faster than other food. Nuts, seeds, and other fatty foods take longer. Ann Wigmore and Victoria Boutenko both teach that greens such as kale, romaine, spinach, chard, dandelions, and collards should be a separate food group from vegetables. They can be blended and digested perfectly with fruit or any other food.[147]

Timing is important, too. Raw organic local dairy foods might be okay early on, but most will eliminate eggs and dairy eventually. Early in transition, eating a lot of nuts is common, but later most find they feel better with fewer. Fasting, juicing, and drinking wheatgrass juice (squeezed from young wheat plants), might be important for some when actively detoxing.

Opinions can vary wildly. Tea sparks discussion as do soy bean products, for a variety of reasons (GMO, digestibility, heated,

---

147 Victoria Boutenko, *Green for Life,* (Ashland, OR: Raw Family Publishing, 2005), 39.

etc.). Raw cacao, or chocolate powder is a valuable "super food" for some; toxic and only for special occasions for others who substitute carob powder. Unpasteurized, organically-produced wine might be acceptable on occasion; or considered toxic. Onion and garlic, too, are controversial—opinions range from 'off limits' to calling them 'super foods.'

Raw fooders can be over-zealous and all people have a plethora of reasons for clinging to the diet they have chosen. Like people on SAD, they will go to great lengths to defend it. Religion and diet are not necessarily one size fits all, no matter how fervent the evangelist. The problem is how to teach about raw food without creating karma for teacher and listener. There are no universal rules, for it is impossible to know the spiritual path of another. It could be that some souls need to experience a lesson of illness, war, violence, or despair in order to turn to the light. Respect your body and the intelligence of others. The best advice about a particular food is: find it in its best form (like organic, whole grain, non-GMO, etc.) then if you want it cooked, do it yourself and do it minimally at the lowest possible temperature, without fat. Try it, be honest, and keep a detailed journal.

FOOD PREPARATION

There are lots of ways to prepare food that leave it alive. Sitting in the garden is best, but from there it gets complicated in different ways. Freshly chopped or blended are better than fermented (uses salt), frozen, or dehydrated; but all are considered alive if the temperature and storage time are not excessive. Heated seeds will not grow but many that have been frozen or dried will sprout and bloom, even after long periods of time.

Try it, be honest, and keep a detailed journal.

> A friend of mine forgot her flax crackers in the turned off dehydrator and was surprised to open the door and find the seeds were growing right out of the cracker, even after they had been thoroughly dried (drew moisture from the air). (I have successfully sprouted lentils that were eight years old.)

Raw chefs can create nearly any cooked dish craved by modern Americans—in living form. There are all levels of preparation, from fancy cakes to simple salads. Raw food is made from the same basic ingredients as cooked food, but some dishes can be made of surprising ingredients. For example, figs and zucchini can be found in moist chocolate cake; cauliflower can be turned into Spanish 'rice,' mashed 'potatoes,' or 'popcorn;' eggplant makes the most delicious lasagna, vegan 'bacon,' or pizza crust. The uses for almonds are endless.

People who are new to raw (and making ongoing adjustments) might be eager to make fancy dishes, but as the body gets purer, the palate follows suit. Raw prepared food can be made using less salt and seasoning because natural food has much more flavor.

> Cooked food must be heavily salted—try eating a baked potato or boiled pasta without salt!

Even raw food recipes can be progressively adjusted to lower salt, nuts, and oils—all of which often *improve* the flavor.

Learning to prepare tasty raw vegan food takes time. It is a little like moving to a foreign country and learning to cook all over again. Raw diet equipment consists mostly of three appliances: a high power blender, a food processor, and a dehydrator. A good sharp knife, lemon and garlic squeezers, and a vegetable peeler are nice, too. It will take some time, but recipes can be found (or created) that are quick, easy, super tasty, and satisfy the deepest hunger. The best dishes use the fewest ingredients. Guiltless meals will not block up the chakras and will still glow in the body the next morning. Raw foodists are usually overjoyed to teach. The same as with cooked food, some rich raw creations are best served only occasionally, too.

The best dishes use the fewest ingredients.

Another issue when 'going raw' is that fewer people in general prepare their own food nowadays. For example, boiling spaghetti and opening a jar of sauce passes for "home cooking." Raw recipes can be overwhelming and off-putting. They often contain exotic ingredients like baby coconut, which, in Minnesota, is a foreign object. Many people don't have the faintest idea of where to start in a kitchen, let alone how to turn a pile of spinach, a box of mushrooms, and a cup of nuts into a raw quiche. Most raw dishes like soups, casseroles, and patés can be made ahead, freeze nicely, and simply need to be warmed. Lots of raw food can be made in big batches, frozen or dried, sealed in a jar, and kept a long time. A quick supper can be fermented food and crackers, blender soup, granola and nut milk, or roll some paté and veggies in a nori wrap or cabbage leaf. Hours of preparation time is strictly optional.

Hours of preparation time is strictly optional.

For dedicated raw foodies, the optimal diet is CLOVER—Complete, Local, Organic, Vegan, Exquisite and Raw. Preparation methods and choice of ingredients are individual. These are only a few preparation ideas. Everyone makes, changes, and breaks their own diet rules as they wish.

Everyone makes, changes, and breaks their own diet rules as they wish.

'EXPERTS' IN NUTRITION

The U. S. government has been giving people advice on what to eat for more than a century, arranged in neat sound bites that change from decade to decade. The results of these recommendations are then reflected in the health issues that appear later in the population. Colorful posters in the classrooms, provided by the food industry, never mention how the food is prepared. While most nutritionists, doctors, and other health care professionals are good people and teach honestly what they have been taught, they are often unaware of the influences political and industrial interests had on those official recommendations and the content of their classes.

In her book, *Food Politics,* nutrition professor Marion Nestle, outlines the procedure that the government follows in issuing the *Dietary Guidelines* now called *The Food Guide Pyramid.* She also reveals the affiliations of members of the advisory committees that develop these guidelines. Food corporations fund research and influence government nutritional policies in a variety of ways. Nestle says that advising people to eat less of anything runs counter to the interests of food producers. Small organic farmers do not hire lobbyists to influence the recommendations of the experts in favor of their products, but such organizations as the big national 'councils' and 'boards' provide grants and exert other financial pressures. Nutrition and public health are not the job of lobbyists and corporate executives whose focus is on making money for their stockholders. Nestle writes, "Food companies will make and market any product that sells, regardless of its food value or effect on health."[148] It is therefore up to the consumer to be aware.

Food corporations fund research and influence government nutritional policies in a variety of ways.

CONVENTIONAL CONTROVERSIES

Protein

Some protein is necessary in the human diet, but the amount is far less than imagined. Proteins are made up of long chains of amino acids, and there are 15 to 20 different kinds of amino acids. Eight of these amino acids are not made in our bodies and must be supplied in food. Food made from parts and products of animals do contain

Some protein is necessary in the human diet, but the amount is far less than imagined.

148 Marion Nestle, *Food Politics,* (Berkeley, CA: University of California Press, 2002), viii.

all the needed amino acids, but as discussed in Chapter 8, cooking denatures them.

T. Colin Campbell writes, "Plant proteins may be lacking in one or more of the essential amino acids, [but] as a group they *do* contain all of them. There is a mountain of compelling research showing that 'low-quality' plant protein, which allows for slow but steady synthesis of new proteins [in our bodies], is the healthiest type of protein [for humans]."[149] Campbell's research found that humans need only 5–6% [of total calorie intake] dietary protein to replace the protein regularly excreted by the body but the government recommendations has been as high as 35%. As also mentioned in Chapter 8, Campbell found animal protein implicated in heart disease, cancer, diabetes, autoimmune disease, and diseases of the kidneys, bones and brain.

Fitness expert Douglas Graham writes, "Mother's [human] milk provides on average approximately 6% (of calories) from protein for growing infants (USDA nutrient database for Standard Reference, Release 18)."[150] According to the diet analysis chart in his book, most fruit contain between 4–8% protein and vegetables have 10–20%. Graham declares, "All plant foods contain protein," and the body recycles most of its own protein, so combining amino acids in a meal to make complete proteins is not necessary.

Another way to measure nutrients is by weight—grams of protein per specific measurement of food. The following is from The NutriBase Nutrition Facts Desk Reference:

- ♥ 1 cup human milk contains 3 grams of protein
- ♥ ¼ cup shelled sunflower seeds contains 6 grams of protein
- ♥ 1 cup sprouted wheat contains 8 grams of protein
- ♥ 1 cup raw chopped broccoli contains 3 grams of protein
- ♥ 1 cup fresh raw raspberries contains 1 gram of protein

---

149 T. Colin Campbell, Ph.D., *The China Study,* (Dallas, TX: Benbella Books, 2004), 30.

150 Dr. Douglas N. Graham, *80/10/10,* (Key Largo, FL: FoodnSport Press, 2006), 99–104.

- ♥ 1 cup mashed raw banana contains 2 grams of protein
- ♥ 1 cup fresh cubed avocado contains 3 grams of protein
- ♥ 3 oz. raw spinach contains 3 grams of protein[151]

Gabriel Cousens puts it this way: "Expert research around the world suggests that the real protein requirement is closer to 25-35 grams [for adults], and less if the protein we eat comes from live foods. Excess protein in the diet does not 'burn cleanly' and has been associated with creating an over-acid system and contributes to such diseases as arthritis, kidney damage, schizophrenia, osteoporosis, atherosclerosis, heart disease, and cancer." He says *all* eight essential amino acids are found in all leafy green vegetables and most fruits and seeds. He, too, mentions human milk, saying, "The average protein concentration in mother's milk is just 1. 4 percent (by weight), sufficient to supply the human organism with all the essential amino acids and protein needed during the period of most rapid growth and brain development. Apes live on a fruitarian diet that averages between .2 and 2.2 percent protein."[152] Cousens suggests, "An excess of protein slows the flow of the spiritualizing energy." Do adult humans need more protein than a newborn or an ape?

Micronutrient Controversies

Many people have been found to be deficient in Vitamin B12. But it is not just raw vegans who have vitamin B12 problems; it is cooked flesh eaters as well. This micronutrient is made by microorganisms found in the soil and intestines of animals. All agree that the amount needed in the human diet is very tiny and that it is easily destroyed by heat. It is doubtful that the cooked food in the Standard American Diet provides much Vitamin B12, either. Some experts feel raw foodists and vegetarians need less vitamin B12 (in their diet), perhaps

---

151 CyberSoft, Inc., *NutriBase Nutrition Facts Desk Reference—2nd ed.* (New York, NY: Penguin Putnam), 2001.

152 Gabriel Cousens, M.D., *Spiritual Nutrition,* (Berkeley, CA: North Atlantic Books, 2005), 269-272.

because they are better at producing it in the mouth and other places. There are lots of reasons for B12 deficiencies; depleted soil where the microorganisms have been destroyed, over-washing and cooking of produce, and conditions in the body like ingested drugs, and certain medical conditions. T. Colin Campbell writes, "Plants grown in healthy soil that has a good concentration of vitamin B12 will readily absorb this nutrient. However, plants grown in 'lifeless' soil (non-organic) may be deficient in vitamin B12."[153] Some feel it can be obtained from food like nutritional yeast, sea vegetables, algae, or live fermented foods (like raw sauerkraut). If a person feels uneasy, she should do the research and perhaps take a good supplement of B12.

Fear around vitamins D and A, essential fatty acids, and Omega 3 also exist for people who eat fewer animal products. Vitamin A is found in the most delicious of plants—the orange ones, such as carrots, mangos, apricots and cantaloupe. It is also found in red sweet pepper, broccoli, and deep green leafy vegetables. Vitamin D comes from the sun and involves the interaction of many vitamins and minerals.

Calcium, as with all minerals, must be converted into a small, water-soluble, compound in order to be absorbed by humans. [154] Animals are unable to use minerals directly from the soil as plants do. Calcium is 32% destroyed by heating above 150° F and can be found in great abundance in raw green leafy vegetables, rhubarb stalks, most seeds, nuts, and grains especially sesame seeds.

Some raw food vegans take manufactured supplements. Others feel their needs will be met by following instinctual eating of a large variety of foods. Some get tested on a regular basis. Since most research is done on content of diet (ignoring production and preparation methods), evaluation of the uncooked vegan diet is rare. Mother

---

153 T. Colin Campbell, Ph.D.., *The China Study,* (Dallas, TX: BenBella Books, 2004), 232.

154 Gabriel Cousens, M.D., *Spiritual Nutrition,* (Berkeley, CA: North Atlantic Books, 2005), 415.

Nature supplies all nutrients in combination with macronutrients and micronutrients known only to her. She does not wrap each one alone in capsule or pill. Raw vegans should do whatever eliminates their nutritional fears.

Raw Pyramid *

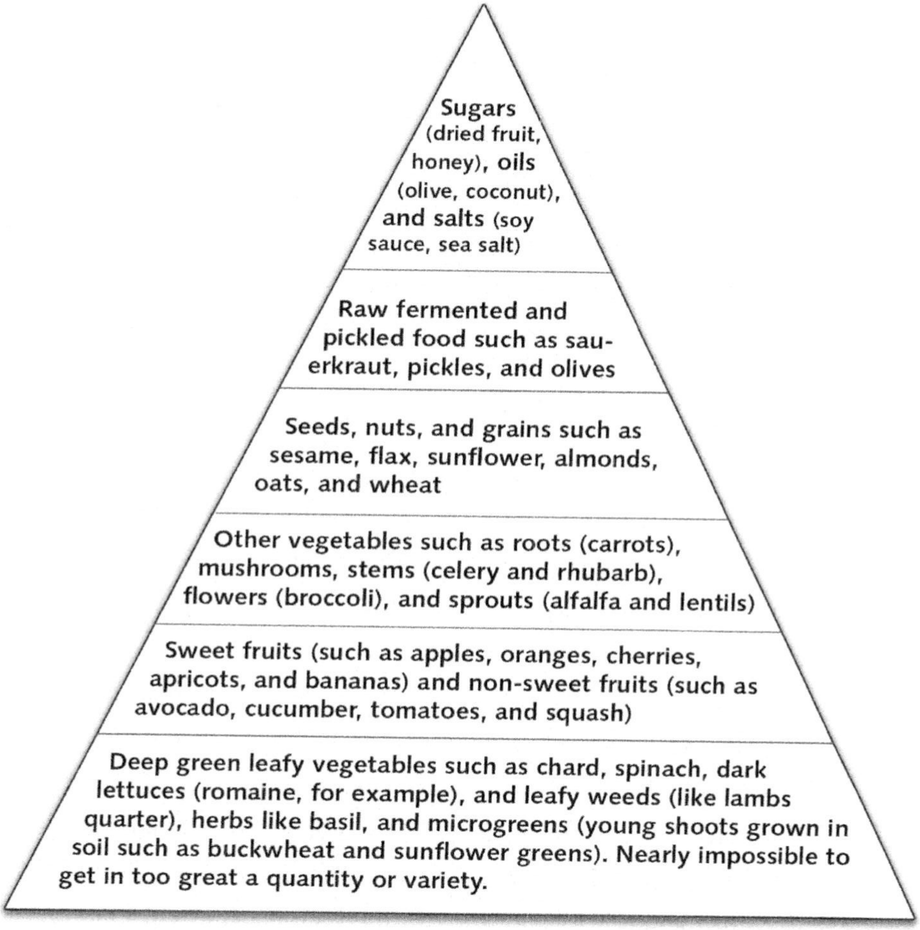
Sugars (dried fruit, honey), oils (olive, coconut), and salts (soy sauce, sea salt)
Raw fermented and pickled food such as sauerkraut, pickles, and olives
Seeds, nuts, and grains such as sesame, flax, sunflower, almonds, oats, and wheat
Other vegetables such as roots (carrots), mushrooms, stems (celery and rhubarb), flowers (broccoli), and sprouts (alfalfa and lentils)
Sweet fruits (such as apples, oranges, cherries, apricots, and bananas) and non-sweet fruits (such as avocado, cucumber, tomatoes, and squash)
Deep green leafy vegetables such as chard, spinach, dark lettuces (romaine, for example), and leafy weeds (like lambs quarter), herbs like basil, and microgreens (young shoots grown in soil such as buckwheat and sunflower greens). Nearly impossible to get in too great a quantity or variety.

**There probably is not a raw vegan anywhere who eats this perfectly or even totally agrees.*

PROBLEMS WITH COOKED FOOD

An 'embalmed' commercial cupcake will stay soft and look fresh for years, but is deadly.

As discussed in Chapter 8, cooking food destroys enzymes, life force energy, natural microorganisms, many nutrients, and most of the flavor it contains. Cooking may have evolved as a means to preserve food such as in canning (all canned food is heated to a high temperature to sterilize it and to seal the jars). Most cooked food (without preservatives, canning or freezing) spoils more quickly than fresh, because its 'life' has been destroyed. Cooked grain rots almost immediately. Humanity has survived because fresh food—such as apples, potatoes, carrots and turnips could be stored in a cool place (like underground) for months. Dry grains and beans will keep for years if perfectly dry. Sauerkraut with its living enzymes and microorganisms also stays fresh and delicious in a cool place for months. An 'embalmed' commercial cupcake will stay soft and look fresh for years, but is deadly.

Microorganisms are destroyed when food is cooked or washed in disinfectants. Sterilized food will not ferment because fermentation depends on these tiny living friends. Bacteria are essential in the human gastrointestinal tract. We know vitamins are made by friendly organisms, and it is impossible to know what else they do. It seems nature intended us to live together.

Cooking food in these modern times has an added danger because the heat changes agricultural poisons, making them even more toxic. For example, tomatoes which have been sprayed with a fungicide contain from ten to ninety times more carcinogenic substances after cooking than raw ones from the same chemically grown plant.[155]

A further problem with cooking food is the loss of flavor. A plain baked potato is hardly worth eating without the butter, salt, pepper, chives, and sour cream. Cooked carrots, broccoli, and spinach are

---

155 Gabriel Cousens, M.D., *Spiritual Nutrition,* (Berkeley, CA: North Atlantic Books, 2005), 289.

nearly inedible. It is no wonder that kids won't eat vegetables! A baked apple is mush that cries for sugar and cinnamon, while a plain blended raw apple is ambrosia to the tongue. Live food does not need added sugar, salt, or fats to delight the nose and mouth.

CHOOSING A DIET

Each person gets to choose how 'clean' and 'pure' she wants her body and mind—how healthy is healthy *enough*? A seeker reads what the experts say about nutrition, considers the *motives* behind the recommendations (who is trying to sell you what), and then picks the spot on their own pyramid that fits their level of consciousness. Scientists may be light years away from being able to describe all the nutrients and the interrelationships between food, people, and the cosmos. The inner wisdom of the Self knows what is needed in each moment—an on-board 'nutritional expert.'

Each person gets to choose how 'clean' and 'pure' she wants her body and mind—how healthy is healthy enough?

> Next time you sit down at a meal take a minute and *really* look at the food in front of you (you won't starve in one minute). What did it look like when it was alive? Where did it grow up? How did it go from its original form to your plate?

There are no shortages of 'expert' formulas and books on diet. The ancient Hindu Ayurveda system divides people into their natural 'energy' categories. Some dietary formulas explore a person's blood-type, recommending a different diet for each one. Sometimes metabolism is evaluated, or personality traits. The bottom line is what makes each person feel like a healthy, alert child, filled with curiosity—free to be who she is, painlessly running all day, squealing with delight, seeing the *truth* in relationships and situations, and sleeping soundly at appropriate times. The right diet will joyfully sustain you day after day, year after year.

By overcoming physical habits, mental 'tricks', addictions, and emotional attachments, each person uses her body as a laboratory. If conflicted about a food item, consult your inner wisdom, eat it and then remember what happens afterwards.

The right diet will joyfully sustain you day after day, year after year.

Keep a 'diet journal' and write everything you eat and drink and how it was prepared in one column with the date and time. In another column write date and time and how you are feeling physically, mentally, and emotionally. Also record your gastrointestinal symptoms such as heartburn and quality of bowel movements ('poop' is just recycled food!). Compare over hours, days, and weeks.

As the cells are cleared of debris, old food choices will likely be replaced with new ones. The same food at one time is delicious and sweet, but at a different time is repulsive and bitter. The cleaner the body, the purer the food desired. If it tastes bitter or distasteful, don't eat it. It all shows up in the body, and *the body does not lie!*

It might be helpful to make a list of existing health and emotional issues when you begin your healthy raw food journey, because when that aching knee feels perfect again it is easy to forget it ever hurt at all. Be sure to keep checking with a health provider on serious conditions such as diabetes, because as the blood sugar corrects itself, the medication requirements will change. Physical ailments have been known to spontaneous heal—for example, a small cut on your finger.

It all shows up in the body, and the body does not lie!

The really good news about the CLOVER diet is people can eat as much and as often as they want from Earth's salad bar—the plethora of raw plants. Eat five apples, or three avocados, or a whole quart of strawberries for a meal; it does not matter. It is not necessary to ever be hungry. But hunger, too can become exciting and enjoyable if thought of as anticipation of the pure delicious treats awaiting your mouth.

Hunger makes everything taste much better! Oh, and humans can eat real *CLOVER* too, like the rest of the herbivores on the planet—clover seed sprouts for salad, dried clover blossoms for tea.

THE MENU AT OUR HOUSE

On our farm (Hygieia Homestead) we usually eat a very simple diet, adjusted for the season and who is present for the meal. Meals are often prepared together. But on special occasions, we experiment with fancy foods. Ordinarily for breakfast a green smoothie is quick, delicious, can be made ahead, and at the time of day when energy is needed, it provides plenty of carbohydrates (and protein). This thick drink is usually made by blending at least two kinds of fruit (a sweeter one and a tart one) with fresh deep green leafy vegetable (or dried greens in winter). A simple recipe is one orange, two apples, and a big handful of greens (as much as can be grasped) with a little water to blend. The smoothie will look green, but it tastes only of fruit. There are an endless variety of smoothie greens like kale, chard, spinach, and dandelions. This combination seems to agree well with the body and sets up a healthy vigor for the day's work, whether physical such as gardening, or mental, such as writing.

Hunger makes everything taste much better!

Smoothies may be made up to three days in advance and refrigerated, (such as for a trip). If there is not time for a smoothie, then several pieces of fruit can be grabbed and eaten en route to the garden or appointment. Sometimes breakfast is simply grapefruit or melon, which should be eaten alone. A special breakfast for birthdays and holidays is a durian (large prickly tropical fruit that tastes like vanilla custard), which can be kept for months in the freezer and thawed slowly for a real treat.

A more traditional breakfast—oatmeal—can be made from soaked steel-cut whole groats (rolled oats are not raw). Delicious milk can be made from soaked seeds such as sesame or almonds and blended with a small amount of water until *very* creamy; then adding honey, salt, vanilla, and more water as desired (no need to strain out the healthy fiber). Granola can be made from dried fruit and dried sprouted seeds and grains. There is no juicer in our house—the only juice is hand squeezed from lemons for recipes.

Lunch is almost always an elaborate green salad unless there are leftovers. Whatever is in season is piled into the bowl, always a beautiful and large variety. We start with tender savory deep green leafy vegetables, such as lettuce, arugula, basil, spinach, etc.—as fresh as possible, washed in pure water and spun dry. On this pretty bed might be shredded roots like carrots, parsnips, beets, radishes, or turnips. We might add sprouts that have been grown in a jar. Usually there is something fermented like sauerkraut or pickles that go wonderfully on a salad, adding bacteria that is good for the gut. We often include shredded or chopped cabbage, broccoli, cucumber, tomatoes, onion (red, white, yellow, or green), sliced celery, kohlrabi, shredded winter or summer squash, or ripe sweet peppers (never green ones). Even peas, asparagus, green beans, and sweet corn can go on a salad in its natural raw state. Although our goal is to grow most of our food, we still buy and chop avocados, olives and mushrooms. Edible flowers such as chive are also pretty. Dressing is usually half olive oil, half apple cider vinegar with lots of garlic and nutritional yeast shaken together. The really big advantage of eating salad is that you need to look at it, pay attention to it (to select your next morsel), chew it (as life energy absorbs into your mouth membranes), and connect with it, unlike many sandwiches consumed in five bites while hurtling down the highway.

Whatever is in season is piled into the bowl, always a beautiful and large variety.

Many days we eat only twice, but a third meal might be a simple supper or a more elaborate 'dinner.' It can be a different salad such as coleslaw with a creamy nut mayonnaise. Supper might be a warm casserole, lasagna, soup, sandwich, burger, pate, or raw pizza.

For holidays like Thanksgiving we prepare a 'traditional' raw meal together—a nut pate, 'mashed potatoes' (cauliflower) with mushroom gravy, 'unbaked' squash, cranberry relish, and raw apple crisp with surprisingly similar taste and appearance to their cooked cousins. Raw pumpkin pie is delicious and cashews make a 'whipped topping' to live for.

The really big advantage of eating salad is that you need to look at it, pay attention to it (to select your next morsel), chew it (as life energy absorbs into your mouth membranes), and connect with it, unlike many sandwiches consumed in five bites while hurtling down the highway.

Even on regular days, we almost always have a delicious dessert. Gooey cakes, chocolate brownies, many kinds of pudding, ice cream, pies, cookies, and shakes. In fact chocolate shakes appear almost every evening.

GROWING FOOD

If you have access to a small patch of Earth where food could be grown, then go to a used book store and get a book (or three) on gardening and start planning right after Christmas if you live in the north (anytime, if you live in the south). Some plants (like people) prefer hot and some like cool weather. There are lots of seed companies that offer organic and heirloom seeds. When planting seeds, space them in consideration of how large the plant will be when mature. Growing on trellises for tomatoes, cucumbers, beans and peas offers more food per square foot. A recent article in *Mother Earth News* tells of a woman who raised what she figured was $700 worth of food in just 100 square feet (10 x 10 plot)—an impressive use of lawn space, indeed. If your laws don't allow lawn gardens—get them changed! Be careful of chemicals that were used in your garden space in the past. A small cold frame or green house can produce a lot of live food. As with humans and pets, plants will thrive with attention, water, love, and conversation.

Forest gardening incorporates fruiting trees and bushes into the plan to efficiently utilize the ground space and sunshine. It is interesting, that growing all or most of one's own food supply also supplies just the right amount of exercise with an invigorating dose of fresh air and sunshine to stay healthy. Isn't nature marvelous?

As with humans and pets, plants will thrive with attention, water, love, and conversation.

Pots of tomatoes, and peppers (they need to be pollinated by an insect), can be put on door steps and balconies. Join or plan a neighborhood garden which turns vacant lots into organic gardens. Organic regulations are a positive step toward world health, but anyone can grow some of their own organic food. Get acquainted with a local organic farmer and support them.

Learn to compost kitchen scraps, lawn and garden clippings, and weeds (anything that was once a plant). A basic recipe is to alternate a dry layer (leaves, for example), then a wet or green layer (like weeds or pits and peels from the kitchen), then a "bacteria" layer like manure or soil, and repeat layering it lasagna-style. It can be a pile in the yard or a fancy worm composter in the garage. There is no odor if it is watered and aerated regularly. Composting toilets are available to compost humanure, which can be used on trees and flowers.

INDOOR GARDENING

Growing sprouts and shoots (we call 'greenies') indoors drastically stretches food dollars. Seeds are inexpensive and glass jars can be found for free.

Soak the seeds in pure water; in general, the larger the seed, the more that is used for a quart of sprouts, and the longer the soak time. For a quart of alfalfa sprouts (tiny seeds) use two tablespoons of seeds and soak six hours. For mung beans, use a half-cup of seeds and soak for 12 hours. Stir and pour off the 'floaters' (they won't sprout). Then fasten a piece of mesh nylon fabric on the top with a rubber band (or get a sprouting lid made for this purpose) and leave resting at an angle in a dish drainer, allowing air to reach the seeds. Rinse with pure water twice a day and start enjoying when they sprout. Put them in the refrigerator to slow the growth.

Lentils, clover or alfalfa, and mung beans are the easiest to sprout. Dry seeds keep a long time in jars (get glass gallons at pubs), take up little space (cool and dry), and is a good way to prepare for times of food scarcity (no need to refrigerate dry seeds).

Shoots or micro greens are young plants grown in a nursery tray containing about an inch of organic potting soil which are cut when they are about four to five inches tall. They are grown from seeds with hulls still on them and are a great addition to smoothies, soups, casseroles, and salads when the cold winds blow. Favorites include sunflower (sunnies), buckwheat (buckies), and field peas. The trays, found at any garden supply store, must have drain holes and, of course, a pan for catching the drained water (you can probably find them recycled). Sow the seeds thickly over the soil and cover with a little more soil, place in a sunny place, and keep the soil slightly moist, and in about 10 days there will be fresh greens.

WHAT THE LIVE VEGAN DIET IS NOT

Diet, of course, is not a panacea. It will not clear the body's energy if it is done against the will, with grumbling, resistance, and cheating—

although that is a learning experience, too. Attitude still trumps diet. If attitude toward food is improved, live food will enhance attitude.

Attitude still trumps diet.

The living vegan diet is not alternative medicine. It is a lifestyle that works magic, not a short term 'treatment' or temporary fix. Some call this 'prevention.' If treated like a therapy, symptoms will return when the SAD is resumed. Any attempt to change your diet to CLOVER will bring benefits, even buying one item organic or switching to whole grain. Food and thoughts affect how you feel in five minutes, five days, *and* five years. The choice of lifestyle must be followed for life if the lightness of body and clearness of mind are to be maintained. Your subconscious mind hears and believes every word and action and stores the information according to your directions.

Any attempt to change your diet to CLOVER will bring benefits, even buying one item organic or switching to whole grain.

Diet is not the whole key to anything sublime. Lots of people have reached high levels of consciousness on cooked meat, white flour, and sugar. One cannot become spiritually enlightened simply by manipulating the diet, for there must be engagement in devotional practices, deeds of compassion, and a sincere, sustained desire to learn your truth. Nevertheless, it does happen that when a person who has been on a degenerative diet adapts to a healthful one, she discovers that her entire functional mind is changed. All the mechanisms that feed the brain and transfer nerve energy are purified, intensified, and rejuvenated. When the secret of happiness is discovered, a way of life is taken up that allows the body-mind to be surrendered into the universal river of life. No, diet is not a panacea, nor does it create instant higher consciousness. It just makes the path easier. That is the key—it makes everything easier!

It just makes the path easier. That is the key—it makes everything easier!

TRANSITION TO LIVE FOOD

In general, when people feel the urgent need to transition quickly they have probably been given a serious diagnosis. These people can start with a fast or a modified fast such as blended green drinks, temporary juicing, or other raw liquid diet. Fasting is a good way to speed the detoxification, but it is best to consult someone familiar with the practice. This type of transition is best done under the supervision of an experienced teacher.

Most people choose a gradual change when there are no acute conditions. Once the decision is made and actions are taken to begin the journey, assistance can be obtained from other raw foodies, live food centers, books, raw restaurants, websites, raw food gatherings, and one's own body signals. Many start by eliminating one food at a time such as meat, alcohol, sugar, white flour, soda pop, or fried foods. Or they start buying their usual foods but in organic form (they are available). Some start each day raw and stay that way as long as they can. Eating is a social event in this culture and a raw foodist will need to plan ahead.

Eating is a social event in this culture and a raw foodist will need to plan ahead.

Food preparation will take more time *in the beginning* because it is unfamiliar. (Later it is much faster than cooking.) Most raw cookbooks give suggestions about how to start your diet transition. Mix up a big batch of something like a pate or crackers when there is extra time and freeze it. As with playing the piano, it gets easier the longer you do it!

Each in-season food can be preserved for later and, you can take advantage of specials (dry some mushrooms when they are fresh and cheap). In the fall, cabbage forms beautiful heads, which can be made into sauerkraut for the winter. Greens and many other fruit and vegetables can be dehydrated when they are in abundance for winter smoothies, soups, and casseroles.

Keep prewashed food handy for snack attacks. Dried fruit may not be at the base of the food pyramid, but it is a darn sight better than a candy bar (dry dates are very much like caramel with fiber). It is also helpful to trade food preparation with another raw foodie for a special treat or on a regular basis—one making raw cookies and the other raw crackers for example, and dividing the goodies between you.

THE RAW PATH

As the body gets cleaner and regains its vitality, food preferences will automatically change, and what sounded and tasted delicious one week will taste bitter or seem repulsive the next, and vice versa. The quantity of food will probably decrease as the body becomes healthier (it might temporarily increase first). Food preparation and planning takes less and less time as favorite recipes are adapted.

> When experimenting with a new recipe, always write down exactly what you put in so you can replicate. After you eat it note suggestions for what to do next time to improve it (less salt etc.) Also jot down how much of it you ate for future reference.

Interests change as well, and raw cookbooks and websites suddenly become fascinating reading. At first it may seem like food is more expensive, since things like really raw cashews need to be special ordered. But as one's tastes are refined, the high fat and high protein foods (seeds and nuts) become less palatable and less expensive foods (romaine and carrots) become most appetizing.

But as one's tastes are refined, the high fat and high protein foods (seeds and nuts) become less palatable and less expensive foods (romaine and carrots) become most appetizing.

Besides supreme health, glowing skin, good figure, shiny hair, comfortable joints, clear peaceful thoughts, and a new awareness of SELF as a spark of the divine, there are other more mundane benefits on the raw path. Meals are simpler, as is clean up after a meal. Healthy people have more energy for relationships, career, and projects. Your new energy seeps out to assist others in the family, the community, and the world. Service to humanity is the main point of living, and raw energy lights a spark within that spreads to ignite those around you.

The aspirant learns the difference between the grip of cooked food addictions and real wholesome hunger. The subtle pleasure of anticipation, such as the aroma of onion or red pepper being chopped and lemons being squeezed fills the air (instead of the smell of scorching pancakes).

Service to humanity is the main point of living, and raw energy lights a spark within that spreads to ignite those around you.

COST

Even though cost and availability are often cited as excuses to eat junk, Ann Wigmore estimated that the raw food diet actually decreased food expenses as much as 80%. This is because a raw foodist eats less and unprocessed food is cheaper in the long run. A pound of carrots is considerably cheaper than a half pound of potato chips, for example. A day's supply of nuts is cheaper than a carnivore's purchase of hamburger.

Once a diet decision is made, ordering in bulk saves money. Buy a case of fresh fruit and split it with a friend, dry or freeze it—ripe bananas to make ice cream, for example. Farmer's markets, volunteering at organic farms, and joining a CSA (community supported agriculture) where the consumer pays in the early part of the year for a share of each week's harvest can be fun ways to get really healthy food cheaper. Buying clubs and coops exist all over the country and save money on healthier foods. Always comparison shop and keep track.

Even though cost and availability are often cited as excuses to eat junk, Ann Wigmore estimated that the raw food diet actually decreased food expenses as much as 80%.

TIME

A simple CLOVER diet takes far less time to prepare. Green smoothies and salads are easier than microwaving a pizza. Shopping is easier and quicker as well—you only have to visit the produce section. Shred or chop one vegetable a day and keep in a bowl in the refrigerator covered with a clean cloth. Clean up is quicker, too. When you have seasonal excess from the garden or farmer's market, it is much quicker to dehydrate, ferment, and just freeze as compared to canning and blanching. I have been there, too.

WHEN FEELING ILL

While toxins are being ushered out of the body by the living fiber in the colon, mucous in the throat, eruptions through the skin, breath from the lungs, and water through the kidneys, there might be temporary times of lower energy, even lethargy. Sometimes there are flu-like symptoms, aches in various parts of the body. Bowels may move in a new way or more often. These are detoxification (withdrawal) symptoms and are not the same for each person, since diet history, as well as mental attitude, are different for each person.

These are detoxification (withdrawal) symptoms and are not the same for each person, since diet history, as well as mental attitude, are different for each person.

Of course, if symptoms are acute or if your inner guides direct it, see a medical provider. Remember that pills are toxic; and while they perhaps might help relieve symptoms for a while, they will ultimately slow the detoxification process. Another plan might be to slowly drink a quart of water (over an hour) and see if that helps. Water is amazingly healing. Sometimes the body needs rest from food and physical and mental activity. This is the time to sleep, keeping a note pad, pen, and light by the bed to record what great intuitive wisdom comes during the 'twilight time' before, after, and in between sleeps. Be extra careful when getting out of bed, as you might be dizzy or weak. If this happens, arrange a friend to be with you, eat a little more or temporarily add foods you are planning to eliminate, like plain cooked grain or steamed vegetables (not a donut!).

The point is that *feeling* ill doesn't necessarily mean you *are* ill. It is more likely the body is demonstrating its vitality and willingness to clear itself. The irony is that the more toxins in the diet, the more the person is able to tolerate them. But the more toxins that are taken in, the more they accumulate in the tissues, thus increasing the threat of long-term illness. Fear of illness is pervasive in this society—a popular topic of conversation but we don't need to join the dialog. According to the law of attraction, what is focused upon will come in greater profusion, so focus on wellness and healing. Remember to keep drinking water.

Moving the body will assist it to remove toxins easier. So even when it might be tempting to sleep all day, a gentle walk around the block will assist the circulation, which in turn removes toxins. It is also cleansing to be outside in the sun and fresh air. Looking at any sort of nature is grounding and uplifting. Take a beginning yoga class, turn on music and gently dance alone, or get some house cleaning done while your body cleans. Remember to drink water.

Moving the body will assist it to remove toxins easier.

MENTAL/EMOTIONAL PURIFICATION

Emotional changes are also signs of detoxification—like a deep longing, anger, sadness, or weepiness. This is also part of the withdrawal and purification process. Paying attention to these symptoms can lead to resolution of long buried hurts and resentments. Like an alcoholic who begins to stay sober, the issues that were being avoided by the ingestion of mind-dulling substances (i.e. cooked food) will still be there waiting when the 'buzz' goes away. The same suggestions given for physical withdrawal symptoms will work for the emotional healing crises. It is good time to sleep or meditate, be in nature, exercise. Ponder whatever comes up. Record your insights and what you think they mean—whether they are about past memories or 'resolutions' for the future. It is a transition time of cleansing and important changes.

Emotions are the result of thoughts. Thoughts are affected by the vibration of food and the level of physical toxicity. So changing to a

Emotions are the result of thoughts.

raw diet may allow negative emotions to surface where they can be analyzed and cleared. Raw food enhances the ability to think, discern, and be in the moment, like a child. Now that you are a powerful adult, you can become very honest when looking in the mirror—notice the beauty instead of only the pimples. The raw journey helps change the way you look at the world and at yourSELF.

STRUGGLES WITH ADDICTION AND WITHDRAWAL

Addiction is the continued use of a substance or practice of a behavior despite adverse consequences. Addicts seem to have impaired control over their addictions, which typically have short-term rewards and long-term costs. They are preoccupied with the substance or behavior despite their damaging consequences, and often exhibit denial concerning their addiction. Physiological dependence occurs when the body adjusts to the substance by incorporating it into normal functioning, creating both tolerance and withdrawal symptoms if it is discontinued.[156]

The seduction of flesh and other cooked food can be compared or equated with other addictions—a craving for an effect that suppresses thoughts or emotions. Also, people actually seem to miss the feeling of being overfull and slightly ill after eating, depressed and achy in the morning, and a vague fatigue and mental fog most of the time. They sometimes deliberately sabotage themselves by eating sugary, GMO treats despite the symptoms they know will come. Or they deny the painful knee has anything to do with the six cookies eaten the day before. Food is another way to 'self-medicate' yourself.

Food is another way to 'self-medicate' yourself.

A human baby, given an apple and a small live rabbit will likely eat the apple and play with the rabbit—not the other way around, like a dog might. Babies are then conditioned at a young age to eat

156 "Addiction," from Wikipedia, February 8, 2013.

cooked food, animal products, and sugar. Modern children are often given very limited food choices, which leads to believing that sugar, cooked flesh, and white flour is food. It is hard to tell when addiction begins.

One of the major struggles for those aspiring to adopt a raw food diet is that, along with the general population, medical and nutrition experts are also addicted to cooked food and *don't realize it*. 'Comfort food' is attached to mother-love and smells from childhood, so the roots in all of us are deep. It is a human urge to want to fit in with the group. There is a price to pay for going against the crowd, your doctor, your family, television, and your childhood habits. It is hard to believe it is an addiction if everyone does it.

Sometimes people say they need meat to be 'grounded,' but this too is addiction to the sleepy feeling that comes after eating it—similar to the after-effects of using recreational drugs. What is mistaken for protein insufficiency is usually a lack of natural sugar, good fat, or simply dehydration. Amino acids are rarely in short supply. The body does not naturally cry for transfats, caffeine, alcohol, preservatives, drugs, and sugar.

The body does not naturally cry for transfats, caffeine, alcohol, preservatives, drugs, and sugar.

Temptation is likely when energy is blocked in some area of the body. That part will feel hollow with a subtle ache, making the person long for an 'unknown something.' Accustomed to avoiding discomfort, people reach for food to fill the hole; but indulging in the toxic substance results in building even more blocks in both body and mind. The heart (inner wisdom) says live food is better, but the addiction is powerful.

Most find the hardest part of the raw vegan diet is avoiding familiar comfort foods that everyone else is eating. In order to enjoy a social gathering where others will be eating the SAD, carry something fresh and really delicious along. It is better to be a little hungry than sick, but keep nuts and dried fruit nearby. If someone asks about it, you can say you are on a 'special diet' (more socially accepted than "I want to be healthy"). Or there might be a person who really wants to learn and will keep asking questions. Answer the questions but don't preach.

Being too rigid in the transition, before the will is strong, can lead to a breakdown in resolve when an emotional event occurs or the desire is overwhelming. Different people crave different things. Acknowledge the craving and plan ahead regarding what you will allow yourself to eat. It is better to eat something if you really desire it than to feel deprived; but find an organic version before indulging. One idea is to 'reward' yourself with something organic and cooked. For example, "if I stay raw for three days I can have (organic whole grain) pasta on Saturday." If cooked food is eaten, it might lower resistance, as with the alcoholic. But it also produces a return of subtle symptoms whose absence had gone unnoticed (like intestinal gas or underarm odor). What used to hurt begins to hurt again, and the mind plays games.

It usually takes three days for the effects of cooked or non-organic food to resolve. Observe how the body reacts and allow it to recover. One donut or a few chemical sprayed strawberries, eaten by a person that is pretty well cleared, for example, might give her quite severe flu symptoms for three days to a week.

The Standard American Diet acts as its own natural aversion therapy—the after-effects impress upon the subconscious mind not to do that again.

'Aversion therapy' is where something negative or uncomfortable is paired with an activity for the purpose of discontinuing it—an electric shock when lighting a cigarette, for example. There are drugs that make a person violently ill if alcohol is ingested. The Standard American Diet acts as its own natural aversion therapy—the after-effects impress upon the subconscious mind not to do *that* again.

WILLPOWER

It is well understood and accepted that people control their own actions; but thoughts are *also* controllable (despite attempts by the media to direct your thoughts, emotions, and desires). Although we often abdicate our personal responsibility over our thoughts, when we think the same thought over and over it becomes a habit, wearing a neuropathway 'groove' in the brain—it becomes 'our story.' Each of us must mentally *decide* which habits to keep. Substituting a different thought will push the 'delete' button for the old one, because it is possible to think only one thought at a time. Habits *are* changeable—with time and willpower.

The best way to divert attention from food obsessions or withdrawal symptoms of detoxification is by distraction. At a relaxed time make a mental list of enjoyable activities that could be employed at a time of 'weakness.' Walk in nature; watch a video on raw food preparation. Read a spiritually inspiring book. Find something that is indulgent, like a swim, to divert attention. Satisfy hunger by eating something healthy and delicious and don't go grocery shopping! Get involved in an uplifting movie, visit a positive friend, or take up a hobby, like knitting, where your hands are kept busy. Avoid dwelling on what is undesired and focus attention instead on benefits being realized. Most important is to plan ahead what you *will* eat.

Another plan to avoid eating cooked food is to not have any available. If it must be had, it will take some effort to get it. Keep salad and smoothie ingredients on hand. Fresh fruit, nuts, dehydrated snacks, and cut up vegetables are easy to keep handy. Treat yourself to raw organic things you love.

Take the positive approach—think ahead so that a meal plan is always in mind and there is a delicious vision to anticipate. This is called 'prepaving' and it tells your subconscious mind what you expect to happen. Think of what the day's menu will be and take steps to prepare it. For example, if a pate is desired for nori rolls at supper, put the nuts or seeds to soak in the morning. Freeze bananas for ice cream or shakes. This is now something to look forward to all day. Whenever there is extra time, make cookies, crackers, granola and other snack foods, so that there is always something special, delicious, and healthy available. As with other diets, plan your menu before shopping. And then adapt it at the store according to what is available. At first, carrying a recipe book to the market might be a good idea.

When a physical act is carried out, a powerful message is sent to the impressionable inner child. Shredding carrots sends the message to the body and mind that a lunch will be a delicious salad. An act is a very loud thought.

An act is a very loud thought.

In the book *Willpower,* the authors discuss the importance of exercising your will, but not over-doing it.[157] They suggest choosing which decisions are most important and working on those first. Like a muscle, the will gets stronger with use, but gets fatigued if forced to operate beyond its strength for too long. That is when lapses occur. The book discusses the famous study where four-year-olds were offered an extra marshmallow if they did not eat the first one when left alone for a time. The ones that resisted and got the reward did so by distracting themselves. Later, these strong-willed resisters did better in school, earned higher salaries, and were less prone to weight gain and problems with drug abuse. In other words a strong will leads to success in other areas of life, not just marshmallow resisting.

If there is a lapse resulting in 'eaters regret,' take responsibility.

If there is a lapse resulting in 'eaters regret,' take responsibility. Begin to drink extra water until the tissues clear. Then make a new plan for the next time. As with smoking cessation, the temptations get fewer and weaker as time goes on.

157 Roy F. Baumeister & John Tierney, *Willpower,* (New York, NY: Penguin Press, 2011).

Always carry water, preferably in a glass container, and when tempted, drink a quart over an hour or so. Often thirst feels like hunger, so this will help resist the bad food. Also drink a quart of water in the morning before eating any food to hydrate the cells and clear the urinary and intestinal tracts. A goal for daily water consumption for an adult is a gallon a day.

Like trying to overcome any addiction, most people need support of some type. Maybe someday there will be cooked-food anonymous groups. Victoria Boutenko recommends at least having a raw-food buddy to call when temptation hits. Find a friend with similar goals and prepare food together. Agree to be willing to discuss a temptation by phone with the raw-buddy and be ready to make a suggestion for her. She can also lend a listening ear when emotional cleansing prompts a need to vent. We can help strengthen each other's willpower.

TRAVELING RAW

Traveling on any diet takes some preparation, even if it is just a toothbrush in your purse. Air travel has become more difficult for raw foodies but is still manageable. Some are concerned about the screening irradiation at airports, which could be a reason to drive or find another mode of transportation. If you have to fly, it is doable, even with new airline rules. Dried food in plastic bags in a carry-on can be hand searched (nuts, fruit, raw crackers, and cookies for example). Insulated shoulder bags can be a personal item with fresh fruit and vegetables. Water filter bottles are allowed empty through check points, and can be filled before boarding. Upon arrival head for a food co-op or health food store with the cloth shopping bags you brought along.

Even long distances can be challenging, but definitely possible. In 2006 we traveled to Seattle and Okinawa for 10 days. The airlines took our honey, but we stayed raw, purchasing only fresh fruit and salad greens. Our food took as many bags as our clothes but how many outfits do you need when your body looks great, your hair is shiny, your eyes are glowing, and you are full of energy and enthusiasm?

Fresh produce is bulky and needs refrigeration, but there is no problem stashing a cooler in a car. There is a relatively inexpensive cooler that plugs into the car lighter, or with an adaptor, into a motel room outlet. Make jars of green smoothies. Keep narrow mouth jars of water and wide mouth jars of crackers near the driver. Always bless any food before eating.

Others have traveled taking *all* their foods in dehydrated form, needing only water at the destination, which can be filtered for further purity. Dried greens and dried fruit can be made into a tasty smoothie if there is a blender available. Dried veggies and herbs can be easily mixed with water and warmed for a short time to make a delicious soup. Crackers, cookies, trail mix, marinated dried veggies for snacks all keep without refrigeration for several weeks. It takes time to prepare to leave but once on the road, all food issues are covered and the time can be spent meeting, loving, and watching new people and places.

EATING OUT

Eating out usually means eating nonorganic food, but the positive social and psychological benefits might outweigh this drawback. Seek a restaurant with a nice salad bar, preferably with deep green leafy lettuce, and build from the other raw things found there. Many restaurants will have a Caesar salad on the menu that can be ordered without animal products. Ask for no meat, dairy, or croutons. They can add whatever they have raw in the kitchen. We have enjoyed many happy meals without attracting too much attention by carrying a 3 x 5 card for the wait-person which says:

> I am a raw (not ever heated) vegetarian.
>
> Please bring me a salad of deep green lettuce or spinach and any of the following: tomato, cucumber, onion, avocado, broccoli, cauliflower, mushrooms, carrot, peppers, asparagus, cabbage, kale, radishes, fresh or dry fruit.
>
> No: canned food, croutons, chips, cooked beans, corn, dairy, or meat.

We have never been disappointed with the dish we are served using this card. It is not usually organic—bless it before eating. It is easy to carry a small pouch of nuts or dried fruit in pocket or purse and discreetly add them to the salad or nibble on after the salad is eaten while others are eating dessert.

If the 'mean hunger' grabs you while grocery shopping, it helps to carry a small bottle of raw dressing (or settle for a bottle of organic). Pick up a plastic container of prewashed salad greens, cherry tomatoes, avocado, baby carrots, or cucumber, whatever there is in the organic section. Rush through the check-out counter. Then circle around to the deli area, grab a plastic fork and knife. Open the salad container, cut up the avocado and cucumber with the knife, pour on a little dressing, and feast your mouth on healthy food, feeling grateful to the vegetable divas! Sometimes we even plan to 'dine' out at the super market.

MODERN RAW FOOD MOVEMENT—WHERE TO FIND SUPPORT

There are literally hundreds of restaurants and online sites offering a plethora of raw ingredients, ready-made products, and advice. See if there is a raw food group nearby or join a group website. There are hundreds of raw recipe books. Some focus on fancy recipes made with lots of nuts and oils and baby coconut, but they can be modified as needs and tastes change. Librarians might not be able to help you fix raw food, but they sure can find books on it.

Join or (after confidence has grown in 'uncooking' skills) start a raw food potluck. It could be in a home or another space like a church. Invite a speaker to teach raw food preparation or another healthy topic.

SOME PITFALLS TO AVOID

Some people who adopt a live vegan diet become overly zealous. Besides getting too picky with food, they also anxiously watch body functions. They focus on negative symptoms, as if they were terminally ill instead of becoming more and more vibrant. They get a little crazy if they happen to eat something off the approved menu or if they miss a day of sunbathing. They examine their skin and stools for evidence of illness or a problem. They have missed the lesson on positive thoughts and the Law of Attraction.

Sometimes raw foodists also turn off SAD people by trying to convert them. They are as annoying as religious know-it-alls who shame others with a holier-than-thou attitude. The diet is obvious and if someone is interested, they will ask. Diet can turn into a glamour or maya (an emotional illusion), misleading a person to believe it will bring security or survival. This can either blind a person to her spiritual path or perhaps serve as another learning opportunity. Eating can become a rigidly-followed 'religion' or a joyful spiritual path.

Judging others might also become an issue. It is hard to watch a loved one unknowingly 'dig their own grave with their forks' when you know that most common chronic illnesses improve on CLOVER. Diabetes, heart diseases, and cancer, commonly linked with decreased life span have been the subject of testimonials of reversal on CLOVER. Aside from asking if they are interested, serving as a good role model, and professing love for them; there is nothing more to do. They cannot know what they do not know. Silently bless them and visualize abundant health and light upon their path, which is a powerful healing.

They cannot know what they do not know.

THE ESSENCE OF THE PREMISE

Eating can either be an unconscious choice that pollutes your body or a beautiful dance with divine love. Instruction on the raw living food diet, however, is not the ultimate aim of this book. The point is not what *is* eaten but what is *not* eaten. The emphasis on diet is simply to *avoid* toxic food in the SAD; more than willpower, it requires 'won't power'. There are many kinds of tempting 'candy' that will take away the responsibility, pain, and fear, blocking the energy of body and mind. Learning to make fancy raw food won't help unless the ingestion of toxic substances is intentionally stopped. The small salad won't balance out the spaghetti and meatballs. The essence of the premise of this book is: the body can and will heal itself on all levels, if the energy blocks are removed and the toxins are discontinued. The best way to 'detox' is to quit 'toxing.'

The point is not what is eaten but what is not eaten.

The essence of the premise of this book is: the body can and will heal itself on all levels, if the energy blocks are removed and the toxins are discontinued.

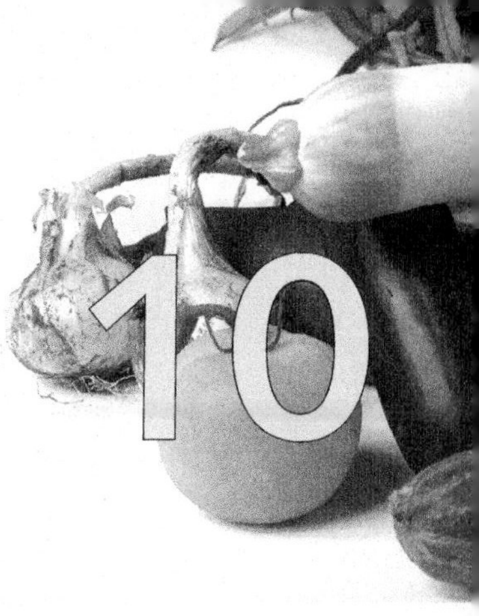

Additional New Age Preparations

Grace falls like rain on everyone but, also like rain, it can only be received by a vessel properly prepared to catch it.

— John White

This book emphasizes that purifying the physical body by discontinuing the intake of toxic substances enables easier access to spiritual inspiration. There are, however, other practices that can enhance wellness of body, mind, and spirit in preparation for enlightenment. The material world is part of the spiritual universe, so anything that purifies the body or resolves an emotional issue will raise spiritual consciousness.

It is difficult to dispel the centuries-old illusion that adding a substance (such as a vitamin or a chemical) into the body will cure disease. Since most illnesses are a result of toxicity, adding more toxins cannot possibly address the underlying cause. The only thing that will ultimately make a body healthy is to purify it. Attempts at purification can be complicated or sabotaged by toxic thoughts, but physical cleansing is a good place to start. The best way to detox is to stop toxing!

The best way to detox is to stop toxing!

STOP INTENTIONALLY "TOXING" THE BODY

Besides the SAD diet, the public gets conflicting messages about many toxic, addictive substances. Most people know alcohol affects all parts of the body, effectively destroying the brain and liver, yet experts continue to say a certain quantity is healthy. Illicit mind-altering substances, natural or manufactured, like marijuana and methamphetamine are considered toxic, but many people think prescription drugs are safer. Sugar (and especially its substitutes) and caffeine beverages are among the most poisonous of what is considered 'food,' yet people are persuaded to buy them. How can there be a 'safe dose' of a deadly toxin?

As mentioned earlier in this book, medically prescribed treatments are the highest cause of death in the United States. This is not referring to overdoses and mistakes, but rather to drugs and other treatments taken intentionally and exactly as prescribed. All drugs *are* toxic, despite belief to the contrary. In a healthy body with clean energy circuits, drugs are not only unnecessary but can be mortally poisonous. Headaches and depression are not caused by a drug deficiency.

Some household products are more toxic than others, of course, but the Earth and our grandchildren will appreciate each conscious decision to choose less toxic brands. Bug sprays, cleaning supplies, body soaps and lotions, deodorizers for air and armpits, make-up, and lawn and garden chemicals are but a few products made by corporations who do not have the health of the consumer in mind. Clothing made of petroleum plastic interferes with the flow of body energy, as do chemicals used in conventionally grown natural fibers like cotton. If absolutely necessary to dry clean something, then the garment should hang outside for at least a day or two, allowing the toxins to dissipate. Plastic food containers are another source of contamination—glass should be substituted whenever possible.

Headaches and depression are not caused by a drug deficiency.

Showering in hot chlorinated water is especially toxic, because the heat disperses chlorine and other volatile toxins into its gaseous form. They absorb easily through warm naked skin, with pores wide open. The lungs breathe in and absorb chlorine-laden steam. Skin and lungs are both so good at absorbing medication administered this way. Again, how can there be a 'safe dose' of a deadly toxin?

Electromagnetic fields include everything from radio waves, ordinary light, and the waves from every electrical and electronic device, such as microwave ovens and cell phones. There is debate about how much and which ones are harmful. Follow nature's lead and get into nature as much as possible and keep electrical and electronic devices away from your body.

Again, how can there be a 'safe dose' of a deadly toxin?

LIFE DETOXIFIED

♥ Exercise

It is well known that exercise is good for health. It moves the muscles, joints, and other tissue, loosening and removing impurities stored there. Walking, jogging, or other 'jostling,' like on a trampoline, also moves the fluids in the body to help clear toxins from tissues. Dead foreign substances must be released from the cells and moved into blood and lymph vessels for transportation. They are then removed through the skin, colon, lymph nodes, lungs, kidneys, and other less obvious portals. *So move it!*

Walking, jogging, or other 'jostling,' like on a trampoline, also moves the fluids in the body to help clear toxins from tissues.

♥ Skin Brushing

Brushing the skin with a moderately stiff brush before bathing assists the skin to eliminate toxins, especially before sweating in a hot tub or sauna. Each stroke should be made toward the heart, giving loving attention and gratitude to each part. Begin with the face and brush downward to the neck and chest. Use a long-handled brush to stroke the back. Then begin at the hands, brushing upward to the armpit and then down the body, getting well into the underarm area to awaken the lymph channels. Breasts love to be brushed. The belly and back below the waist should be brushed upward. Then start on the bottoms of the feet, the tops of the feet and up the legs toward the heart. Feel the tingle of 'petting' yourself. No wonder pets love to be brushed!

♥ Scalp Massage

Massage the scalp and then brush both hair and scalp. It stimulates circulation to the follicles which will make hair thicker and healthier. It distributes the scalp oils to the drier ends of the hair. It is good to bend over and lower the head below heart level if possible, which brings blood to your brain, too. Headaches *might* be caused by a lack of brushing.

♥ Showering

Showering before bed (with a water filter and using safe biodegradable soap) not only keeps the bed clothes clean, reducing the need to use water, electricity, and soap to wash them; but it also energetically removes the day's negative energy from the body, as well. It is a good way to gently close contact with the physical world and prepare for spiritual learning on the inner planes. A short shower works as well as a long one and catch the first cold water in a pail to water plants. Be conscious of water usage and reuse the shower water (as well as water from the washer and sink) however you can with a gray water recycling plan to get it to plants that need it.

♥ Pure Air

Air pollution can be a major contributor to the toxic load in your body. Move to cleaner air, if possible, but at least investigate air purifiers for the home, especially in the bedroom. Trees and plants clean the air, so go for long walks in parks and get out to cleaner air as often as possible. Check out the air filtering system at work and improve it however possible Trees and plants in the home will please both lungs and senses. They are inexpensive and are nature's filters—a good place to use your 'graywater.'

♥ Moisturizing

Pure raw foodists have no body odor at all, so deodorant is totally unnecessary. Their feces don't stink, either. They rarely have very dry skin, but if needed, good natural moisturizers are cacao butter and olive and coconut oil, which can be blended with essential oils and beeswax. Lips are best left alone to toughen, which takes a week or so of cold weather.

♥ Chewing

The enjoyable exercise of chewing not only breaks up the food into tiny particles for better digestion, it also releases life-force and natural enzymes found in the cells of living food and infuses them with moisture and salivary enzymes. A lot of digestion takes place in the mouth. Chewing also allows time for vital life energy to be absorbed through the tissues of the mouth into the energy system of the body. Teeth are *meant* to chew on substantial, fibrous substances, stimulating the roots of the teeth, in much the same way lifting weights and walking stress the bones which keep them healthy. Chewing gum is good, too. Lying on the couch, eating soft, cooked food produces weak teeth as well as soft bones. Chew each mouthful 30 times—straight up and down, not with a grinding motion. Savor the flavor.

Chew each mouthful 30 times—straight up and down, not with a grinding motion.

♥ Teeth Care

Flossing after chewing any food not only removes debris but sends loving *attention* to them. A simple tooth powder can be made from non-aluminum baking soda and bentonite clay powder. Floss after meals, 'swish' with peroxide, and brush every day for at least three minutes before bed. Metaphysically, teeth are about decisions—be decisive and pay attention to messages coming from the teeth if they hurt, or are loose—ask them what they need.

♥ Drinking Water

Drink lots of pure water—approximately a gallon a day is about right for an average adult. Investigate to find the most efficient water filter; expensive is not necessarily the best. Start by drinking three or four cups upon awakening before eating anything, to get the tissues hydrated for the day. It helps wash out the toxins ingested the day before. Whenever feeling achy or sluggish, it is probably time for another cup or three. It requires being aware of the precious body and its signals. Sometimes it feels like hunger when it is really thirst.

Drink lots of pure water—approximately a gallon a day is about right for an average adult.

♥ Colon Care

Especially in the early phases of detoxification, it is a good idea to cleanse the lower colon with enemas or even colonics, which are enemas that go higher and are administered by trained colon therapists. Colonics remove very old accumulated debris which can become even more toxic if not removed. This helps the colon to resume the natural habits that babies are born with, before cooked and refined food. Simple water enemas can be self-administered, following instructions using equipment found at any pharmacy. The raw high-fiber diet with its living intelligence will speed the evacuation of the colon as well and eventually make enemas unnecessary.

♥ Stretching

Yoga is a form of stretching that can involve meditation, but any stretching is good. It is easy to see how yoga, at any level, helps the body stay flexible and get rid of waste in the tissues. What a pleasant experience to hear a whispered "thank you" from the stretched part. Watch a dog or cat after a nap and imitate them. Doing yoga on a regular basis shows up in your posture, health, and whole countenance.

♥ Professional Massage

Yoga is a form of stretching that can involve meditation, but any stretching is good.

A soothing or deep massage, too, will assist the tissues to release their toxins by moving fluid through the flesh. A good masseuse will always push the tissue in the direction of the blood returning toward the heart. This makes sure the tiny valves located in the vessels will not be stressed and fluid from around the cells can be removed and taken by the blood and lymph systems to be purified in the kidneys, lymph nodes, etc. Drink lots of water after a massage.

♥ Productive Repetition

Find a repetitive hobby like knitting or playing an instrument and do it regularly which will both satisfy the need to create and put the mind in a peaceful state. Playing computer games is repetitive but results in no warm winter hat to wear or give away.

♥ Sleep

During the mysterious process known as sleep, much more is being done than simply resting the body. It is thought to be a time of reconnection with the real truth of existence. Most people find that after just a few weeks on the raw vegan diet, sleep becomes much deeper and more beneficial. Sometimes people find they actually need less sleep as they become physically and emotionally cleared. But during periods of emotional cleansing, more sleep might be required. Keep a journal nearby to catch the elusive wisps of wisdom before they flutter away.

♥ Environmental Awareness

Use organic, environmentally safe biodegradable laundry, dish, and body soaps, toilet paper and other paper goods. Minimize use of plastic by storing food in glass jars and bowls using a plate for a lid. Ask your local bar to save glass jars and offer to pay. A glass canning jar makes a very acceptable drinking glass of sufficient volume. Pay attention to labels at the store before buying anything, food or household products.

SUNLIGHT

Sunlight is good for skin and energy, but has been discouraged by fear-based science. Expensive toxic sunscreens are absorbed through the skin and should be avoided. It is never good, of course, to burn the skin by any means, but if one begins with very short periods of sun exposure and increases until burning is no longer a worry, the sun is a direct way to energize the cells of the body. The sun benefits the body by the manufacture of vitamin D (necessary for healthy bones, etc.), boosts the mood (even for those without a diagnosis), and stimulates normal hormone production. There are many studies linking various types of cancer with a lack of sunshine. Sunbathing nude is best, but according to existing societal norms, a bikini is usually needed. We are solar-powered beings!

We are solar-powered beings!

According to Gabriel Cousens, "The proper microelectrical potential gives cells the power to rid themselves of toxins and maintain the selective capacity to bring in the appropriate nutrients and oxygen supplies."[158] He goes on to explain that a drop in the electrical potential is the first step in disease, putting people in a state of subclinical 'dis-ease.' He believes a live food diet raises the microelectrical potential of the cells. Cousens also writes, "Sunlight is the nutrient of life. The sun is an outer manifestation of our inner light." He says we need about 30 minutes of sun a day, which is absorbed through the eyes and possibly directly through the capillaries at the surface of the skin. He cautions that we should use intelligent moderation when exposing our bodies to the sun's rays.

Pioneer in the use of light and color therapy Jacob Liberman writes, "Light is the basic component from which all life originates, develops, heals, and evolves. The human body is truly a living photocell that is energized by the sun's light, the nutrient of human kind."[159] He says anything that can be accomplished outdoors should not be done indoors. Liberman also found a direct correlation between decreased exposure to sunlight and higher incidence of irritability, fatigue, illness, insomnia, depression, alcoholism, and suicide.

OTHER ENERGY-ENHANCING HABITS

♥ Sweating

Sun bathing can lead to sweating, which is also greatly beneficial in detoxifying the body and cleansing the skin. Other means of inducing a good healthy sweat are sauna, hot tub, hot bathing, and just plain old-fashioned hard *work*. The sweat should be rinsed off before the toxins reabsorb. Be sure to drink lots of pure water when sweating.

Be sure to drink lots of pure water when sweating.

158 Gabriel Cousens, M.D., *Conscious Eating,* (Berkeley, CA: North Atlantic Books, 2000), 571.

159 Jacob Liberman, O. D., Ph.D., *Light: Medicine of the Future,* (Santa Fe, NM: Bear & Company, 1991), 11.

♥ Walking

Take a walk. A walking meditation offers a variety of simultaneous benefits: exercise, deep breathing, looking at nature, a 'break' from life, and smiles from other people. Take extra deep breaths when exercising, especially outdoors. Swing your arms when walking; whistle or sing; talk to a squirrel or a tree. It is amazing how a smile can enhance both physical and mental energy. A smile changes the energy of the 'smiler' and lifts the mood of others. People feel much more confident when they stand, walk, and sit tall. Hips were not meant to always operate in a semi-flexed position. Raise your eyes above the horizon (you won't stumble). That simple act elevates mood and measurably increases the chi in and around the body. Instead of thinking about how dreadful life is, ask "How could things get any better?" Enjoy *life.*

♥ Eye Exercise

The muscles of the eye also need attention and exercise. Blink frequently and move your head around, relaxing the neck muscles. Practice looking at far and near objects at intervals. Go without corrective lenses as often as possible and avoid sunglasses unless it is an absolutely necessity. Eyes need light just as teeth need chewing and legs need walking. Eyes drink in beauty and it is safe to see the world as it really is.

♥ Facial Exercise

Exercise and stretch the muscles of the face to keep the underlying tone and avoid wrinkles. Expressions get etched and frozen so make faces in the mirror and pick one out and practice it often. How do you want to be remembered?

FENG SHUI

The quality of the energy in people and animals is affected by their physical environment. Feng Shui is the Chinese study of the flow of energy (or "chi") in a space and how it can be enhanced to create harmony and balance. Subtle reaction to placement, structure, decor, and arrangement of a home or business affects the energy of occupants. Changing even the smallest detail of decorative colors, furniture, or outdoor plantings can change the subtle energy of a place and affect our peace of mind, health, relationships, longevity, and even the flow of abundance. Feng Shui is concerned with architecture as well as interior and landscape design and can be used both in commercial and private settings. It assists humans to integrate with nature and achieve love and prosperity. Be aware of the clutter in your surroundings and extend your energy to clean it or make it more peaceful in some way. How does your office, bedroom, or dining room make you *feel* when you are there?

The quality of the energy in people and animals is affected by their physical environment.

MENTAL DISCIPLINE AND CHOICE

A life without discipline is chaotic. Discipline involves both right and left brained activities and is far more than schedules and rules. Have the courage to make a decision based upon the urgings of your heart; and then to *do* the right thing. Discipline can be flexible, but there must be guidelines for weighing each choice. Everything that shows up in your life is a result of a choice that was made earlier, either consciously or by default (which is also a choice).

Everything that shows up in your life is a result of a choice that was made earlier, either consciously or by default (which is also a choice).

All actions, even a person's appearance, are outward evidence of choices that have been made inwardly. Actions speak loudly to your own subconscious self and affect the vibration of others. Your home, car, clothing, health, and even your handwriting give clues to inner attitudes. Actions are loud thoughts so be careful choosing thoughts. If choices are always left to those in authority—your doctor, preacher, boss or spouse, politicians, TV ads, or the USDA—that is a choice you have made to live in bondage.

Choices extend to every thought and action allowed—which friends to choose, which house to buy, what food goes into your mouth, and the music and programs listened to on the radio or TV. Consider what activities happen before bed and choose something peaceful (not the tragic news of the day). Be aware of the 'energy' of games and particularly of movies that are chosen. Uplifting, truth-seeking movies are out there by the thousands. Use inner wisdom before clicking the play button. Pay attention to where your attention is being paid.

The mind can actually be disciplined to regularly allow the feeling of joy. Visualize the "Christmas morning" feeling from childhood—the thrill and giddiness of anticipation. Let joy invade and embrace you whenever it wants. There will be an instant change in things you experience, from getting the right card in a solitaire game to the behavior and attitude of other people. The trick is to remember to take a deep breath when shame, anger, or fear threatens to overtake you. When late for work, when a spouse is angry, when there is an accident of any sort—remember all creatures are divine. A lost job often leads to a much better one. A relationship could have ended for the spiritual growth of all concerned. Even the seeming tragedy of a death can be an awakening in the consciousness of those left behind (and perhaps the one who has passed, as well). Humans are all here to assist each other even when, in the physical world, it seems to be a 'mistake.' All is in divine order moving gently toward enlightenment of all.

Pay attention to where your attention is being paid.

There is evidence that by changing the chemistry of your body, thoughts, or habits your physiology will change—even personality, health conditions, and attitude can change. Detoxify your body and clean up your thinking and watch what happens. Caroline Myss, energy medicine pioneer, says, "Keep in mind at all times that your

All is in divine order moving gently toward enlightenment of all.

biography becomes your biology."[160] Candice Pert says, "Your body IS your subconscious mind."[161]

BREATH CONTROL

It is good to take a deep breath periodically, especially when feeling stressed. Breathe in through the nose, raising the chest, straightening the spine, and pushing down the diaphragm, which moves the abdomen out. Then expel every bit through the mouth, uttering a pleasant sound or "om," (if in an appropriate place). Pull in the abdominal muscles to drain the lungs. Deep breathing might at first cause lightheadedness, but this is good. Oxygen carries love.

It is known to health care providers that a rapid respiration rate is a sign of ill health, but it is also a sign of a frantic mind. Breathing through your nose is calming, warms the air, and slows the flow. There is a lot written about breathing exercises because controlling your breath is to some extent being in control of your state of mind. Yoga instructor Richard Hittleman writes, "In classical Yoga texts the breath is spoken of as 'the string which controls the kite'"—the kite being the mind, and as the string (breath) moves so moves the mind. If breathing is short and rapid, your mind will work nervously, agitatedly. If your breathing is erratic, your mind must be disturbed and anxious. But if your breathing is long, slow, smooth and even, the wildly racing mechanical nature of your mind will become tranquil and peaceful."[162]

Yogis believe breath is prana and is more easily absorbed through the nose. Yogic breathing is intended to revitalize the body, calm the emotions, and clear the mind. Its focus is not only on breathing deeply, filling the lungs using the diaphragm and abdominal muscles, but

---

160 Caroline Myss, Ph.D., *Anatomy of the Spirit,* (New York, NY: Three Rivers Press, 1996), 58.

161 Candace Pert, Ph.D., "Your Body Is Your Subconscious Mind," 2004, Audio tape from Sounds True.

162 Richard Hittleman, *Guide to Yoga Meditation,* (New York, NY: Bantam Books, 1969), 79.

also exhaling completely and allowing periods of holding the breath both on inhale and exhale phases of breath. Square breathing is one example and can be done in any position. It is also good while doing a walking meditation which combines three disciplines (exercise, meditation, and breath control).

> 'Square Breathing:' Breathe in deeply for a count of four, hold your breath for another four, breathe out completely for the next count of four and then hold for a final count of four. Repeat.

Natural living advocate Steven Capeder explains in depth why it is important not to over-breathe. He writes, "While oxygen is the energizer of the body, CO_2 is the source of life and serves to regenerate many functions in the body. One of the most important functions of CO_2, is its role in helping the body release oxygen into our tissues, and when we over-breathe, we actually reduce the amount of oxygen that gets into our bodies."[163]

MEDITATION

Meditation does for the mind what CLOVER (complete, local, organic, exquisite and raw) diet does for the body. It cleanses it. Meditation allows the negative thought-habits to be noticed and deleted like junk-files on a computer, because negative thoughts slow the functioning of your mind and body like computer trash slows a computer. It 'defrags' your mind. With SIN (Self-Inflicted Nonsense) thoughts eliminated, joy (our true natural state) can dominate. Meditation can be likened to intoxication without drugs or alcohol. As the body gets purer, it is easier to steer the power of mind toward positive desires, and your heart's real intentions will be naturally

Meditation does for the mind what CLOVER (complete, local, organic, exquisite and raw) diet does for the body.

163 Steven Capeder, *The Four Seasons Diet,* (Duvall, WA: Therapeutae Publishing, 2012), 320.

drawn to you, like a magnet. Meditation and CLOVER both change the energy of the body cells.

Meditation can be likened to intoxication without drugs or alcohol.

Meditating is a habit worth adopting faithfully. Find time to just *be*, in silence, with the mental chatter (called monkey-mind) turned off. Do it in the bathroom, while waiting in lines, during muted commercials, and so on. Meditation is making a conscious intent to *not* think with the rational left brain. When the reasoning mind is 'on,' it cannot hear the wisdom of the soul. Meditation is a simple thing, but not easy. It is an important key to effecting positive changes for the planet. Thoughts that come from the intuitive right mind can be profound, so keep a notepad and pencil nearby. Meditation is being in your 'right mind.'

Meditation is a simple thing, but not easy.

Meditation is very important in these times of changing energies. The only task during this time is to *understand*—to be an open chalice receiving the droplets of new wisdom in each moment. Group meditation is especially helpful in these times, because that helps peaceful energy spread more quickly. Silent reflection requires discipline and improved discipline will be helpful in all areas of life—diet, sex, and patience, for example.

Meditation is being in your 'right mind.'

SUGGESTIONS FOR MEDITATING

♥ Preparation

There are many techniques for getting in the 'meditation-mood,' such as posture and music. Regularity trains the subconscious mind. Before sleep is a good time to meditate or before (or after) a stressful task. Put the body in the same posture, in the same place, following the same ritual (prayer shawl or pillows, for example). Perhaps lighting a candle, removing shoes, and turning off the phone will be helpful. Find a safe and private location (at least for beginners).

♥ Position

When sitting for meditation you should be in a comfortable position—either in a chair or cross-legged on a pillow or bed, keeping a straight spine, which turns the boney column into an 'antenna.' Holding the hands comfortably with palms up symbolically 'catches' the incoming messages. Stretch your shoulders and neck gently for a few minutes, and then turn inward. It is okay to meditate sitting, lying down, in a head stand, fetal, or any other position. If you are still breathing, it is possible to meditate.

♥ Enhancers

It helps *greatly* to turn the eyes upward (even though closed). It changes the vibration of your very being (try it!). A slight smile raises vibration, too. Think of something that causes good feelings—a loved one, a happy event, a time of delight. Chant a mantra (a phrase that has positive meaning in any language), a name (a person you love or deeply admire or especially effective is to use your own name), or sing a hymn or meaningful song and see what feelings are evoked. Visualize a beautiful flower or better yet, gaze at a real flower. Visualize something that is desired, like a better relationship, a new car, or peace on Earth.

Think of a time of serious stress when the problem was resolved, like waiting for someone to drive home in a snowstorm and the feeling of deep relief when the car lights turned into the driveway and she opened the door smiling with arms wide. Remember that "whew," "perfect," or "yes!" feeling. Notice the vibration and then find a word that evokes that same feeling like: "There!" "Good!" or "All right!" Repeat these words to uplift yourSELF anytime when stressed.

♥ Focus and Attention

After you are seated and before meditation, 'untie the knot' in the solar chakra by putting your attention on the triangle just above the belly button between the lower ribs and consciously relax the 'knot' you will usually find there. Focus on each body part and ask it to relax, allowing chi to flow freely from toes to crown. Visualize light coming into the top of the head or by way of a silver thread directly into the heart. Focus on your breath—pretend the incoming breath is peace, and breathing out tensions. Or silently think a positive phrase like "I am love". Send love and good wishes to all distressed people of the world, and to yourself. Then close those thoughts and be silent.

Although they may appear the same to an observer, meditation is the opposite of sleeping. The senses are enhanced during meditation, so there is awareness that is not noticed in waking life and even during sleep. Conversely, we deliberately ignore everyday noises such as traffic or the refrigerator clicking on. The intuitive right brain can be 'heard' above the cacophony of the left brain and the outside world. With eyes closed there can be glorious brilliant color light show playing behind the eyelids. This delight of connecting to the core of love becomes as eagerly anticipated as retiring to bed at the end of a day of honest labor—peacefully 'at home.'

Perhaps it is clear from the above discussion that it does not matter exactly how you meditate (or where). The point is to stop thinking, so intuition can break through over the chatter, allowing the meditator to remember who she *really* is. A few minutes of blessed silence each day is truly needed to realize that each of us is part of the divine *and* the divine plan. The ultimate goal is to get so familiar with this deep peace that it is carried within, even in the most distressing places—an airport, the stock market, or the bustle of a supermarket will not disturb this peace and connection with the 'river of love.'

The point is to stop thinking, so intuition can break through over the chatter, allowing the meditator to remember who she really is.

Chant: I am ready, Radiant Light, enter in.

Touch my eyes with Holy Sight, Enter in, enter in.

Light the corners of my night, Cleanse and purify my sight.

Enter in, enter in.[164]

BENEFITS OF MEDITATION

In 1988 Michael Murphy and Steven Donovan did a comprehensive review of contemporary meditation research sponsored by the Esalen Institute. They concluded that meditation effectively does the following:

- Slows heart rate
- Increases blood flow to muscles and skin
- Lowers blood pressure in people who are normal or moderately hypertensive
- Increases alpha activity on EEG (brain waves associated with a state of relaxation),
- Lowers respiration rate
- Reduces muscle tension
- Lowers anxiety as measured by galvanic skin response
- Reduces pain associated with migraine, dysmenorrhea, muscle-tension, and angina
- Increased alertness, resulting in improvement of reaction time
- Relieves both acute and chronic anxiety
- Helps relieve addiction, neurosis, obesity, and claustrophobia
- Reduces insomnia
- Decreases smoking, marijuana, and alcohol use

164 Light of Christ Community Church and Seminary, *Songs and Chants for Meditation, Inspiration and Praise.* Sparrow Hawk Village, Tahlequah, OK.

Deepak Chopra teaches that a daily practice of meditation provides greater levels of intuition and creativity, relief from stress and anxiety, a more restful sleep, an increasing inner calm and innumerable health benefits. In fact, meditation is more restful than even deep sleep. It improves the flow of chi in the cells and of fluids through the tissues. Reducing chronic muscle clenching and increasing the flow of energy through the body enhances the immune system, improves breathing, and even decreases both signs and symptoms of aging. Meditation shortens recovery time from a trauma or illness and decreases the need for pain medication. It increases self-confidence, mental clarity, problem solving ability, and the feeling of empathy for others. Often creative ideas are born during meditation.

Training the mind to be quiet, using the intention of the will, increases will-power in other areas of life, like overcoming addictions, and creating good habits. It also improves memory, organizational skills, and the ability to focus. Deep meditation allows a meditator to become aware that nature includes *each* human—all of us together. No one achieves consciousness without helping their siblings grow as well. It puts the divine SELF in control of the child self. This is higher consciousness.

No one achieves consciousness without helping their siblings grow as well.

Psychotherapist and meditation teacher Lawrence LeShan describes "two major psychological effects of consistent meditation: the attainment of another way of perceiving and relating to reality and a greater efficiency and enthusiasm in everyday life."[165] Meditation has been found to improve relationships on all levels. It is a great aid to sexual enjoyment, which is similar to the union felt in yogic ecstasy and kundalini rising. There are no negative side effects from meditation—only lots of positive ones. It requires no special equipment and is simple to learn. It can be practiced anywhere, any time and is not

There are no negative side effects from meditation—only lots of positive ones.

165 Lawrence LeShan, *How to Meditate,* (Boston, MA: Little, Brown & Company, 1974), 19.

time consuming (15 to 20 minutes is good). Oh, and by the way it is completely free!

> Try this: Sit outside in the sun in meditation (before eating). Let a mosquito, or other biting insect light on your skin. Notice when your mind is focused upon love and gratitude, the bug will not bite and almost seems to be caressing you. As soon as thoughts slip into looking for what is wrong—anger, fear, shame, etc.,—bugs seem more likely to dig in their little proboscises (which only increases your negative emotions). Coincidence? Maybe.

MEDITATION AND FOOD

One of the most important aids to meditation is an organic live vegan diet. Eating a diet filled with light enhances health on all levels. When food is pure, the mind is pure; when the mind is pure, concentration is steady; when concentration is achieved, it loosens the knots that bind the heart. The mind and the body are organically interrelated and bodily conditions strongly influence thoughts. When the body ails, the soul, too, is obscured, making it more difficult to pray or meditate. A body full of toxins hinders reaching a state of SELF-realization. The thoughts of those who grow, gather, prepare, and serve the food affect the subtle quality of the one who eats it, so try singing when working in the garden and the kitchen. A spiritual diet ultimately creates a quiet mind.

A spiritual diet ultimately creates a quiet mind.

FASTING

There are hundreds of books written about fasting, which simply means abstaining from something—usually food and drink. It can mean ingesting nothing at all, or drinking water only, water with lemon or vinegar and honey or maple syrup, or a fruit drink. Some even refer to a simple diet of drinks of blended greens and fruit as fasting. It is considered to be a way to cleanse the colon and thus all the tissues of the body. Fasting develops will, clears the digestive tract, and has been known to save lives.

Fasting is used for many purposes, such as restoring physical health, enhancing mental clarity, and achieving spiritual awareness. It is also an exercise in discipline. It takes will power to fast for the first few days, but after that, many fasters report no longer feeling hungry. A feeling of peace, pride, and mental clarity sets in. Fasting seems to direct the energy inward, thus resolving emotional issues. The benefits reported by fasters are evidence of the negative effect food has on body-mind. Fasting is mentioned frequently in many religious writings and some describe that it gives a 'glow to the skin of your face,' possibly referring to enlightenment.

All things in moderation, as the saying goes, and fasting in excess can become unhealthy, perhaps depending on the faster's attitude. If you have a medical condition, consult a health provider before fasting. There are many centers where supervised fasting is offered. It would be better to be supervised if you are fasting for more than a few days or have a serious illness.

THE ART OF PONDERING

Pondering is using the logical mind, and at the same time, noticing intuitive feelings about the issue. Inner wisdom can come as the deep inner knowing that relentlessly nags at the gut until the wrong is righted (sometimes referred to as 'guilt'). Inner wisdom knows things the logical mind would rather not acknowledge. By using both logic and intuition, a wiser and more balanced decision can be made. If thinking about someone or something provokes negative feelings, ponder what past events might have been buried that now evokes the same feelings in you. Send love to the person or situation and visualize light on their path and the problem, clearing the energy blocks.

Conscious pondering is not simply running the same fear-based head-decisions over and over without benefit of the heart-intuitive influence. In the film, *Anne of a Thousand Days,* based on Maxwell Anderson's 1948 play which tells the story of Anne Boleyn, King Henry VIII thinks about beheading his wife so he can have another woman who has caught his eye. He says "God wouldn't let me have these thoughts if they were not the right thing to do." Common sense and compassion reveal the fallacy in his thinking.

Consciousness is not something that falls from the sky like grace or rain. It must be earned and it takes hard work. In fact, it may be the hardest work, since mind-clouds (errors in thinking) are the very issues folks have avoided and guarded against for years, perhaps lifetimes. We protect 'our story' and our 'righteous' position by looking for shreds of information that back us up. They are our personal fantasies and fallacies, SINs (Self-Inflicted Nonsense) and we all have them. It is by far easier to see another's thought errors than our own. The truth is: everyone is lovable, loved, loving, and in fact, made of pure love. It is the work of each person at every age and in every age to really *know* this.

Life is a mirror that gives not only clues, but a direct image of what is going on inside, both consciously and unconsciously. People around you are good 'sounding boards' to see what echoes back. The physical body is also a mirror—both internally and externally. What shows up in the tissues is what has been allowed to be believed in the mind. If you are not content then the higher, wiser, divine aspect of yourself has been pushed aside in preference for dark, destructive thoughts and beliefs. One thought won't create a disease, but a habit

Life is a mirror that gives not only clues, but a direct image of what is going on inside, both consciously and unconsciously.

of toxic thoughts, words, or deeds *will*. Words and deeds are very loud thoughts.

BODY MESSAGES

Make a habit of checking body posture, tension, and clenched muscles. These symptoms are sure signs that a body part (or several of them) is 'holding its breath.' Energy is choked off from reaching those parts. A headache may be the brain 'holding its breath.' Once again, pay attention to where attention is being paid. What is focused upon will manifest; look closely to see if that is what you really want. If you are making negative statements about health, aging, the circumstances of life, or the world in general to yourself, begin to send positive blessings to the body part or situation that were being disparaged.

Since the body is also sending *you* messages, try speaking back directly to the intelligence (energy) of area or function of the body. If the part hurts or does not function correctly, chances are it is hiding pain, toxins, or is filled with fear. Tell your shoulder or your liver that all is well, it is safe, and that it can return to perfect function now. Be sure to thank your beautiful body.

Each body function represents an aspect of your beliefs and serves as a reservoir for unresolved emotional issues. When an area of the body develops a disease, it means there are blocks in energy on some level. It does not usually happen suddenly, so errors might be detected and corrected before serious things, like cancer, set in. Louise Hay and others have written about what each body area represents and why a disease might be developing there.

ALLERGIES

Allergies are body messages that tell of a mental/emotional issue. An allergic reaction is a physical manifestation of a body memory. For example, a woman came to a hypnosis clinic for relief of an allergy to cats. In an altered state, she recalled having found a litter of kittens in the barn when she was a very small girl. She had put the kittens in a box under her bed to 'save' them. When her mother found the kittens, she told the girl to return them to the barn because the mother cat would come back to them. As she approached the barn, the girl was spotted, attacked, and severely scratched by the mother cat. More importantly, the girl was terrified and traumatized by this experience. The patient had not consciously remembered the incident, but when assured under hypnosis that she herself had unwittingly caused the problem and cats do not normally pose a threat, the allergy was completely cleared.

Allergies are body messages that tell of a mental/emotional issue.

We can convince ourselves that anything is dangerous or toxic, and a sliver of truth can be magnified into a debilitating handicap, causing untold hardship and expense. Many people drive themselves mad trying to avoid environmental allergens like plastic. It is true, plastic has toxic elements; but to uproot one's whole lifestyle to avoid any chemical is irrational, unnecessary, and probably impossible.

The problem, however, is almost never what the conscious mind would guess it to be; and there is always *another* layer to peel away! Often, both the unconscious and subconscious mind needs to be accessed in indirect ways. Allergies are one of those clues to the hidden issues.

CRYING

Crying is cleansing, whether it springs from happiness or sadness. Real crying should not be stifled. As with anything, there is the possibility of getting into a habit of crying almost to the point of addiction; but if there is cleansing going on and progress is being made, crying is generally good for mental *and* physical health. Sometimes it takes years of vigorous crying to get to buried hurts that

Crying is cleansing, whether it springs from happiness or sadness.

have been denied by the adult mind, in order to find the child who needs to be hugged and reassured.

> If tears well up, find a quiet place, and see if the pain, event, or abuse lying buried beneath the tears can be unearthed. Try to really feel the emotion behind the tears. Many times it stems from what you tell yourself about yourself—your story. It might be a familiar phrase repeated mentally over and over like, a variation of "I am not good enough," or "I will probably be ignored."

Again, crying too can be overdone. When tears are used as a tool to manipulate others, for example, they are not real. Sometimes friends get tired of hearing the same sob story over and over, and the crier needs to decide if there is actually something else behind the 'story' that has not been touched. Or maybe it is time to decide to let go of the issue and move on. Tears are clues to yourSELF and they are cleansing—so let them flow!

THERAPIES

All therapies involve energy—some are in harmony with life force and some are not. They can enhance the flow of energy in and around the body or block it. Medications, radiation, and surgery might be needed in emergency situations, but they kill cells and drain the body's energy. The word 'antibiotic' means against life!

All therapies involve energy—some are in harmony with life force and some are not.

♥ Aroma Therapy

On the other hand there are therapies that assist the normal flow of chi. One means of enhancing energy is aromatherapy, which uses essential oil from plants and each high-quality oil has unique energies. Administered by inhaling, skin application, or taken internally, oils clear energy blocks and promote healing in various ways.

♥ Herbs

Herbal therapy uses energy from plants, too. A preparation is made from flowers, berries, leaves or other parts of vegetation that assists in toxin removal and energy enhancement.

♥ Music & Dance

Music changes the energy of the body and can be either soothing or fear-inducing. Dancing is an ancient way of raising chi, perhaps by increasing respiration; oxygen therapy itself has recently become popular.

♥ Magnets, Gemstones & Crystals

Magnets are another therapy that stimulates the flow of energy, relieving pain-causing congestion. Gemstones, crystals and other "rocks" found on and in mother earth carry a magical subtle energy that can enhance intuition and overcome negative energies. Always trust your inner wisdom when you choose a stone that will enhance your energy.

♥ Centers & Pathways

Acupuncture and acupressure involve the stimulation of energy points on the body by a trained practitioner or when self-administered. Centers and pathways are stimulated in massage and acupressure, which frees them to carry energy easier like clearing a log jam from a river.

♥ Mind

Mental therapists facilitate healing by uncovering the mental causes of energy blocks. This might be the traditional talk-therapy where the patient attempts to explain her feelings and the therapist points out possible connections. It also includes altered states therapies like hypnosis and guided imagery.

There are many therapies from which to choose, conventional and otherwise. Consult your own heart and inner wisdom before seeking advice from a therapist. The energy you seek to enhance is yours. Therapists can have vested interests elsewhere.

SPIRITUAL OR ENERGY HEALING

Spiritual healing is not about healing the spirit, because spirit does not need healing. There is no actual 'healing' either, but rather more an *allowing* of the flow of sacred presence, which facilitates healing. Healers help move needed energy toward dark places and calm distorted or congested areas in a client, whether the source of the problem is from outside or within.

Spiritual healing is not about healing the spirit, because spirit does not need healing.

All subtle energy treatment techniques performed by energy therapists have a similar underlying premise—to infuse love where it is lacking. The therapist uses her intuitive senses to scan and identify problems in the flow of energy in and around the body of a client. Using loving intent, she invokes metaphysical helpers and intelligent divine energy to assist in dispersing the blocks. The treatment comes from a higher vibration than that of the healer, but it flows through her, raising the vibration of both healer and healee. Both get a 'treatment.'

Seers can find areas of blockage and congestion within the body and sometimes determine ailments—even the cause of the disease. All humans have this receiving and transmitting power to heal themselves and others. Some understand this naturally, while others seek teachers to help them contact their own 'inner knower.' Everyone is always receiving and transmitting energy, often without being aware of the power they possess. Energy follows intent. Examples of energy or spiritual healing methods are:

The treatment comes from a higher vibration than that of the healer, but it flows through her, raising the vibration of both healer and healee.

- Esoteric Healing
- Reiki
- Craniosacral Therapy
- Therapeutic Touch

Energy follows intent.

Energy healers' bodies act like a crystal antenna attracting cosmic energy, and their minds consciously direct it to places where it is needed. This energy is intelligent and will follow the intent of the healer who works for the highest good of all. Clearing congested or blocked energy can relieve symptoms for a time and is very helpful. Ultimate permanent restoration of health, though, depends upon the owner of the body correcting the habits of thought and action which created the block. The healing, like most therapies, only acts as a temporary bridge.

Early Christians called spiritual or energy healing "laying on of hands"; however such healing can be done without touching or even being near the person being treated, because this vital life 'juice' can be directed with intent from anywhere to anywhere. Energy treatments can be both requested and given remotely, because energy follows intent, no matter the distance. Thoughts constantly direct energy. Prayer is a form of energy healing, and all thoughts are prayers.

Truly loving another may soften their energy.

People who have adopted the living vegan diet report that when they receive energy treatments, these therapies seem to have greater effect than when they were eating cooked food. This makes sense because the 'electric circuits' will be cleaner and more able to tolerate the 'current' being delivered by the practitioner. When physical and emotional blocks are loosened or are being removed by unseen helpers inside the body, love being directed through human helpers will more easily break through. Truly loving another may soften their energy. Joy is contagious!

Energy healings often facilitate clearer thinking, relieve physical discomfort, and bring peace and calming. It is, however, unethical to alter the energy of another without permission. Energy healing must only be done with the permission of the recipient (or guardian). It constitutes violation of the karma of both the healer and healee if energy of another is changed with selfish motives or against the will of the person. Each must walk alone the dark valleys that are found on the path. One cannot help others unless they wish to be helped, since it is the *asking* that really switches on the 'call light' which attracts assistance.

One cannot help others unless they wish to be helped, since it is the asking that really switches on the 'call light' which attracts assistance.

Without permission, however, we can send rainbows of love to a person or situation, making it easier for them to find their path and resolution. Hold a vision of them whole and at peace, for one person cannot know what 'healed' means for another. Treatments can be offered, but avoid pressure to accept. It is another example of why we are here at this time together, both to comfort and confront each other.

It is another example of why we are here at this time together, both to comfort and confront each other.

Alice Bailey wrote that all disease is the result of inhibited soul life. She declared that "the art of the healer consists in releasing the soul so that its life can flow through the aggregate of organisms which constitute any particular form."[166] Her writings have awakened the healer in many aspirants.

CONNECT WITH NATURE

Nature is everywhere, constantly seeking to reclaim the cement and broken glass left behind by civilization. It is easy to connect with her by paying attention to her.

166 Alice Bailey, *Esoteric Healing,* (New York, NY: Lucis Press, 1953), 532.

> Look out the window, gaze at the sky, a tree, or any flower. It is not necessary to own the land or the flower shop; just walk in and 'feel' the flowers. Walk barefoot on unpolluted Earth and take a moment to feel her breathing under your feet. Feel 'life' pulsing there, rising into everything. Find a place to hug a tree or run barefoot in unsprayed grass or sand.

Grow a garden, even if it is in a pot in the window. Talk to your plants and the divas that are also tending them. Thank the garden for each fruit or flower and bless it as you leave. There are few pleasures that can compare to fasting and meditating while sitting on the ground in the garden bathed with sunlight.

Watch a wood fire dancing and crackling. Sleep near one if possible. Talk to the fire and get lost in the light. It is also not necessary to own the fireplace.

A good reason to have a pet is the energy they bring. They seem to want to be fed but perhaps it is really the attention they are craving. They respond to your intent. Natural born healers, animals have been shown to 'know' what part of their owner's body is ill and often lay over the cancerous breast or painful stomach. Animals understand about energy; they communicate that way. They know what you are saying and they answer energetically. Explain to them why something must be done in clear verbal and non-verbal language. Sitting in the hay cradling a baby goat (or a cat in the lap) is supremely grounding and totally peaceful. If you can't 'own' a pet, volunteer at an animal shelter. Nature (god) is free.

CONNECT WITH OTHER PEOPLE

Hugs are essential and enormously healing. Always ask first if the other person wants the hug and respect the answer. Hugs, by definition, are an equal exchange—give one and get one...for free! Sincere hugs are supremely healing.

> The perfect hug: Always make eye contact first and get permission with words or a nod. Raise your left arm instead of the usual right arm so that your hearts will be next to each other during the hug. The taller person should bend her knees to make height more even. It should last 4 or 5 seconds while you concentrate completely on the person you are hugging. Break if and when the other person wants to. Make eye contact again.

Sincere hugs are supremely healing.

Smile at people in public while making eye contact; usually a smile comes back to you in return. When asking for help, a smile goes a long way to facilitate getting it. Cheering others brings back blessings, too. Keep a sense of humor. Admire someone's hair or clothes. Find a common thread with everyone and focus on similarities. There is nothing in the universe except love and the fear that blocks it.

Make love with someone. This can be either sexually or simply with your eyes or fingers. Babies die without touch. So do adults! Dancing can be a form of making love, as can gardening, painting, preparing food, or eating together. Making love is an exchange of divine energy channeled through living angels and animals to other divine bodies.

There is nothing in the universe except love and the fear that blocks it.

CONNECT WITH YOURSELF

Each person is a part of loving, peaceful nature and can reconnect with it. There are many ways to connect with yourSELF. Dancing does not require a partner; nor even music. Find an uplifting song or melody in your mind and smile, swaying gently alone, or vigorously pump your blood with your feet and body in rhythm with a faster beat.

Singing raises your energy level whether alone or in a group. Sing with the radio or make something up. Sometimes subconscious messages are revealed by what song comes to mind. "Slip out the back Jack." "Oh, what a beautiful morning!" "You are beautiful, just the way you are." "I'm on top of the world, looking down on creation." Are the lyrics telling you something?

SILENCE

Once a day, allow the luxury of a few minutes (or longer) of complete silence (or as close as can be managed). In the city, the middle of the night offers the best opportunity. Just breathe in the quiet without attempting to meditate or employ any other discipline except to resist turning on the various noise-makers always close at hand. Many people find silence causes panic as memories, worry, or self-deprecating thoughts come back that had been held at bay by the incessant noise. Feel the vibration of the fear and ponder from whence it came. Perhaps there is something that must be done to make things right. Make a plan to do that. The heart tells the truth in the silence. Let the negative thoughts sit as long as they wish and then watch them go—for they are not real, but only a habit that was taken on voluntarily. Watch them break up and dissolve like asking a fluffy cloud to dissipate (which works, by the way).

Each individual has a body, but she is not that body. Every person has thoughts, but she is not those thoughts. Thoughts produce emotions, but the 'feeler' is not her emotions. You have a body, thoughts and emotions but they are not the *real* you. Body, mind, and emotions belong to the soul, who uses them to learn universal truths. In many spiritual traditions it is taught that the way to peace is to know thySELF. Being still allows this. Silence is truly golden and is a good thing to do before you meditate or go to sleep.

MAKE YOUR OWN HEALTHY RULES

A personal program of health includes rules concerning: food, exercise, meditation, sunshine, hygiene, and environment. Take charge of yourSELF. Set in your mind what you will and won't eat and under what circumstances and see how your body and mind respond. Be ready to modify your rules to include or exclude anything as you see necessary. Your schedule might allow exercise only at certain times, for example. As a practical matter this is a list of easy-to-implement daily rules from discussions in this chapter that some people have found worked for them at one time or another on their healthy journey. Setting your own rules gives you a routine that is health-affirming that might steer your decisions when you don't feel like thinking about it; for example, when out to eat with friends. Rules might keep you from slipping back into habits that you want to change. Reward yourself with healthy food, going on the Internet, and sleep.

AN EXAMPLE OF A PERSONAL HEALTH PROGRAM

1. Drink a gallon of pure water a day.

Drink at least a quart before eating anything in the morning.

2. Do yoga-like stretches for at least 15 minutes every day

Make a rule to stretch before going on the Internet.

3. Diet 95% C.L.O.V.E.R. (Or whatever number you choose today)

No flesh of any kind.

If eating something cooked it has to be organic. If not organic it has to be raw.

Keep quiet about it.

4. Exercise at least a half hour a day

No supper before getting out of breath with increased heart rate for half an hour.

5. Floss and brush teeth at least 3 minutes a day

Never go to sleep until this is done.

6. Shower every night (short and warm)

Brush skin before showering at least once a week and always shower before bed.

7. Meditate 15 minutes every day

8. Live sustainably

Ask the question, "If everyone lived this way would the world be a better place?"

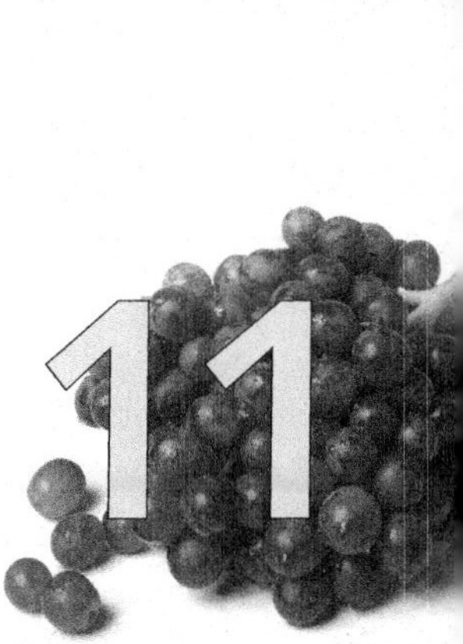

Spiritual Ecology—Effects on the Planet

Reversing the spread of hunger will mean learning to create a world based on cooperation and on the affirmation of the human spirit.

— John Robbins

The Earth is an intelligent, vibrant entity—as an organism herself, she *feels* the attitude of humans who dwell upon her. She, too, is undergoing a major transition. Our mother is having a Near Death Experience (NDE). When humans come close to dying, whether from being gravely ill, after a serious accident, or when they actually die for a period of time it is called an NDE. People often gain great insights about the meaning of life and their individual place in it during an NDE. The Earth, like humanity, is currently making a major decision to continue living and trying to heal herself or to let her systems break down and become overwhelmed with toxins. Human disrespect for the living planet has put her in the same situation as SAD has put people—starved for divine love.

The Earth has energy centers (analogous to human chakras) called 'vortices,' and like our blood and lymph vessels, her rivers and streams carry life-giving fluids. She has cleansing organs called 'wetlands,' similar to our own liver and kidneys. Plants serve as protective clothing to her delicate skin. Trees reach deep into her heart and give shelter, sustenance, and oxygen to the animal 'kindom' (all are kin). Humanity has blocked and diverted her rivers and lakes,

Human disrespect for the living planet has put her in the same situation as SAD has put people—starved for divine love.

unbalancing and starving her tissues of energy, like cholesterol blocks human arteries. Mankind has polluted and drained the marshlands so they barely function as filters. Our earth mother loves, feeds, and protects her children. It is time to return the favor.

Spreading concentrated fertilizer on plants is the same as feeding a child high fructose corn syrup—lots of kindling, no real fuel or building blocks. Everyone knows that children need more than sugar to grow healthy and conscious. The growth is unsustainable. After the initial boost, chemical fertilizer ultimately weakens the plant. Pests are attracted to unhealthy plants because the function of insects and microorganisms in nature is to clean up dead and dying tissue. Chemical farmers must then kill the pests with poison in order to 'save' the crop. Plants and children need lots of nutrients to be healthy. Well-nourished plants do not interest insects. Healthy plants are better able to withstand harsh, overly wet, or dry conditions. Children and other animals fed nutritious food grow strong, healthy, resilient, and wise.

Humanity is past the time when the citizens of Earth can stand by, focused on war and weapons of mass distraction, lamenting that the president is not doing enough about climate change. Disciplined actions of even one person can begin ripples of change that could save the planet. In this time of New Age energies, conscious stewardship can assist the transition of the Earth as she hovers on the brink. The raw, bloodless diet can be a major factor benefiting Earth and humanity. If the transformation is to be right here (not in a mythical heaven), then it must be realized that all humanity will benefit if humans behave more humanely. In addition, according to the Law of Attraction, sharing resources with others will bring riches to oneself. Restoring mother earth will bring prosperity to *all* her inhabitants.

DIET ECOLOGY AND WORLD HUNGER

Human diets play a major role in the preservation or destruction of the planet in several ways. Resources used to produce the SAD are far more wasteful than for a raw vegan diet. For example, food produced by cycling grain through livestock wastes 90% of the protein, 96% of the calories, and 100% of its fiber and carbohydrates (compared to eating the grain ourselves).[167] In other words, we are losing most of our investment, and meanwhile we are starving. If Americans would decrease their meat consumption by just 10%, enough grain would be saved to feed 60 million people, approximately the number of people who die of hunger related diseases each year.[168] Food needs to be ethically distributed, too. There are 1.2 billion *underfed* and malnourished people in the world and about the same number of people *overfed* and *still* malnourished.[169] People in rich countries can afford to eat toxic animal products, but all of Earth's children need to act responsibly so that everyone is adequately nourished. We must learn to feed each other.

Restoring mother earth will bring prosperity to all her inhabitants.

The following chart compares the amount of land need to support a SAD eater and a person who abstains from animal products.

This is the number of people whose food energy needs can be met by the food produced on 2.5 acres of land:

* Cabbage–23 people
* Potatoes–22 people
* Rice–19 people
* Corn–17 people
* Wheat–15 people
* Chicken–2 people
* Milk–2 people
* Eggs–1 person
* Beef–1 person.[170]

167 John Robbins, *Diet for a New America,* (Tiburon, CA: HJ Kramer, 1987), 352.
168 John Robbins, *May All Be Fed,* (New York, NY: William Morrow, 1992), 35.
169 John Robbins, *The Food Revolution,* (Berkeley, CA: Conari Press, 2001), 290.
170 John Robbins, *The Food Revolution,* (Berkeley, CA: Conari Press, 2001), 294.

John Robbins wrote twenty-five years ago that it takes three and a quarter acres of land to supply food for one flesh eater for a year while a pure vegetarian requires only one sixth of an acre. In other words, a given amount of our Earth's surface can feed almost twenty times as many people eating a pure vegetarian diet. A raw vegan would require even less. Livestock consume enough grain and beans to feed *over five times the entire human population.* One acre can grow 20,000 pounds of potatoes or 165 pounds of beef.[171]

Somewhat more recently, Robbins reported that 70% of the grain and cereals grown in the U. S. are fed to livestock. It takes 17 pounds of grain to produce one pound of beef flesh and half of the Earth's land mass is used as pasture for livestock.[172] Cattle and hogs are huge animals and require great quantities of food. They cannot subsist on marginal land. They will destroy a wetland if allowed to plunder it. Overgrazed and mismanaged pastures and fields lead to deserts and dustbowls.

In answer to what will become of the animals—stop breeding them, let them die naturally, and add their bodies to the compost pile along with pits, peels, leaves, hulls, and stalks from plants. The compost will then enrich the soil to grow better vegetables and fruit. The land that was used to graze these huge animals could return to oxygen-giving forests. We can live peacefully with animals. In the wild, nature keeps their numbers in check. They give us their manure for our fruits and vegetables, love us, and some even protect us (there are stories of dogs, dolphins, sea turtles, pigs, and even canaries saving humans). They pull our plows, give us their extra fleece coats, and trust us with their babies. There is no need to kill them.

Peace will come only when all people are treated equally and have enough nutritious food to eat. A hungry person can think of nothing

171 John Robbins, Diet *for a New America,* (Tiburon, CA: HJ Kramer, 1987), 352–353.

172 John Robbins, *The Food Revolution,* (Berkeley, CA: Conari Press, 2001), 290–293.

else. No one reaches enlightenment until we extend a hand to all the others. That doesn't mean giving them free charity. Just give everyone an equal chance to feed themselves, enough water to grow a garden, and enough love to want to live. There is abundance for all if we have the courage to share.

TOPSOIL

The Earth suffers in other ways from providing large numbers of flesh entrées and other animal products in human diets. The SAD has directly or indirectly contributed to the pollution of the Earth's surface with pesticides and the loss of almost three quarters of the topsoil that was here when 'civilization' arrived. There was twenty-one inches of humus-rich topsoil two hundred years ago. Today there is an average of only six inches. It takes nature 500 years to build one inch of topsoil.[173]

Topsoil depletion and loss have been due to several factors. The unnatural practice of mono-cropping, (the planting of only one type of plant) on hundreds of acres, (mostly growing grain for animal feed) depletes the soil of crucial nutrients. Modern agriculture practices have also left the irrigated fields laden with salt and polluted with chemical fertilizers and pesticides. Mother earth never leaves herself naked for long—if the soil is good enough, a crop of weeds soon springs up which enrich the soil and are often edible for animals. Natural events destroy plants and animals but according to U. S Geological Survey and Washington State University, life usually springs back soon after volcanoes, windstorms, and wildfires—enhancing biodiversity and enriching the soil. Human destruction takes much longer to heal.

It takes nature 500 years to build one inch of topsoil.

Conventional agriculture and clear-cutting forests, on the other hand, remove huge sections of mother's covering, leaving her precious topsoil exposed—lying open, to 'bleed' away nutrients and tiny living

173 John Robbins, *Diet for a New America,* (Tiburon, CA: HJ Kramer, 1987), 357.

creatures. Without vegetation, topsoil washes away with heavy rain or blows away with the wind. Carrying toxic chemical fertilizers and pesticides, this precious topsoil is washed into rivers and ultimately forms "dead zones" at the point where the river drains into the sea. The chemicals cause the oxygen to be depleted, which kills all plants and animals that would normally be found there. There are over 400 such zones; some are thousands of miles square.[174]

POLLUTION AND CLIMATE CHANGE

Climate change is a term given to a set of key indicators: carbon dioxide concentration, global surface temperature, arctic sea ice, land ice, and sea level. These changes are thought to be caused by increased gases (carbon dioxide, methane, water vapor, nitrous oxide, and chlorofluorocarbons) in the atmosphere, causing a "greenhouse effect"—the trapping of the sun's heat near the surface of the Earth. Burning of fossil fuels, confined animal feed operations (CAFO), and the destruction of forests—especially the tropical rainforests—produce these gasses. In the last 40 years human activity has raised the level of carbon dioxide in the atmosphere by 25%.[175] According to the Intergovernmental Panel on Climate Change (IPPC), which includes more than 1,300 scientists from the around the world, atmospheric temperature is expected (and already is beginning) to rise from 2. 5 to 10 degrees. 2012 surpassed the record for the hottest year (set in 1998) by one whole degree.[176] This warming leads to higher sea levels, intense rainfall events, and longer periods of drought.

The warmer temperatures are critical as the topsoil disappears and becomes less fertile with conventional farming methods. Hybrid and genetically modified plants cannot withstand extreme changes. Organically farmed land, on the other hand, absorbs water more easily with less 'run-off,' because it is rich in humus and filled with

174 Wikipedia, *Dead Zone (ecology)* March 5, 2013.

175 John Robbins, *The Food Revolution,* (Berkeley, CA: Conari Press, 2001), 259.

176 *New York Times,* "Global Warming & Climate Change," Wednesday, March 6, 2013.

tunnels made by deep-rooted cover crops like clover and by worms fed by with compost and mulch left on the surface. Food shortages are a real possibility as global warming progresses. We choose to survive by buying sustainably grown food.

There are more than three times as many animals on planet Earth as there are humans.[177] Animals raised for food produce 130 times more excrement than the entire human population. The animal manure produces methane, thought to be a major contributor to global warming. These mountains of manure, concentrated in small areas because of CAFOs, which if used in small amounts would enrich the soil, all too often end up destroying plant and animal life in the ponds and rivers they ultimately enter. To make matters worse, the manure contains concentrated amounts of antibiotics, pesticides, and hormones given to conventionally raised animals to keep them alive until they are killed.

Global warming in turn is responsible for turbulent weather-related disasters which destroy crops and cropland. Floods wash away acres of topsoil in one day. Drought allows the wind to remove and scatter unanchored soil. It is a full circle from flesh eating to mono-cropping, to global warming, to floods and loss of topsoil. Lush plants are needed to build and hold topsoil in place. Eat more plants!

RAINFORESTS

Tropical rainforests are precious Earth resources, providing a major source of oxygen and diverse plant and animal life, yet every second an acre (the size of a football field) of it is destroyed to feed cattle for American burgers.[178] It has been said that each person who becomes a vegetarian will personally be responsible for saving an acre of rainforest. For *every* quarter-pound burger made of rainforest beef, 55 square feet of tropical rainforest (a small kitchen) is turned into

Eat more plants!

177 John Robbins, *The Food Revolution,* (Berkeley, CA: Conari Press), 2001), 234.

178 John Robbins, *The Food Revolution,* (Berkeley, CA: Conari Press), 2001), 255.

desert, causing the loss of over a pound of topsoil and destroying over 150 different plant, insect and animal species.[179] We will never know what gifts these natural creatures had to give.

FOOD SHORTAGES AND FUEL

Wherever it is produced, meat consumption directly leads to depletion of fossil fuels. It takes twenty times as much fossil fuel to produce one calorie of protein from flesh as from plant sources, as illustrated in the following chart.

Number of calories of fossil fuel used to produce one calorie of food protein from:

* Soybeans - 2
* Corn or wheat–3
* Beef - 54[180]

In addition, conventional crops use petroleum for fertilizer as well for as powering farm equipment and shipping. The average head of lettuce travels 1,000 miles before it is eaten. What will happen when we are past "peak oil" and the supplies dwindle? Will it become more important to have pineapple for breakfast in northern climates or to heat your house?

CLOVER uses far less fuel from soil to plate. The food for a living diet is harvested, refrigerated, transported, and stored—usually loose in large boxes. It has not been processed into pizza or canned soup, for example. SAD packaging uses tons of paper, cans, and plastic. Packaging must be shipped and stored with the food and is later added to the growing masses of landfill. Most of the waste in a raw kitchen is compostable—using very little packaging (much of which can be reused or recycled). Cooking also uses lots of energy.

---

179 Rainforest Action Network, Student Fact Sheet 8, "Seven Things You Can Do to Save the Rainforest," www.ran.org, March, 4, 2013.

180 John Robbins, *The Food Revolution*, (Berkeley, CA: Conari Press, 2001), 266.

When everyone grows a kitchen garden or has a garden plot like the dachas in Russia (small private homes with gardens that grow around half of the country's food), the food will merely require a walk in the fresh air and sunshine to transport. A raw foodist will take seasonal fresh food (ideally from a reusable basket at a farmer's market) and freeze, ferment, or dehydrate it. After drying, dehydrated food uses no refrigeration and takes up very little space.

Burning of fossil fuels to cook food not only destroys the nutrients in the food, but destroys the atmosphere as well. The cost of fuel for cooking (virtually all the food for the SAD) has to be significant. The Hunza people do not cook their food because of the scarcity of fuel and they live long, healthy lives. With the reports of fuel shortages and soaring prices, isn't it time to encourage everyone to do the same? CLOVER clears the mind of mind-clouds that declare that destroying the planet, torturing animals, and allowing children in the world to starve is OK. Living on live food, a person turns toward the light, like a living plant.

WATER

We are currently experiencing the beginnings of a global water crisis of near disaster proportion that is predicted to worsen as climate changes progress. Every day the privatization of water causes poor people to go without this most basic of human needs, while the rich and politically savvy compete for the rights to sell this precious 'blue gold' to the poorest of the Earth who cannot afford it. What water is still available is likely to become contaminated in a disruption of the natural balance of life, which diminishes its healing energy. There is already a war over water.

Living on live food, a person turns toward the light, like a living plant.

Water can be conserved and kept from contamination by adopting a CLOVER diet. Juicy fruits, vegetables, and living seeds directly from the Earth require far less water to produce than food taken from the bodies of animals.

1 pound of lettuce	23 gallons
1 pound of tomatoes	23 gallons
1 pound of potatoes	24 gallons
1 pound of wheat	25 gallons
1 pound of carrots	33 gallons
1 pound of apples	49 gallons
1 pound of chicken	815 gallons
1 pound of pork	1,630 gallons
1 pound of beef	5,214 gallons
7 minute shower daily for a year	5,200 gallons

Food production figures from Soil and Water specialists at University of California Agricultural Extension working with livestock farm advisors.[181]

The vast aquifers that made the United States wealthy in food production are drying up along with the depleted soils they irrigated. Animals raised for meat are not only drinking, but they are also contaminating the precious water upon which all life depends. Chickens, hogs, cattle and other meat animals are the primary consumers of water in the U. S. ; one pig drinks 21 gallons of water a day while a dairy cow consumes 50 gallons.[182] Humans drink about a gallon of water a day.

We have diverted many natural waterways, causing unknown changes to the balance of the Earth. It is difficult to put that back. People whose careers depend on selling animal products tend to underestimate the water issue and the government favors these big agribusinesses. But it is the "99 percent" who will go without.

---

181 Schulback, Herb, et al., in *Soil and Water* 38 (Fall 1978). In John Robbins, *The Food Revolution,* (Berkeley, CA: Conari Press, 2001), 236.

182 PETA, "Vegetarianism and the Environment," found on www.PETA.org, March 11, 2013.

GMO: DON'T MESS WITH MOTHER NATURE

Genetically modified organisms (GMO) are those created through genetic engineering (GE), sometimes referred to as "Franken foods" (referring to the story of Frankenstein—science gone badly). It involves taking genes from one species and inserting them artificially into another, genetically crossing unrelated organisms (such as microorganisms with plants) which would never cross-breed in nature, creating unpredictable effects. This is done for a variety of reasons, chiefly to make the plants resistant to certain chemicals which can then be used on the crop to kill weeds. The company can then patent the new organism and prosecute anyone found to have that genetic material on their property, no matter how it got there.[183] All research on the safety of GMO food has been done by the biotech companies themselves, who are not required to produce evidence from human trials on either toxicity or allergies. Currently GMO food is not required to be labeled as such in most areas of the United States (but that may be changing). These artificially altered foods are thought to affect both the DNA of human bodies and of the bacteria in human intestines. Once released, GE organisms become part of the environment.

No more nutritious than conventionally grown food, it clearly has the potential to be toxic and a threat to human health. It also threatens a gardener's way of life by making it illegal or difficult to reuse her own seed.

Ironically, GMO farmers must ultimately use even more pesticides, because GMO plants cross with weeds, making them also resistant to the effects of herbicides. The chemicals often cost farmers more than the crop is worth. Patenting seeds has deprived third world farmers (as well as those from the first and second worlds) of their native right to save their own seeds, which is a detriment to world plant diversity.

---

183 Deborah Koons Garcia, movie "The Future of Food", 2004.

When genes are more diverse, they are more robust. Plants with reduced genetic diversity cannot handle drought and disease nearly as well as natural plants, as evidenced during the 1845 potato famine in Ireland which was caused by growing only one variety.[184] When that variety was destroyed by a season of disease, the people starved.

On December 14, 1999, two hundred and thirty-one scientists from thirty-one countries published an "Open Letter to All Governments" calling for a global moratorium on all genetically engineered foods and crops. This has been robustly resisted by the producers of the altered seeds and the chemicals that are designed to be used with them. Although GE plants dominate the farmlands of the U. S. and Canada, parts of many countries require labeling or have banned them all together. The United States does neither—yet.

Spiritual seers have speculated that nature will restore genes to a natural state as soon as humans stop messing with mother nature. Carol Parrish-Harra has said that Mad Cow disease may be animals choosing to leave the Earth rather than be treated so badly. Plants and animals are conscious, know they are being betrayed, and ultimately they will obey the laws of nature. Nature will win.

WAR

John Robbins wrote, "Meat eating contributes to the fear in the world by putting us in a position in which there is not enough to go around." He goes on to say that today's animals are almost guaranteed to die in terror, which infuses the eater with that panic. This expresses itself in war and the violence seen daily in many lives.[185] War benefits only corporate finances.

Nature will win.

In order to condition small children to tolerate the Standard American Diet, society is required to desensitize them to their inborn essential feelings and awareness. This is more than sad, because it is

184 Ronnie Cummins and Ben Lilliston, *Genetically Engineered Food,* (New York, NY: Marlowe & Company, 2004), 3.

185 Robbins, John, *Diet for a New America,* (Tiburon, CA: HJ Kramer, 1987), 356.

this same erosion of compassion that allows these precious children to dehumanize an enemy, a member of their own family (the human race), and kill without a second thought. This unnatural act causes untold misery to the soldier and her family as well as the family of the dead. Adoption of a compassionate diet fosters evolution to a state of consciousness where peace and freedom are possible.

War benefits only corporate finances.

The threat of military Armageddon can only be removed when people really *think* about what they are doing. They must be conscious enough to resist following a charismatic leader into a war from which no living thing survives or thrives.

Adoption of a compassionate diet fosters evolution to a state of consciousness where peace and freedom are possible.

"As long as men massacre animals, they will kill each other."

—Pythagoras.

ORGANIC FARMING

Like our bodies, mother earth will heal herself if loving energy is restored. She wants humans to stop toxing her with chemical fertilizers, bug sprays, weed killers, and genetically modified organisms. Like our skin, mother's wounds need to be dressed with mulch and cover crops. Crops are even happier when farmers avoid over-tilling, which kills earthworms and microorganisms necessary for soil fertility. The dreaded insects eating the crops are smart enough to evolve and become immune to the sprays just like the 'pathogens' in our bodies learn to resist stronger and stronger antibiotics. But most important is the life in the soil, which is unable to be seen even by a microscope and is, as yet, unidentified by science—*life force energy*. Love your mother because like all organisms, mother earth needs the love of her children.

Love your mother because like all organisms, mother Earth needs the love of her children.

Naturally growing 'weeds' (considered noxious and typically destroyed) are there to protect, heal, and nourish the garden. They also give vital information about the condition of the soil, revealing what is lacking or overabundant. Weeds promote the growth of bacteria and fungi which actively restore the fertility of the soil. And they produce sugar for the tiny microorganisms that in turn produce what the plants need. Some even say that weeds can change one mineral into another one that is lacking in that soil (alchemy). Of course weeds will overtake and kill the garden if not controlled—but it is always good to leave at least some of them around—the more diverse the better. Many are edible, delicious, and super-nutritious for humans. Parts of the milkweed plant are, for example, not only edible for us, but are the primary food for the endangered Monarch butterfly as well (if not sprayed with chemicals).

Plants are highly intelligent living organisms, which display the ability to respond to music, prayer, and thoughts. Using artificial fertilizer (originally discarded from ammunition manufacturing) results in the plants becoming nitrogen addicts like people on steroids—for a while they might appear more robust, but their overall health is at increased risk. The cells are flooded with some nutrients, while others such as iron and selenium go lacking.

Some living creatures in the soil can be seen, like the sacred earthworm (a measure of the soil's health and toxin level)—while other entities, like nematodes, are microscopic. One cup of healthy nourished soil holds more living organisms than there are people on planet Earth! Mother's skin needs carbon and nitrogen in the form of plant and animal bodies, and she will restore herself. Earth, like us, also lives in cycles—daily, yearly, and beyond. She is a wise old lady who has lived in harmony with plants, animals, sun, rain, and earthquakes for untold millennia. Humanity has the intelligence to respect the wisdom of the Earth. When will we have the wisdom to respect her intelligence?

One cup of healthy nourished soil holds more living organisms than there are people on planet Earth!

Organic food is raised according to federal USDA standards. Ironically, no permits, inspections, records, or labels are required for chemical farming; but to use the label "USDA organic" a farmer must comply with all of these regulations, *and* pay a hefty *fee* besides. Shouldn't the fees be levied on the folks who have done the damage? In order to produce healthy food, an organic farmer must pay for the privilege of proving she did *not* use harmful substances. A conventional farmer can use any spray or chemical she wants without disclosing it to anyone. The term "certified organic" means that the farmer followed organic standards, avoided materials considered unsafe, kept careful records, and was properly inspected. Organic crops cannot be grown from GMO seed. This certification gives a consumer some reassurance that toxic substances were not applied to the soil, plant, or used in harvesting.

Humanity has the intelligence to respect the wisdom of the Earth. When will we have the wisdom to respect her intelligence?

In order to produce healthy food, an organic farmer must pay for the privilege of proving she did not use harmful substances.

Not only does organic growing help preserve the planet, but organic food is higher in minerals compared to conventionally grown food. It is 63% higher in calcium, 73% higher in iodine, 59% higher in iron, and 390% higher in selenium.[186] It keeps fresh longer in storage and is usually sweeter. Organic food is safer not only for the consumer and food preparer, but for the farmer and farm laborers as well. Do you want to eat food that has been sprayed with substances that required 'hazmat" protective gear? Support organic farmers, especially your local ones. Volunteer at their farms and watch what they apply to the plants, but if that is not possible then buy organic food at the store. When you vote for 'chemical-free' with your food dollars, eventually organic will be the norm and chemical foods will be more expensive.

In the movie, *Real Dirt on Farmer John*, John Peterson says "This time I was going to farm organically. I think raising crops under the influence of so many chemicals sort of warps or twists the life force

186 John Robbins, *The Food Revolution,* (Berkeley, CA: Conari Press, 2001), 370.

and that shows up in the health of livestock and people, and raises absolute havoc with the planet!"

As more humans adopt a vegan diet, it will lead to the restoration of the soil that has been destroyed by growing great quantities of grain mostly consumed by ruminants (livestock, who by the way, do not naturally eat grain in such large quantity). The spare land could be rotated and tended with mulch, rock powders, sea minerals, and cover crops, thus restoring vital nutrients. Work animals (horses, oxen, and mules), along with sheep and other fiber animals, can provide the small amount of manure needed for vegetables. When people and animals stop ingesting poison medications in a false attempt to be symptom-free, their rich, uncontaminated manure becomes a great source of nourishment for trees, shrubs, and flowers. Healthy weeds might show up to soak up sun and rain for the little microbes, allowing mother nature to work her magic.

FOOD COST

Raw foodists need less food—for several reasons. Fiber fills up the stomach quicker and the natural complex carbohydrates quickly nourish the brain and other cells. Since there are many more vitamins, minerals, and micronutrients in living food, less is needed to satisfy the craving of the body cells, once addictions are overcome. This means fewer calories need to be consumed. People eating processed food tend to overeat because the cells are still starving. Even if fresh organic food *seems* more expensive, it ultimately costs less when all factors are figured. Some of these considerations are:

♥ It is unnecessary to buy expensive food supplements. It makes no sense to cook naturally fermented sauerkraut and buy manufactured probiotics. It also makes no sense to eat meat and take 'fiber' pills.

- ♥ The long-term cost of the damage to the earth will drive up future food prices
- ♥ Health care expenses are greatly reduced when you are healthy.
- ♥ The cost of prescription and over the counter drugs is staggering. Zero for the healthy.
- ♥ Unprocessed produce is naturally cheaper than manufactured products sold for food.
- ♥ It is possible to grow some percentage of your own live food.

Rosalind Creasy, a home gardener, made a 5'x 20' garden—just 100 square feet—which produced an estimated $746.52 dollars' worth of food (in northern California) in one year with a net savings of $683.43 after deducting expenses of seeds, plants, and compost. This was in contrast to buying food in the supermarket. She grew organic tomatoes, peppers, zucchinis, basil, and lettuce.[187] This home-grown food is likely to become even more valuable as petroleum, food, and water prices increase.

The book *Anastasia* mentions the Russian 'dachas' and their importance.[188] 70% of the population grows part of their own food on these small private garden spaces, even the wealthy. There is a short (110 days) growing season in Russia but dachas produced 80% of the fruit and berries, and 66% of the vegetables consumed in Russia in 2011. This number is lower than it had been in previous years. *Mother Earth News* points out that in the United States, lawns take up more than twice the amount of land Russia's gardens do (est. 40-45 million acres). Imagine the impact of an organic home garden revival in the United States, growing foods on previously useless lawn space with no shipping, chemicals, or processing fees to be paid. It could be victory over illness and corporate domination.

---

187 Rosalind Creasy with Cathy Wilkinson Barash, "Grow $700 of Food in 100 Square Feet" in *Mother Earth News*, December 2009/January 2010 Issue 237, 30.

188 Vladimir Megré, *Anastasia, The Ringing Cedar Series, Book One*, (Kahului, HI: Ringing Cedars Press, 1996).

WESTON PRICE, et. al.

During the 1930s, a dentist named Weston Price traveled the world looking for primitive people to study—those who did not eat the over processed food that modern Americans (even in his time) lived on. He searched for those isolated people specifically to correlate their diet with tooth development and condition. He studied 14 groups, photographing their teeth, assessing their longevity and mental status. In his book *Nutrition and Physical Degeneration,* he apparently made only one statement regarding animal products: "It is significant that I have as yet found no group that was building and maintaining good bodies exclusively on plant foods."[189]

It was upon this one statement that many advocates of flesh eating have based their writings. Price's work was not focused upon the vegetarian factor, so he did not explore the diets of vegetarians specifically; and he did not say that there were no healthy vegetarians—only that he did not find any among the 14 primitive groups he studied. This line of thought promotes using animal sources as a means of making up for nutritional deficiencies in the soil. While it is true that the soil is depleted, neither a diet of cooked grain and beans nor one of roasted flesh will add life to either the soil or the human body.

While it is true that the soil is depleted, neither a diet of cooked grain and beans nor one of roasted flesh will add life to either the soil or the human body.

Price and his contemporary, William Albrecht, whose article is included as a chapter in Price's book, both agreed that soil fertility is of urgent importance in human health, with the current diet depleting the soils of the earth faster than they can naturally regenerate. Albrecht, who taught the well-known 'Albrecht method' of soil restoration, classifies man at the top of the biotic pyramid and as separate from carnivore, omnivore, and herbivore. He states that more research is needed as we shift the protein-providing responsibility in our diet away from meats and milk and more toward the foods of distinctly vegetable origin, "thereby a step closer to the soil fertility

189 Weston A. Price, D.D.S. *Nutrition and Physical Degeneration,* (LaMesa, CA: Price-Pottenger Nutrition Foundation, 2003), 282.

as the foundation of the entire biotic pyramid."[190] He praises the lowly microbe, so feared and attacked by modern society, as a major benefactor of the soil and the body. He writes that microbes' entrance into the body is not necessarily attack, but "part of a task of disposal under the beginnings of death recognized earlier by them than by their pseudo-victim."[191] He highly recommends composting of both dead plants and animals as a means of adding organic matter to soil, but warns against over-manuring.

AGRIBUSINESS

Humans survived evolution because nutritious foods were readily available in nature. It is one of the great ironies of nutrition that the traditional plant-based diets, consumed by the poor in many countries, are ideally suited to meeting their nutritional needs. Once people are 'well off,' they begin eating more meat, fat, and processed foods. The result is more obesity and chronic disease. Thanks to the agribusiness corporations, Americans have many kinds of food readily available but are persuaded toward the fatty, sugary, depleted, subsidized, and cheap ones. These food corporations have also caused the number of varieties of each food to diminish. Americans think there are only one or two kinds of cucumber, carrot, potatoes, cherries, and plums, for example, but there used to be thousands of varieties grown.

One result of overabundance is pressure to 'add value' to foods by processing, making it more costly to consumers (compare the cost of a pound of potatoes with a pound of potato chips). The producers of raw food (farmers) receive only a fraction of the price paid at the supermarket when it has gone through a corporate 'embalming ritual.' In 1998, for example, an average of 20% of the retail price of all food was returned to the farmer. With processing, the money is even more

---

190 William A. Albrecht, Ph.D., *The Albrecht Papers,* (Raytown, MO: Acres U.S.A., 1975), 177.

191 William A. Albrecht, Ph.D., *The Albrecht Papers,* (Raytown, MO: Acres U.S.A., 1975), 75.

unequally distributed, with the grower receiving as little as 5%.[192] The remaining 80 to 95% goes to the processor for machinery, buildings, labor, packaging, advertising, and transportation. It is better to buy fresh, organic, and local.

FOOD

Edgar Cayce, the sleeping prophet, frequently advised in his readings to eat food grown nearby, rather than shipped in. He said this will prepare the body systems to acclimate to a given territory more quickly than anything else. It is more important than the specific type of food.[193]

Nourishment is derived, not only from the nutrients in foods, but from their fields of energy as well. The subtle energy of food nourishes the energy field of the eater so it is healthier and less stressful to eat locally grown and seasonal foods whenever possible. As an important link with the environment, plant food harmonizes animals with the larger systems of the universe. Imported food will carry the energy of the environment of origin. Some people have written of the healing powers of such things as honey.

It is better to buy fresh, organic, and local.

NATURAL FOOD

Hybrid foods are a result of pollinating one variety of the same kind of plant with a different variety to strengthen certain characteristics, such as the ability to hold up in shipping. Many of America's favorite vegetables are highly hybridized, which means far fewer varieties now available than generations ago. When seed from a hybridized plant is replanted, it will grow, but is not likely to produce fruit like the plant it came from. These plants have lower life force energy than wild plants. Open-pollinated or heirloom (non-hybrid) produce tastes better.

Nourishment is derived, not only from the nutrients in foods, but from their fields of energy as well.

192 Marion Nestle, *Food Politics,* (Berkeley, CA: University of California Press, 2002), 17.

193 Ann Read, Carol Ilstrup and Margaret Gammon under the editorship of Hugh Lynn Cayce, *Edgar Cayce on Diet and Health,* (New York, NY: Paperback Library, 1969), 24.

Everything is a hybrid, of course. It happens all the time in nature. But humans often do it to breed out the reproductive part of a plant, as with seedless watermelon. This diminishes its vigor and natural urge to reproduce. Nature loves diversity.

SUSTAINABLE AGRICULTURE

At the heart of the New Age movement is a deep concern for the natural world—a sense of communion with the planet that sees it as a living, breathing biosphere deserving care and respect. In his book, *Atlas of the New Age,* Gerry Maguire Thompson writes, "The tree, with its roots deep in the earth, its branches in the air, exchanging spent breath for the life-giving oxygen in symbiosis with animal life, is a powerful symbol of New Age consciousness."[194]

Nature loves diversity.

A gardener does not need to become certified organic or biodynamic, just smarter—by watching what mother nature does. There are easier ways to grow healthier food, and often at less expense. Using old plants (especially hay) for mulch (instead of plastic), for instance, conserves and evens natural rain moisture to the plant root systems, suppresses weeds, and keeps the soil from becoming too compacted when tending and harvesting plants. Natural mulch protects the soil from extremes of temperature, does not pollute, and returns nutrients to the soil, increasing both organic matter and nitrogen in the soil. It feeds earthworms so they can loosen and fertilize the soil. In the spring it can be tilled in or pushed aside to insert new plants. It will be quite decomposed by then. This lowers the expense of watering. Both tiling (placing a network of tiles below the surface of the soil to drain off excess water during wet periods) and artificial watering (irrigating) wash nutrients from the field. Better to build up the soil so it will hold moisture as well as little microorganisms.

---

194 Gerry Maguire Thompson, *Atlas of the New Age,* (Hauppage, NY: Quarto, Inc., 1999), 7.

Crop rotation and planting cover crops assists nature to return nutrients to the soil. Growing heirloom plants and collecting their seeds saves money. It is easy to start plants indoors in early spring and is cheaper than buying from the nursery. It gives greater choice of varieties and can be grown without sprays. Plant a tree, even on someone else's land (with permission) so future generations will have fruit. Anonymous gifts to the future are so fun to give!

One of the great recent tragedies has been the abandoning of farmland by multitudes of farm families. People are healthiest and happiest when physically active outdoors in the sun and fresh air. Growing one's own food is a natural way to do just that. A garden of only two hundred square feet with a six month growing season can grow the yearly amount of vegetables consumed by the average American. According to the Department of Health and Human services the amount of exercise needed for physical, mental, and emotional health is about 20 minutes to a half hour a day. Interesting that the exercise provided by a garden is just about the amount needed for health!

In his book *Spiritual Foundations for the Renewal of Agriculture,* mystic Rudolf Steiner discusses the need to consider the cosmic as well as the earthly elements in restoring the earth for sustainable healthy food production. Biodynamic Agriculture grew from his lectures given in response to farmers who were concerned about the declining vigor of their crops and animals. It addresses the interaction between plants, animals, minerals, and the cosmic forces in this time of transition from the Kali Yuga (dark age) to a new Age of Light. He considers the soil an 'organ' of the Earth "organism."

Interesting that the exercise provided by a garden is just about the amount needed for health!

Biodynamic agriculture teaches us to read from the 'Book of Nature' with her cosmic rhythms and unseen teeming life below the surface of the soil. Beyond organic farming practices, it prescribes placing naturally occurring plant and animal materials, like dandelion blossoms, in natural locations such as in the earth, for a time—to absorb energy. The energized substances, called "preps," are then used in compost or spread directly on the land to assist the life forces of nature. Biodynamically grown food, having greater vital forces, stays fresh longer than the same foods grown by other methods. Studies have shown it to be sweeter and have more iron and other nutrients. It is a step ahead of organic and miles ahead of chemical farming, as it is not only sustainable but *healing* to the Earth.

FOREST GARDENS

The term "forest garden" was coined by Robert Hart to describe a method of producing food modeled upon woodlands with three layers of vegetation: trees, shrubs, and herbaceous plants. The trees put down deep roots, utilize the high sunlight and produce fruits and nuts. The shrubs also produce fruit, and the ground plants produce a diverse variety of vegetables, herbs, and seeds. Each garden is different, blooms in its own season, and strives to be harmonious with the earth and all other living things, especially the tiny life in the soil that turns organic matter back into rich soil. It may or may not contain a greenhouse and is ideal for a city back (or front) yard, roof top, balcony or porch. Forest garden ideas can be used on larger plots growing more food in a diversified and sustainable way.

ACCEPTING RESPONSIBILITY

Realizing that one is in control of what shows up in her life and, to some extent, the direction of all humanity, is an awesome responsibility. We all partake in the decision whether the Earth will return to life or become a barren desert. One person was overheard to say, "I don't want to believe it, because then I have to do something about it." This pretty much sums up a lot of people's attitude. If, however, humanity can learn to grow up and realize that to be really in control is exhilarating, then this life can be a great vacation trip to planet Earth. Don't trash the resort!

Realizing that one is in control of what shows up in her life and, to some extent, the direction of all humanity, is an awesome responsibility.

Nature's purpose is to assist humans to become conscious. Plants and animals have been willing to sacrifice themselves to that end, similar to the sacrifice of a loving parent who is willing to die to protect their young. But as humans have become over-indulgent, animals and plants have developed mysterious diseases, some becoming extinct. Animals have been willing to die to feed us in an emergency, but not to die unnecessarily and in a tormented fashion.

Nature's purpose is to assist humans to become conscious.

Is the environment where we were born to thrive worth decimating to be able to eat dead food that makes humans sick? Humans are part of a whole and when we have defecated in our own food bowl, how will we adapt to conditions of polluted air, soil, water, or food? How will we explain this to our great-grandchildren as they lie starving and anguished? In order to survive, conscious people who take seriously the 'stewards of the Earth' assignment must realize that change is needed. We must reach out to the feminine part of sisters and brothers across the globe and form not only a brotherhood but a sisterhood as well, agreeing to use masculine power only when absolutely necessary. The killing and destructive, abusive hierarchical male dominance must stop. Fear and violence must and will end when humans realize there is plenty of everything for all. We thrive only when we help all others thrive.

IMAGINE

Imagine what the impact of improved health of the population would mean. The resources currently used for sick-care could be redirected to ensuring that healthy food is accessible to all, resulting in a less fearful society. People would have more energy to communicate with each other, grow a garden, and enjoy the beauty of the arts, music, and books.

The Earth too would benefit if allowed to purify herself naturally without overwhelming pollutants. Human manure from drug-free people could safely be used for fertilizer instead of being toxic waste. Natural green skin would cover the nakedness of the Earth, and she could grow proud decorations of trees and flowers. Healthy plants would be more nourishing to animals, making their manure and dead bodies healthier for the soil. Conscious people use resources more wisely. It is necessary to stay warm; but if homes were consciously designed with earth-sheltering techniques, far less fuel would be needed to heat and cool the structure. Passive solar heating is amazingly effective even in very cold climates.

We thrive only when we help all others thrive.

Aging would no longer be synonymous with sickness. Healthy, vigorous elderly people would be perceived as wise and their advice consulted. With less pain, fatigue, illness, and fear in the world, it would be a more beautiful place to live. Dare we refer to it as the heaven described in religious literature?

Imagine the impact of a critical mass of humans who are conscious and physically able to hold the new energies in their bodies. Wisdom writings predict there will be a refreshing surge of peaceful people who have balanced feminine energies of inclusion, intuition, and community with masculine energies of courage, strength, and logic. Perhaps world peace may break out, giving rise to better distribution of the Earth's resources. If *all* children (of every age) were fed and loved, it would most certainly decrease the crime rate, freeing resources for education of children, adults, and elderly

Healthy, vigorous elderly people would be perceived as wise and their advice consulted.

alike. Joy in all types of relationships might be increased as a result of a kinder society.

If all children (of every age) were fed and loved, it would most certainly decrease the crime rate, freeing resources for education of children, adults, and elderly alike.

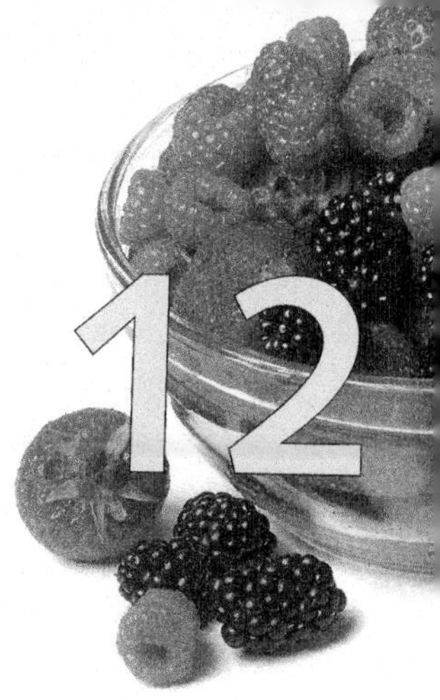

Profound Wisdom of the SELF

Knowledge, like wealth, is intended for use.

— The Kybalion

WE ARE BECOMING A NEW 'RACE'

Alice Bailey wrote, "A new kingdom is coming into being; a fifth kingdom in nature is materializing, and already has a nucleus functioning on earth in physical bodies. We are seeing the birth of a new and deathless race—a race in which the germ of immortality will flower and which divinity can express itself through the transfiguration of mankind."[195] Protestant foremothers sang of "Beulah Land," the "shining glory-shore."[196] Little did they know—it was right here on Earth. Spiritual teachers from all over the world write that with the opening of consciousness comes freedom from prejudices, bias, and fear. Shining glory emerges.

Russian spiritual teacher Helena Roerich writes, "Every epoch has its Call, and the calling foundation of the New Era will be the power of thought."[197] Roerich advises spiritual aspirants to use this attraction of like-minded thought to teach those who are ready

195 Alice A. Bailey, *From Bethlehem to Calvary,* (New York, NY: Lucis Publishing Company, 1965), 254.

196 "Beulah Land" written by Edgar Page Stites and Jno. R. Sweeney.

197 Helena Roerich, *Letters of Helena Roerich 1929–1938, Volume I,* (New York, NY: Agni Yoga Society, 1954), 3.

to accept. When a soul is ready for change, the organism itself will indicate what is required. In order to prepare for the new dimension, physical adjustments will need to be made. These preparations will be on all levels—material, physical, emotional, and thus spiritual. It is time to openly teach the 'Law of Attraction,' the knowledge that thinking is the greatest magnet—that thoughts attract their same vibration. By choosing thoughts, a person chooses what is to be attracted. Humans are one-by-one becoming conscious of their own divinity and immortality.

By choosing thoughts, a person chooses what is to be attracted.

Humans have always had spirit guides moving them toward enlightenment. There were unseen helpers at the signing of the Declaration of Independence, assisting in the Emancipation Proclamation, and the gaining of equality for women. But it must be hard for our 'friends in spiritual light,' with their higher vibration and divine wisdom, to watch as we are painfully slow to cease torturing each other, animals, and the earth. How can our guides have the patience to watch us childishly fight over religion, oil, and water? It must seem absurd to the angels that humans continue to see each other as threats and try to calm themselves by killing those they fear. At least human parents can see their children grow and learn in a few years. Humanity takes millennia!

It must seem absurd to the angels that humans continue to see each other as threats and try to calm themselves by killing those they fear.

A new KIN-dom

It is no longer a male dominated 'kingdom' but a new 'KINdom,' where everyone is a sibling. The masculine energies of competition, mental logic, physical strength, and hierarchy of rank will be balanced with feminine healing, inner wisdom, and inclusion—the return of a golden age of harmony, peace, and equality. The approaching great epoch is closely connected with the ascendancy of woman to her rightful place alongside her eternal fellow traveler and co-worker—

man; for the cosmos is built of dual origin and it is not possible to belittle one element of it. Roerich writes, "spirit has no sex,"[198] The future is equality for all.

Principle of Polarity

"The Hermetic Teachings are to the effect that the difference between things seemingly diametrically opposed to each other is merely a matter of degree [and] pairs of opposites may be reconciled."[199] This is the Principle of Polarity—heat and cold, light and dark, good and evil, love and hate, courage and fear, spirit and matter. The musical scale illustrates the principle of polarity; you start at "C" and move upward to another "C." Each note is the same with a matter of degree of vibration. Fear is only a few degrees from courage.

The future is equality for all.

The two poles may be classified as positive and negative. Love is positive to hate, courage to fear. The positive pole seems to be of a higher order than the negative and readily dominates it. The tendency of nature is in the direction of the dominant activity of the positive pole. Fear may be transmuted into courage and hate can become love by the use of the will. The spiritual universe moves in the direction of higher vibration where love overcomes fear. We will come to realize that fear from outside us cannot harm our love as dark cannot penetrate light. The sun always lights the night.

WHY IS HUMANITY HERE ON EARTH?

Our spiritual predecessors created the Earth of divine energy. Some of our foremothers got lost from the source of light and forgot who they really were. This created the duality of darkness and light, love and fear, which we see presently on Earth. Through the experience of darkness, we begin to long for light. The contrast of fear

The sun always lights the night.

---

198 Helena Roerich, *Letters of Helena Roerich 1935–1939, Volume II,* (New York, NY: Agni Yoga Society, 1967), 358.

199 Three Initiates, *The Kybalion, Heretic Philosophy,* (Chicago, IL: Yogi Publication Society, 1940), 150.

with the sweetness of love brings forth aspirants, seeking truth. But extreme duality need only be as temporary as withdrawal symptoms of detoxification of the body. The Earth is a school for learning to realize who we really are.

We are not here to suffer, however, nor to inflict suffering on other living beings. We were not intended to have short, painfully sad lives. We are here to have fun, to play with the devas (angels) and with each other. Somewhere we got lost in the anger and fear. During the next age, it will be easier to bloom into the flowers and fruit we were intended to be.

We are not here to suffer, however, nor to inflict suffering on other living beings.

Ancient wisdom writings teach that in this New Age of enlightenment, our task as awakening humanity is to "spiritualize matter," which is merely to fully realize that matter and energy are the same. That which is called "God" is simply the same substance of which each human is also made—the same as trees, water, and everything in the universe.

Nature works in magical ways if we stop thwarting her. When weeds reclaim a plowed field, they perform 'alchemy' that restores modified genes, breaks down poison pesticides, and actually creates needed minerals out of the elements that are available, restoring and purifying the soil once again. Nature's energy will likewise reclaim physical human bodies, cleaning the colon, purifying the tissues, and raising the vibration of the cells. Intentionally purifying one's body *is* spiritualizing it. When the physical is spiritualized, the mental tends to become positive with more life-giving conscious thoughts. Nature always moves in the direction of good.

Intentionally purifying one's body is spiritualizing it.

In her book, *New Cells, New Bodies, NEW LIFE!,* New Age spiritual writer Virginia Essene writes that human beings came to planet Earth in a body of dense matter with the intention of raising the planetary vibration to a state of love.[200] Her writings verify that during the energy shift that is occurring, the greatest challenge is to let go of fear. Each of us plays a valuable role in the divine plan for this planet's evolution. She also agrees that meditation is a doorway to self-knowledge ('no ledge—no limit'). According to Essene, many light workers may feel that they do not belong here, but *they are actually* the advanced souls who will lead. Life is an opportunity to demonstrate self-mastery in the use of the mind, for our thoughts serve a purpose higher than just one tiny personality. Negativity is simply useful feedback that you are out of sync with your real SELF. Essene describes our new bodies that are evolving as rainbows, "coats of many colors"—embodied "fountains of youth" sparkling with energy.

According to Essene, many light workers may feel that they do not belong here, but they are actually the advanced souls who will lead.

Humans are the meeting point of the mental and material—pure consciousness, which embraces both physical fruit and spiritual love. Every level of reality exists within each person, and is a fractal (small duplicate of the whole) of the omniverse. Contemplation of the purpose of existence reveals this is all there is! Each tiny fractal of the 'All' merely needs to look in the mirror to see her own inner wisdom. To realize the profundity of a breath, look in the face of any other being, human or animal. John White explains, "we are Spirit materialized, engaged in spiritualizing matter."[201]

Many are awaiting an external deliverer to save them. But New Age transformation is actually in the heart of each human who will personally experience their own intimate divine nature that was there all along. The idea that everything is ultimately connected and eternal is a common one among the great religions of the world. Becoming conscious of this involves effort—some exertion of will on the part of each person. Collective humanity will visualize a harmonious world and then make decisions to move in that direction.

But New Age transformation is actually in the heart of each human who will personally experience their own intimate divine nature that was there all along.

---

200 Virginia Essene, ed., *New Cells, New Bodies, NEW LIFE!,* (Santa Clara, CA: S.E.E. Publishing, 1991), 1–36.

201 John White, *The Meeting of Science and Spirit,* (New York, NY: Paragon House, 1990), xiv.

We are to let go of fear—fear of lack and fear of those whose ways are different.

Present humans are a sacred reflection of the new human species, which will be the embodiment of cosmic wisdom and love upon the living planet of Earth. We are partners with Earth in a cosmic awakening during this energy shift. We are to let go of fear—fear of lack and fear of those whose ways are different. When material possessions become less important, all will be free to explore everything in life: service, relationships, how and where we want to live.

As we relinquish linear time, there is an illusion that time has accelerated, leaving a peculiar feeling. These changes are temporary on our way to reassuming a higher frequency that we had before being birthed into physical bodies. Each person experiences these changes in a slightly different way as we heal and realize that love is all there is. There is an eternity of time.

WHAT WILL HAPPEN IN THE NEW AGE?

The Kybalion sheds more light on what the age of consciousness will look like. The hermetic Principle of Rhythm, states that everything has a forward and backward motion, ebb and flow, but the advanced student learns to polarize herself at the positive pole, refusing to participate in the backward swing. Will is superior to the Principle of Rhythm. The Principle of Cause and Effect states "every cause has its effect; every effect has its cause." But again spiritual aspirants, "knowing the rules of the game, rise above the plane of material life, and placing themselves in touch with the higher powers of their nature, dominate their own moods, characters, qualities, and polarity, as well as the environment surrounding them and thus become Movers in the game, instead of Pawns—Causes instead of Effects."[202] The 'higher' will always prevail against the 'lower.' A serious student of the natural laws will be able to aid others with her knowledge, but

202 Three Initiates, *The Kybalion, Hermetic Philosophy,* (Chicago, IL: Yogi Publication Society, 1940), 164, 165.

until we grasp the 'profound wisdom of our inner self' there will be confusion. "Knowledge, like wealth, is intended for use."[203]

So what is actually happening in this time of transition from Kali Yuga (the iron or dark age), to Satya Yuga (the age of light)? Why does it seem to be so hopeless with terror threats, economic collapse, violent video games, and nasty political campaigns that never seem to end? Even if one is aware that there is light dawning on the horizon, how does a light worker prepare to become a better conductor of divine energy in order to soothe and uplift her human siblings who are drowning in fear? Strong 'cornerstones' of organization are needed who are willing to welcome everyone—each a precious spark—into the New Age community. Feminine views of caring are gently sweeping over frightened, materialistic hierarchical cultures, reminding each person that they are actually made of love. What better purpose is there for being born?

No one seems to know for sure exactly how the New Age will unfold, because the script is impromptu and there are seven billion screenwriters; but it promises to be the best movie ever made. As the consciousness of the 'critical mass' is raised, we realize that we can make this planet into the heaven we seek—when we come to understand that there is no one here to ask but ourselves, no one but us to take over and guide the ship. Earth awaits our decisions but for most of us there is no choice. Love trumps fear.

No one seems to know for sure exactly how the New Age will unfold, because the script is impromptu and there are seven billion screenwriters; but it promises to be the best movie ever made.

Many seers have given descriptions of physical changes expected as the Golden Era begins, possible scenarios involving changes in the way we experience life on earth. Some say we will enter a photon belt, which will temporarily change the hours of night and day. The magnetic field might be altered so that neither electric nor battery-powered appliances work, requiring new (or old) forms of energy to be used. Changes in seismic activity and weather cycles can be expected.

---

203 Three Initiates, *The Kybalion, Hermetic Philosophy,* (Chicago, IL: Yogi Publication society, 1940), 213.

Many of the descriptions resemble commonly recognized events like lightening, earthquakes, volcanoes, and more unusual events related to the sun and moon, such as sunspots. Perhaps such events will last longer, be more intense, or trigger very unusual and unpredictable weather.

As the light gets brighter, shadows appear darker. Fear attracts fearful events; but as with any purification, when the detoxification and adjustment period are over, life will be vastly improved. In addition to the planet, the human body will change down to the very atoms of which it is made. The veil between spirit and matter is dissolving.

As the light gets brighter, shadows appear darker.

There may be physical sensations of being compacted or bloated, and there may be a time of darkness and cold, but this will only last a few days. It is important to remember that we are being assisted by spiritual helpers. Ask for assistance and then be confident of their perpetual love. People will be inclined to offer to assist each other, as they do during holidays or severe snowstorms. This is the dawning of the age of love and equality.

New Age does not mean the end of the world, but the end of an age—an end to the egocentric state of suffering. What will emerge is an awareness of paradise, a super-consciousness, and a peace which "passeth all understanding"—a direct experience of divinity. And it will all be right here!

When fear is dissolved and hearts are opened, grace, like a butterfly, will gently light upon our heads, making forgiveness easy. Really! Peace will seep in like rainwater into soft humus-rich soil. Vultures, flies, germs, and love will invade dead areas, digest the pain and cancers of the past, and restore our bodies, hearts, and minds to wholeness and holiness. The defining essence of the New Age's commencement is that the intense events will change humans from selfish, lonely, corrupt individuals in bondage, into beings of unselfish love and peaceful compassion. There will be a new vision of each of us as a part of the divine whole.

EVIDENCE THAT THE TIME IS NOW

Gregg Braden wrote in *Fractal Time* that the prophecies of Nostradamus, Edgar Cayce, the Aztecs, the Hopi, the Maya, and others point to the current time as the end of two cycles, two giant spirals of time that occasionally intersect.[204] There is strong evidence that this time, around the turn of the millennium, is when the Earth and her busload of passengers will pass through the darkest of times, both in terms of her position in the heavens and in terms of Earth conditions. Remember, these are really big cycles, so 'around' is a long time—hundreds of years! Don't expect exact dates to be predicted.

Liberals and conservatives argue over the cause of the phenomenon called "Earth changes" and both might prove to be right. Humans *have* polluted the soil and the atmosphere, causing deserts and drought, floods and mudslides, illness, and pestilence. That is the human lesson to learn. Nature is also at work assisting humans to purify body and mind by altering the energy stream, a plan already in place for this cycle. No one would refute the Earth changes occurring at this time are significant to life on Earth.

Remember, these are really big cycles, so 'around' is a long time—hundreds of years!

MENTAL AND PHYSICAL TRANSITION OF HUMANS

When knowledge of truth dawns in a person's heart, there is a feeling that all effort toward denial is for naught. The mental wall of resistance crumbles and one stands naked in the light. It often leads to a rearrangement of one's whole life structure—friends, home, partners, occupation, and lifestyle. It could mean risking the loss of approval, ostracism from friends and family, and the disintegration of

204 Gregg Braden, *Fractal Time*, (Carlsbad, CA: Hay House, 2009), 64.

the facade that served as an identity for years or decades. One could think of these times as birth-pains that are shared, each assisting the other to emerge. Like midwives, we help each other out of the darkness into the 'light.'

Like midwives, we help each other out of the darkness into the 'light.'

We and the Earth are in a "cosmic awakening experience" in these times of tremendous energy shift to greater consciousness, explains Virginia Essene.[205] "Physical structures are changing." This affects feelings, which can be unsettling. Illness and pain serve no purpose, however, so humanity must begin its own education about energy. Sending and receiving telepathic thoughts from others—both in this physical Earth and beyond—will be more commonplace. Confusion is expected when leaving the structured realm of third-dimensional consciousness and advancing to the sphere of instant manifestation in the fourth dimension. Essene writes "you are expanding into beings with the great flowing halos you have seen painted by artists of saints and angels."

Satprem was a student of the teacher simply called 'Mother' and her companion Sri Aurobindo. Mother and Aurobindo were pioneers, or experimenters, of the next species, wherein we will not leave matter but will find a new state while still in physical form. Satprem wrote of the journey Mother and Aurobindo traveled to discover how physical substance is evolving and will be capable of bridging the gap between the physical life as we know it and the 'supramental' life that will manifest. Satprem says, "The body is the bridge."[206] We can only truly understand with the whole body, for we are becoming a new species. The body must transform as we move to a new environment, as did the bodies of the primitive ocean species when they walked onto dry land. In the divine state of love, there is an electric, enhanced sense of realization, as the body itself changes consciousness.

---

205 Virginia Essene, ed. *New Cells, New Bodies, NEW LIFE!,* (Santa Clara, CA: S.E.E. Publishing, 1991), 2-10.

206 Satprem, *The Mind of the Cells,* (New York, NY: Institute for Evolutionary Research, 1982), 9.

Satprem concludes, "And yet, dammit, if evolution exists at all, it must take place in matter, in *our* matter."[207] In the new world, the conscious mind has authority over substance. The realization of truth must be done in the dense matter of the body, and the rational mind needs to get out of the way of that realization, for the cells of the body obey that mind.

In the divine state of love, there is an electric, enhanced sense of realization, as the body itself changes consciousness.

There is only one vibration in the universe—love—which is present in varying degrees in everything. This creates 'levels' of vibration that will rise as a person's mind realizes the profound wisdom available to it. This realization can be compared to dawn gradually penetrating the darkness. Consciousness is paying more attention to the love-based ethereal heart-wisdom urges than to the fear-based mental subconscious messages. Love tempts with the carrot, fear threatens with the stick.

Satprem says healing power is not *exerting* a 'higher force' through matter; instead, there is a 'contagion'-like transfer of higher vibration from purified matter to dense matter directly, like one candle lighting another. When the mind is calmed, lowering resistance in the tissues, the physical pain stops. A person can actually be in contact with their own cells, gaining knowledge of the body's consciousness at the cellular level. We can assist each other in healing the body, but consciousness is a matter of will and is a distinctly personal journey.

Love tempts with the carrot, fear threatens with the stick.

A caterpillar goes through a liquid state to become a butterfly. We, too, must 'melt' to find ourselves (perhaps this where the term 'melt-down' comes from). We don't literally melt, of course but it feels like it. We need to 'forget' what we have been taught and have practiced for a lifetime in order to embrace new truths. The universe is consciousness, matter is consciousness—humans are beginning to realize the extent of their own consciousness. We are not human beings; we are 'human becomings.' When the energy of the body is blocked and unbalanced,

---

207 Satprem, *The Mind of the Cells,* (New York, NY: Institute for Evolutionary Research, 1982), 35.

disease and entropy (aging) result. When our cells are in harmony with the rest of the universe, a comfortable transition into the new human species and the new 'KIN-dom' can take place.

Ken Carey, who was given information by "some alien, yet hauntingly familiar, intelligence," wrote the book, *Starseed Transmissions,* which has been described as a classic of intuitive knowledge and offers a new view of human evolution.[208] Carey explains that his messages came from extraterrestrial or angelic realms in non-verbal form to tell us about our true selves. He writes the 'words' of these angels: "There is but the filmiest of screens between your present condition and your true nature." The angel's purpose is to awaken humanity, for all are under a spell. The true nature of humanity is to be mediator between spirit and matter. The angels come to prepare people for an event—an interval of non-time when the "Creator will slip inside Creation." Biological reactions are being triggered by the increasing proximity of spirit within human bodies. There will be a time when the struggling with rational fear-patterns will stop. Each person will let themselves do the divine dance of inner direction, each in their own time. Carey writes, "One's life does indeed begin to change when one decides to work with the approaching forces!"

When our cells are in harmony with the rest of the universe, a comfortable transition into the new human species and the new 'KIN-dom' can take place.

The true nature of humanity is to be mediator between spirit and matter.

The angels predict that there will be increasingly two distinct worlds of consciousness (love and fear) and that this polarization will continue to intensify for a while. Humans have a choice between love and fear, life and death. Most will choose love and life. Angels are calling the awakened to get out of their head and be like little children playing in the wonderland of matter, letting go of guilt and fear by attending to the information coming from the source of infinite knowledge—the whispers in the heart.

It is said that in the near future current technological methods of communication will be rendered obsolete by one far superior:

208 Ken Carey, *The Starseed Transmissions,* (San Francisco, CA: Harper, 1995), 20.

the human mind. It is love that brings the sprouts in the spring, the fruit to the branch, and the transformation that enables humanity to speak with no need for words. It is obvious that animals and plants communicate with nature without fear of punishment from a fearful deity. Humans have even greater potential on the edge of their realization. Many can already feel it. Thoughts and feelings will be known instantly. Distance is no barrier; nor is death. When the emotions and intent of our human 'siblings' and other earthly creatures can be intuitively perceived, there will be no misunderstanding or need to fear each other.

Human beings are in a constant state of spiritual evolution toward expanding the consciousness of their real nature. The change in the air is almost palpable, which makes people nervous and excited at the same time. Humans are like radio receivers, and when the channel is adjusted, truth can be received from the mysterious higher vibration. The ancient Hermetic Principle of Correspondence, "as above, so below" teaches that humans are microcosms of the macrocosm—the universe is in each of us. In essence, we are collectively moving together back into the light—one by one we awaken to who we really are. It is written in both the Old and New Testaments of the Christian *Bible*, "ye are gods." (Psalms 82:6 and John 10:34)

When the emotions and intent of our human 'siblings' and other earthly creatures can be intuitively perceived, there will be no misunderstanding or need to fear each other.

DNA—DEOXYRIBONUCLEIC ACID (ALSO DISCUSSED IN CHAPTER 6)

Many spiritual writers predict that the DNA of our bodies will actually change in the transition to the New Age. DNA is the protein contained in the cells of the body that carries the genetic instructions used in the development and functioning of all living organisms; but it does not seem to have the final authority over our bodies, as was previously assumed. Epigenetics theory studies how genes can be turned on and off by experiences and environmental factors such as stress, toxins, and diet. It dispels the myth that genes account for absolutely everything.[209] Factors such as exposure to plastics, chemical 'fertilizers', medications, detergents, and pesticides that were introduced in the 1940s might explain the surge in obesity, autism and diabetes today, for example. These factors can also influence behavior, physical traits, and illnesses that genes alone cannot explain. Exposure to unnatural substances may alter the DNA a person inherited, changing who she becomes.

Bruce Lipton, a respected cell biologist, revealed in his book *The Biology of Belief* that human DNA can and does change to adapt to the physical and energetic environment. He writes that genes are merely blueprints to bring cells and the resulting tissues and organs into physical existence. These plans *can* be changed. The intelligence of the cell is aware, not only of the environment, but of our reactions toward and beliefs about it. Both our cells and the character of our life are based upon how we perceive them. Our perceptions shape our biology, which ends the myth that we are victims of the genes from our predecessors.[210] Our genes do not dictate our destiny, says Lipton, for nutrition, stress, and emotions are factors that can alter our gene structure. He writes, "Using prescription drugs to silence a body's symptoms enables us to ignore personal involvement we may have with the onset of those symptoms."[211]

Exposure to unnatural substances may alter the DNA a person inherited, changing who she becomes.

Lipton describes the conscious mind as "the creative one, the one that can conjure up positive thoughts," while the subconscious mind is "strictly habitual" and will play its repository of stimulus-response tapes derived from instincts and learned experiences over and over. It is these beliefs, not our genes, which control both our body health and our lives. Our beliefs, in fact, control our genes and DNA. The conscious mind

209 Lena Butler, "What is Epigenetics Theory? Myths and Facts," *Test Country Articles, testcountry.com* January 25, 2013.
210 Bruce Lipton, Ph.D., *The Biology of Belief,* (Carlsbad, CA: Hay House, 2009), xv.
211 Bruce Lipton, Ph.D., *The Biology of Belief,* (Carlsbad, CA: Hay House, 2009), 82.

can decide to change the program. He calls the new age the "return of White Light"—when every human being recognizes every other as part of the whole. Lipton writes, "Our job is to protect and nurture each human frequency so that the White Light can return."[212] This will result in humans who are evolved and come together in a loving global community with co-dominant females and males in charge.

Lewis Thomas, a medical doctor in the last century, writes in *Lives of a Cell*, "Man is embedded in nature."[213] Parts of our cells are actually separate animals that seem to work in our interest. Our DNA has come from all kinds of sources in nature, making us "assemblages of genes, formed by the emergence of mutants." He called viruses "mobile genes" who dart about rearranging the genomes of our DNA. Microorganisms usually happily coexist in a symbiotic relationship with us, and it is our *response* to their presence that creates the disease. Bodies seem to panic in the presence of some bacteria, launching our own explosive arsenal, releasing destructive mechanisms when the bacteria itself is not intrinsically poisonous. Human animals seem to self-destruct in the presence of substances carried by some bacteria, causing fever, hemorrhage, necrosis, and shock.[214]

Our beliefs, in fact, control our genes and DNA.

According to Thomas, we communicate with each other by means of unconscious or subconscious pheromones, sounds, and what he referred to as "collective thinking," much the same as insects. We think our way along, exchanging information and transforming the species collectively. He thought it best that way, for if humans took scientific control, they would lose fallibility, "the unpredictability, and total improbability of our connected minds." Scientists need to keep open all the options, as they have in the past, or risk getting stuck for a millennium. This collective thinking is what the New Age is about.

---

212 Bruce Lipton, Ph.D., *The Biology of Belief*, (Carlsbad, CA: Hay House, 2009), 164.
213 Lewis Thomas, *The Lives of a Cell*, (New York, NY: Penguin Books, 1974), 3.
214 Lewis Thomas, *The Lives of a Cell*, (New York, NY: Penguin Books, 1974), 75–80.

Each human, although in a dense physical body, is a reflection of the new human species, and her genetic patterns are of celestial nature. Each body contains genetic memory codes and intelligence factors to fulfill the evolutionary advancement. The actual physical structure, along with its genetic code, is changing with the powerful energy shift, and one of the greatest challenges is to let go of the fear caused by wanting to hold on to the familiar during the divine transformation. As humans originally descended from a non-physical state into dense flesh, the high frequency energy vibration was reduced, and now that process is being reversed. For this healing of humanity to happen, the cells must receive and retain more light, necessitating release of restrictions—physical conditions, emotional attitudes, and mental perceptions acquired during earthly life. We can trust our cells, for they are actually made of *light*.

This collective thinking is what the New Age is about.

In order for our DNA to change us into 'light bodies,' it is best if the cells are free of destructive substances—anti-life pills, 'cidal' sprays (pesticides, germicides, herbicides), and synthetic 'nutrients' from non-living sources. Living material from plant herbal complexes, like enzymes, are needed to restore energetic organization to the cells and the DNA. Pure, natural water must be present to carry oxygen for DNA production. Gene expression (what the genes tell the body and mind) is profoundly affected by the types and condition of the food we eat. Live, plant-based, organic food tends to turn *on* the 'healthy signal' from the genes inside the cells to the body as a whole.

Live, plant-based, organic food tends to turn on the 'healthy signal' from the genes inside the cells to the body as a whole.

SPIRITUAL TRANSITION

Dark Night of the Soul

Another aspect of the transition of humans is the spiritual 'dark night of the soul," which is similar to the physical 'detoxification withdrawal symptoms' and the mental/emotional 'healing crisis.'

There really is no spiritual detoxification, for when our physical, emotional, and mental issues are faced, resolved, and healed, the spiritual light stands awaiting the arrival of the pure self-actualized soul. But the facing, resolving, and healing take time and effort. It is new territory and always takes a different route for each of us because it is our personal inner darkness.

The point when awareness of spiritual energy begins, when we leave on the journey, is sometimes called the 'dark night of soul.' It can be a very scary process to realize that what is taught by authority figures—parents, teachers, doctors, ministers, and the Internet—is in error. As the spiritual lights 'dawn,' one light bulb at a time, it leads to the next awareness, and the next. Eventually, the dark tunnel which is life on Earth, becomes illuminated—a dazzling and shocking experience. There is no turning back—you cannot become unaware of a profound truth.

Dark nights of the soul are triggered by various events and take different forms. It might be a personal error (Self-Inflicted Nonsense) or a collective hypnosis (unconscious beliefs shared by many) that is coming into conscious awareness to be resolved. The process is leading to the light, but that light cannot be seen from the tunnel. Sensations of unfamiliar energy, waves of apparently 'unprovoked' ("out of nowhere") emotions, behaviors that seem involuntary, and uncanny coincidences are linking the world of inner realities with everyday life. They can be short 'ah-ha moments' or take years to unfold.

There is no turning back—you cannot become unaware of a profound truth.

Similar to what is referred to as a 'religious experience' (but without a denominational motivator), spiritual growth toward consciousness or enlightenment occurs when an aspirant becomes aware of errors in thought, word, or deed and makes an effort to see through the 'clouds' to disperse them, leading to forgiveness. Indeed,

The process is leading to the light, but that light cannot be seen from the tunnel.

sometimes enlightenment means to see that the clouds were placed there *by* religion. This process dissolves the blocks between humans and the bright light—'heaven' or 'nirvana.' Dark nights of the soul may be what are referred to in the Bible as the "valley of the shadow of death." People often describe a sensation similar to dying while awake. There is fear and yet there is not an identifiable stimulus for that fear. The world appears surreal for a while and many go from healer to psychic, to priest, to doctor for assistance. Each person has a unique set of 'clouds' and 'mean-bears' to wrestle, to which she is often *blind*, for she has been vehemently protecting these beliefs her whole life. It is much easier to see the errors in the thought processes of other people. It takes a persistent, willful intent toward achieving mental peace and physical health to dissolve our *own* blind spots. But dissolve they most certainly will.

There is fear and yet there is not an identifiable stimulus for that fear.

In her book, *Frontiers of Health,* medical doctor Christine Page describes "dark night of the soul" as a state of deep depression when consciousness has experienced and observed the different levels of duality of spirit and matter, heaven and Earth. These levels existed all along, but now become obvious. The light of the soul can be seen more clearly, like a candle seems brighter in a darkened room.[215] It can be described as the interim period between one state of being and the next and is often a very confusing time, when previous beliefs and goals are examined and changed.

Carol Parrish explains it further as a time when those seeking higher consciousness "penetrate beyond the realm of knowable things" and into the void or emptiness.[216] It is not really empty, of course; but since it is outside the familiar, material 'known world,' it seems that way. It is a period of transition, often precipitated unexpectedly by

---

215 Dr. Christine R. Page, *Frontiers of Health,* (Essex England: C.W. Daniel Company Limited, 1992), 28.

216 Carol E. Parrish-Harra, Ph.D., *The New Dictionary of Spiritual Thought,* (Tahlequah, OK: Sparrow Hawk Press, 2002), 66.

seemingly unrelated events or actions. Changing to a pure diet can be one of these actions.

It has been suggested that people who seem most vulnerable to over-indulging in mind-altering substances like coffee, alcohol, and drugs—even junk food—may be among the most sensitive of the population. They drink or smoke because they do not understand what is happening, and they find no one with whom they can discuss the frightening experiences. Spiritual teachers are all around but must be solicited, because to interfere unbidden is useless. These teachers are available to assure people who start on any spiritual path that the 'dark night of the soul' happens to all of us, until the darkness burns away, our eyes adjust to the brilliance, and we see the light more clearly. The aspirant then becomes a teacher to others.

The aspirant then becomes a teacher to others.

Psychotherapist Emma Bragdon writes of "dark night of the soul" as a time that often precipitates spiritual awakenings.[217] The experience can happen at any age. Often, when a person acquires the wealth so coveted in this society, there follows a deeper, more profound longing for 'something more.' Such people can experience spontaneous psychic happenings and physical distress such as headaches. Bragdon says the spiritual awakenings ultimately increase compassion and peace of mind. But the process can sometimes be difficult to distinguish from psychological disturbance, which, in contrast, causes people to become increasingly fearful, less energetic, and less interested in life. Bragdon notes how "interesting it is that the other side of seeing that you're not who you think you are is *freedom*." We each have angels to guide us.

Spiritual Emergencies

Profound realizations about the falseness of the beliefs of society can put a person off balance for a while and might even look somewhat

217 Emma Bragdon, Ph.D., *A Sourcebook for Helping People with Spiritual Problems*, (Aptos, CA: Lightening Up Press, 1993), 14, 47, 20.

like mental illness. This personal transformation is really part of the evolution of the consciousness of humanity, but to the individual is a 'spiritual emergency.' It can feel like your sense of identity is breaking down, that old values are no longer true. The ground beneath what was once called 'reality' is radically shifting. This can result in fear, confusion, and tremendous anxiety, causing difficulty in dealing with daily tasks.

Stanislav Grof, M.D., a psychiatrist, and his wife Christina Grof founded the Spiritual Emergence Network, which provides support for individuals undergoing transformative crises. In their book, *Spiritual Emergency,* the Grofs write that some of the dramatic experiences and unusual states of mind that traditional psychiatry diagnoses and treats as mental diseases are actually crises of personal transformation, or "spiritual emergencies." A play on words, it is a term "suggesting both a crisis and an opportunity of rising to a new level of awareness, or 'spiritual emergence.'"[218] The Grofs believe that these dark nights of the soul should be understood and supported instead of being suppressed, and they point out that "no organic basis has yet been found for the majority of problems psychiatrists treat." It is important to take a balanced approach and differentiate spiritual emergencies from genuine psychoses. There are professionals trained to recognize the difference.

Spiritual emergencies and mental health diagnoses can also be difficult to differentiate from a person doing emotional detoxification (healing crisis)—and these states of being are probably all interconnected. People having dark nights of the soul might find medication or other treatments unhelpful, yet are hesitant to dispute professional advice or diagnoses.

In general, spiritual emergence will be steadily leading a person to a more positive attitude and better health, to making better decisions

---

218 Stanislaf Grof, M.D., Christina Grof, ed., *Spiritual Emergency,* (New York, NY: Jeremy P. Tarcher/Putnam, 1989), *x*.

for themselves, and to acting with increasing kindness toward other people and all living things. There will be noticeable anticipatory positive excitement, as occurs, for example, when taking a really important step in life such as communion, being ordained, or falling in love. The mood, while scary, is also extremely positive and loving. Mental illness tends to be the opposite—creating dark, destructive thoughts, self-medicating, neglecting of responsibilities and the care of the body. Inner wisdom will guide both the initiate and those who love her to find the best assistance in any instance, just as it would when help for physical symptoms is needed.

Kundalini

A specific form of spiritual emergency can occur as an experience with kundalini. A yoga term, kundalini is life force energy or prana that is within each human. It is the primal force of the universe which lies in potential form at the base of the spine and, when channeled upward toward the brain, stimulates and purifies each chakra along the spinal canal. This process leads to a state of enlightenment and can be happening on several levels simultaneously. Many accounts are written about the experiences of people when this energy begins to rise, some reporting spontaneous movements and body sensations. Although it can be traumatic in its intensity, kundalini rising brings an awareness of our true nature and the profound greatness of the wisdom of the Self.

The familiar symbol of the medical profession, known as the caduceus, is thought to have evolved from the serpentine drawing of the kundalini and represents the balance toward wellness of spirit and matter. Perhaps the health care system and the spiritually awakened can begin to work together for the good of the whole human community.

WHAT CAN BE DONE TO PREPARE?

Having knowledge of the changes and knowing of the influence of thoughts and diet on energy is not enough. Action must be taken to emphasize any conviction. Whatever earth changes are coming, our preparations must, however, be positive and of both a mental and a physical nature. Acting upon a thought impresses its importance on the lower and higher selves who will then work to assist you. Talking about it is not enough.

> Take whatever action and make whatever material preparations you need to in order to calm your fears. Do all activities with love in mind, and prepare to assist your siblings. Guns will be useless and incite fear that is not valid. It might be helpful to have some extra clothing, dried food, water, and candles handy if you feel the need for physical preparation. Money and gold won't be of much use either, but hand gardening tools like shovels, and food preparation equipment like a hand grinder might be valuable. Organic open-pollinated (non-hybrid) garden seeds might be worth more than gold, kept in a cool, dry place and rotated yearly. Get a warm coat and fill some glass or food-grade plastic containers with water and perhaps a water filter. Seeds for sprouting and dried fruit and vegetables take up little space. This may serve to calm fears if done with a positive intent—"I am ready to embrace love and help others."

Take whatever action and make whatever material preparations you need to in order to calm your fears.

Read spiritual, love-filled material that attracts your curiosity. If reading a particular book scares you, put it down. Support causes that promote love and peace. Be prepared to assist others by dispelling fear. Each aspirant will become a little lighthouse of compassion. Accept and appreciate all others on your path. They, too, will bloom. In times past, aging was considered a good thing and will again be

Read spiritual, love-filled material that attracts your curiosity.

a goal worthy of admiration. People gain wisdom and do their best work after the children are grown. If you are an older person, lovingly offer your wisdom to others.

But the most important way a human can prepare for the new Golden Age is to focus on love. Fear is a block and is truly False Evidence Appearing Real and Self-Inflicted Nonsense (SIN). There is no need for it. When we love, our senses become honed like a fine-tuned radio which intuits the truth even when a person is speaking fear. We can see the blind spots and have compassion, which sends waves of healing. Visualize your human sibling bathed in love—especially if she passes into spirit in a mood of fear or despair, for growth continues after this slight change of clothes called 'death.' We are never really gone. Where would we go? We are all peacemakers and will band together—living and dead—to laugh, dance, sing, love, and breathe!

If you get the urge that it is necessary to change where you live or where you are standing *in each moment*, you will also know intuitively when, where to go, what to take, and how to get there. Intuitive aspirants will know how to tell others truths of love and peace without inciting alarm. The preparations are mostly internal and personal. The wisdom of the cells of the body will guide your path.

In preparation for the New Age, meditation is the most important fear-dispelling activity (see chapter 10). It is the key to accessing the right side of the brain. We put the body and mind in a state of restful watching and are thus able to wait until the harmonious universal intelligence begins to reveal her truth. Life begins to be seen through a different lens with full color and in 5D (fifth dimension—beyond matter). Our wiser, older self begins to take over and we simply soak up the love and pass it along. Meditation restores peace and harmony to our DNA as we dip our toes into the 'collective river of love.' Meditation aligns the physical, mental, and emotional aspects of

In preparation for the New Age, meditation is the most important fear-dispelling activity.

our being with cosmic prana. The living diet makes meditation occur much easier.

Service

The activities needed for transition to consciousness are a three-legged stool—education, meditation, and service. At some point spiritual aspirants discover a true and burning desire to be of service. In every relationship, *both* participants are the teacher *and* the student. We are here to be of service to our siblings—to comfort or to confront!

The living diet makes meditation occur much easier.

At every age a person learns valuable lessons that are then passed on to the next generations. It is natural evolution—cycles of life are continually repeated, adding new insights. Wisdom is a parent's ongoing gift to their child, and it does not end when they move out. Each phase of life embraces more difficult conditions—children at each new age master more complex ideas, sometimes from watching their elders and often by trial and error. Though not discussed as much after adulthood, this mastering continues to the end of life. Through service to others, both older and younger than ourselves, we learn compassion for each other and the planet. Take a child to your garden. Ask an elder for advice.

We are here to be of service to our siblings—to comfort or to confront!

Even a person who is totally physically paralyzed can render supreme service by spending their time and intention shining light on the path for other individuals, sending love energy where there is fear, and visualizing a world at peace. It is of the highest service to sit with a fearful person as they journey the "valley of the shadow," holding a mental 'flashlight' for them. We can act as a powerful battery, radiating love to that person—steadying her step, while *she does the climbing.* It does not matter if she is above or below you on the mountain, you can be there for her.

Service is best when there is an equal exchange of some sort of energy, money, information, or labor. The possibilities for 'fair-trade' deals are endless and not necessarily material. The service must be balanced. Even the most enlightened person still has lessons to learn, chores to be done, services they need, and still needs the prayers and love of others. Some of us need to learn to give and others need, *just as desperately*, to learn to receive. Very few have reached a balance. It is a dilemma: what is the right price to charge for a service? If, on the other hand, I take 'care' of another who is capable of caring for herself, I damage both of us. If I give without receiving it is as unbalanced as receiving without giving. And if you take a tax deduction, *that* is your reward.

If I give without receiving it is as unbalanced as receiving without giving.

Sacrifice

The word 'sacrifice' simply means "to make sacred."In other words, when we make a sacrifice for the right reasons, we turn fear into love—we change 'scared' into 'sacred.' Any time we give of ourselves in love, we create ripples of positive vibration that affect everyone. Similar to 'service,' sacrifice can be any form of energy, time, money, love, labor, or a material item. It might be a thoughtful gift, a tithe sent anonymously to a positive cause, volunteering to help someone learn to read, or just sitting with another in the shadow of the valley, either in person or energetically. It is a conscious choice to help. Sacrifice does not mean abusing yourself or letting others take advantage of you. It is not noble or necessary to suffer or worry, nor does it bring anyone closer to enlightenment.

According to New Age philosopher, Torkom Saraydarian, "to sacrifice means to do everything possible to bring cooperation, peace, and unity on earth and to reveal the divinity, latent in human beings."[219] He writes that to do this, an aspirant must develop intellect, love, and willpower. Willpower makes one the master of her physical, emotional, and mental nature and no longer victim of blind urges, drives, glamours, fear, anger, greed, or illusions. Saraydarian goes on to say that the purer our nature, the clearer will be the reception and translation from higher sources. A person whose physical, emotional, and mental 'bodies' are full of impurities will change the nature of a spiritual impression and might even misuse it.

The individual's role in the New Age is to turn her own body into a cup (chalice) by purifying herself so that she is able to hold the purer energies that are coming. We, too will discover what Ann Wigmore did: that we are all commissioned to build our own bodies into holy temples—'The Temples of the Soul'.[220] We begin to make our bodies sacred by purifying them of toxic food, drink, and other substances.

Discipline

Discipline is a funny thing. It can seem like a punishment or a chore or obligation if imposed by a person in authority who is ruled by fear. Sometimes a person has not been taught self-discipline or self-respect and needs to be controlled, even punished by society to protect others; but it should be done with love. Chores need to be done and we do have certain obligations to those who love us. This is not a discussion of control imposed by others like a spouse, a criminal, or a sexual or emotional abuser who 'disciplines' the other with fear. It is also not about institutional sets of rules that are fear-driven. To be dominated or repressed from outside yourself is not self-discipline; rather, true self-discipline is where you alone decide what truth is and how you want your life to be. We are discussing here the discipline of the SELF fueled by love, not fear.

---

219 Torkom Saraydarian, *Breakthrough to Higher Psychism,* (Cave Creek, AZ: T.S.G. Publishing, 1990), 9–10.

220 Ann Wigmore, *Be Your Own Doctor,* (Wayne, NJ: Avery Publishing Group, 1982), 25.

In disciplining one's SELF, it seems an obligation *only if it is not in alignment with one's own soul's purpose.* We have been taught to look for what is wrong with ourselves and the world, but all that is necessary to turn our lives around is to pay attention to what is right in our lives—the benefits, the delights of health, love, sunshine, and the inherent good of all people. What do you want to leave as your legacy? Who knows—while you are looking for good health and joy, you might get rich, find a soul mate, and become younger and more beautiful!

In disciplining one's SELF, it seems an obligation only if it is not in alignment with one's own soul's purpose.

Jill Bolte Taylor's stroke was on the left side of her brain—the rational, grounded, detail and time-oriented side and she was spared the intuitive right side, which observed her recovery. She tells of feeling at 'one with the universe' and learning that the state of Nirvana exists in the consciousness of our right hemisphere and that at any moment we can choose to hook into that part of the brain and experience bliss. She drew on the positive energy of people around her, but knew that how she chose to perceive each new experience was entirely up to her and that nothing external to herself could ever have the power to take away her peace of heart and mind. She identifies the goal as a healthy balance between the right and left brains and that the attention we give to a specific thought creates more impetus to those circuits to run again with minimal external stimulation (pathways). She writes, "We are designed to focus in on whatever we are looking for."[221] She stresses the importance of discipline and censorship, lest our minds run rampant on automatic. We must constantly tend the "garden of our mind," and it takes discipline to stay focused, for "the focused human mind is the most powerful instrument in the universe."[222] Most important, she states, "Our desire for peace must be stronger than our attachment to our misery."[223] Are you in your right mind?

---

221 Jill Bolte Taylor, Ph.D., *My Stroke of Insight,* (New York, NY: Viking, 2006), 139.
222 Jill Bolte Taylor, Ph.D., *My Stroke of Insight,* (New York, NY: Viking, 2006), 157.
223 Jill Bolte Taylor, Ph.D., *My Stroke of Insight,* (New York, NY: Viking, 2006), 171.

The joys of discipline are never tasted by the instant-gratification approach of undisciplined people. Of course, one can be disciplined to the point of rigidity, but the middle ground of discipline is useful in many aspects of life: diet, sex, meditation, study, and relationships. Parents with no discipline themselves raise unhappy, spoiled adult children. When will is strengthened by discipline, it gets stronger.

The Role of Diet

Almost without exception, spiritual writers who write about changes in consciousness of the New Age suggest focusing upon raw, fresh fruit in the diet to evolve a lighter body which will accommodate the higher energies expected in this time of transition. They also mention that *undue or excessive* attention to this aspect is not necessary and diverts the mental attention away from meditation and open receptiveness needed in this time of awakening.

When will is strengthened by discipline, it gets stronger.

Alice Bailey writes in *Esoteric Psychology*, "It is known esoterically that the vegetable kingdom is the transmitter and the transformer of the vital pranic fluid to the other forms of life on our planet. That is its divine and unique function."[224] She says those who endeavor to work upon the higher spiritual planes without doing harm, and to study the reflection of events in the spiritual light correctly, have to be, without exception, strict vegetarians. Only those who have been strict vegetarians for ten years can accurately work in the light. Their link with the vegetable kingdom is then very close and unbreakable and will lead them to the "scene of their investigations." But Bailey also cautions that unless a person has the goal to be of spiritual service it is futile to follow this form of diet.

Virginia Essene teaches that foods are thought-forms just like our body, and humans have the potential ability to transform any

224 Alice Bailey, *Esoteric Psychology I*, (New York, NY: Lucius Publishing, 1962) 241–267.

food, with thought, love, and intention, to a frequency that is totally beneficial to our bodies. But until humankind is fully empowered in this ability, our bodies will love some foods more than others. She explains that raw and organic fruits, flowers, vegetables, green leaves, roots, stems, soaked nuts, and sprouted seeds hold the greatest natural light and contain the elements that future humans will need for their evolution.[225]

In *Survival in the 21st Century* Viktoras Kulvinskas writes that "you become what you want to become" and that changing to a light, sunshine-filled, juicy-foods diet will lessen psychological, social, and physiological discomforts of the new changes.[226] But he cautions to be gentle and "construct a diet as good as your head can tolerate without losing the joy of living." We are all on the journey of enlightenment together and the right food can help reach that light.

Gastrosophy, a term coined by natural food pioneer Herbert Shelton, means the "wisdom of the stomach." It is the harmonious interlocking of production, preparation, and consumption of food. It is the grand field where the labors and arts of the garden, kitchen, orchards, vineyards, and conservatories all meet and mingle, and where the luxury of appreciation has been earned by the labors which have preceded it.[227] Eating a variety from the huge bounty of mother earth's buffet, alive with the love of the sun and the kisses of the Earth, helps the cells of the stomach and all the other cells come more alive. It is important to pay attention to the needs of the body as therein lie many spiritual blocks. The body and its components have sacred intelligences which are connected to each other.

We are all on the journey of enlightenment together and the right food can help reach that light.

Helena Roerich writes in her letters that it is important to eat a healthy vegetarian diet in order to remain able to do the work

225 Virginia Essene, *New Cells, New Bodies, New Life!,* (Santa Clara, CA: S.E.E. Publishing, 1991), 8, 60, 113.

226 Viktoras Kulvinskas, *Survival in the 21st Century,* (Hot Springs, AR: 21st Century Publishers, 2002), 21.

227 Herbert Shelton, *Superior Nutrition,* (San Antonio, TX: Willow Publishing, 1994), 167.

that is required for transition. She says that smoking as well as the immoderate use of alcohol will cause damage. Meat is harmful, as it fills the organism with decayed particles.[228]

When one pursues a diet of clean wholesome foods eaten in their natural live state, the sensibilities become keener and more delicate, the temperament becomes more flexible and tolerant, the mind emerges more alert and receptive to new ideas. The character becomes nobler and the soul more exalted. It is almost impossible to communicate the lightness of a living diet to a person who doesn't know she is barely surviving on cooked foods until she tries it. Like the Law of Attraction, it draws us to the best life possible in all ways.

EFFECTS OF NEW ENERGIES ON WORLD EVENTS

History shows there have always been 'fear parties'—groups of huddled, frightened 'sheeple'—factions of the population who, out of fear, seek to enact laws compelling people to follow their specific beliefs, or restricting the rights of another group. They mindlessly will resort to violence in order to squelch opposition because fear always blurs thinking. Spiritually conscious aspirants understand that fear comes from 'ignore-ance' of truth, and from being in a state of 'stupor' from toxic substances. Frightened children need to be loved. Love is the only way to soothe the angry, frantic and violent mobs, too scared to look beyond the tiny circle of like-minded people leading the attack. Always adjust your own oxygen mask before assisting others in a dark and fearful world. Light workers serve as peacemakers and teachers by *example* to the sick, depressed, and violent masses.

It is almost impossible to communicate the lightness of a living diet to a person who doesn't know she is barely surviving on cooked foods until she tries it.

Light workers serve as peacemakers and teachers by example to the sick, depressed, and violent masses.

In general the less attention that is paid to the screaming frightened parties, the sooner they will realize the folly of fear. Campaigns of 'fight against' (cancer, crime, drugs, terror, for example) merely serve

228 Helena Roerich, *Letters of Helena Roerich 1929–1938 Volume I,* (New York, NY: Agni Yoga Society, 1954), 145.

to magnify the problem. If you must walk the streets with a placard, make it a positive one like "wage peace." Humorists are vital keys in the defusing of frantic alarmist rhetoric. Both laughter and tears are purifying to mind and body. Do both with *gusto*, whenever possible.

As the light gets brighter, the shadows, by contrast, seem darker. When one spends a week at a spiritual retreat, the cacophony of the airport on the way home is unbearable. When one has been raised on mutual respect and compassion, abuse is abhorrent. Disrespect can only be tolerated by a person with a belief that it is 'normal.' As spiritual aspirants discover the power of love, it makes the fear-sellers *seem* louder, in contrast. Remember, fear is False Evidence Appearing Real—an illusion.

Highly evolved people will eventually occupy key posts in government and local and world organizations. Important changes will be enacted by awakened government and cooperative religious leaders operating from their higher spiritual consciousness. In fact, American philosopher, Henry Thoreau, who influenced such peacemakers as Mahatma Gandhi and Martin Luther King, wrote, "This I believe, 'That government is best which governs not at all'; and when men are prepared for it, that will be the kind of government which they will have."[229]

Sensitive people are becoming aware of the light and love presence that is being radiated to mankind. There is change and transfiguration occurring because "new wine cannot be put into old bottles." Enlightened spiritual leaders will come from surprising backgrounds. These quiet leaders will be ridiculed and opposed but will prevail as humanity awakens. The attributes of love and peace will unite all women and men of goodwill throughout the world. There will eventually be a physical sharing of all world resources so bountifully

---

229 Henry D. Thoreau, (Edited by Oscar Cargill), *Henry D. Thoreau, Selected Writings on Nature and Liberty,* "Civil Disobedience," (New York, NY: Liberal Arts Press, 1952), 10.

provided by nature, and all forms of malnutrition and starvation will disappear. The movement toward a living food diet and sustainable agriculture are part of these changes.

HEALING IN THE NEW AGE

The movement toward a living food diet and sustainable agriculture are part of these changes.

In ancient Greece, some four centuries before the time of Jesus, doctors practiced a different kind of medicine. A sick person would go to a temple, make an offering to the gods, and then purify themselves with diet, baths, and abstinence. The temple, where they would sleep as part of the healing process, was open on all sides to fresh air. During sleep Asclepius (translation: "cut-up"), the god of medicine in Greek mythology, would come and remove the disease or give instructions for healing. The patient needed to ask, to believe in the power of the 'prescription', and take the action necessary for healing.

Nonphysical spiritual healers are still here and more willing than ever to assist us to heal our physical bodies. Perhaps Asclepius himself is still 'practicing.' We must do our part by making the decision to be supremely healthy, wealthy, and wise—ask for assistance, do the purification that seals the intention, and then allow the mysterious restoration to take place. You can trust your heart and your body.

You can trust your heart and your body.

Hygieia, Asclepius' daughter and the goddess of health, was celebrated for promoting health as the natural order of things. Health is a positive attribute to which people are entitled if they govern their lives according to the laws of nature. She believed sins against nature are inexcusable and the inevitable 'law of compensation' [karma] must be obeyed. Your body gets what you give it. Maybe we can consult with Hygieia, too.

Many spiritual writers imply that once a person realizes that 'all is one,' it is not necessary to die any more. Death is but a group agreement that people believe has to happen; they even set an approximate time frame for its occurrence. Breaking away from the group won't be easy for modern people with their ingrained habits of living and thought, but ancient writings say that with the new energies, we *can* return to the paradise we originally inhabited. We have the genetic possibility. This current body can last forever if we wish it so—perfectly healthy and happy by living according to the laws of nature. Nature tends to flow in the direction of the dominate positive pole, and the advanced student learns to polarize herself at the positive pole, refusing to participate in the negativity that seems to dominate society.

Just as each person has a unique fingerprint, each also has a different soul purpose, history, lesson plan, and path to follow. This may include disease, war, violence and other extremely difficult experiences. As confounding as it is to find your own personal goal, so much the harder is it to figure out another person's path. Sometimes, however, an intuitive message will come that is for another person and can be of profound assistance, if shared with love. Generally, individual paths are left to the aspirant herself to discover. Since we cannot pretend to know what is right for someone else in any particular time (even our own children), it is inappropriate to pray for a specific outcome for them. It is best to send love to light their path so they may see clearly for themselves. We can assess the energies of another but cannot attempt to alter them or heal them without permission or request.

This current body can last forever if we wish it so—perfectly healthy and happy by living according to the laws of nature.

THE NEW ROLE OF COMMUNITY

Spiritual writers also emphasize that we are to work together in groups in order to enhance contact with spiritual helpers and inner wisdom. This New Age is the 'age of community.' We become transparent to each other with new mental telepathy. Children have always had this ability but learn to deny the truth to please grown-ups. In a way, when each of us gains new insight, we all gain. Spirit then,

This New Age is the 'age of community.'

is a collective—a co-op dealing in all commodities of truth and love. We work like a team moving the ball of awakening up the mountain of knowledge. Some souls carry the ball longer and for the steeper climbs than others, but we all get to enjoy the view. It is impossible to leave anyone behind, for all are equally important.

Aart Jurriaanse, writes that an "overwhelming spirit of goodwill," an increased magnetic force, is now in the process of streaming in from the spiritual hierarchy.[230] This is creating a metamorphosis in those who are sensitive, no matter what religion or ritual is practiced. Dark or fearful people of hate, selfishness, ignorance, sarcasm, and greed will need assistance to adjust to love energies. He writes, "The etheric atmosphere is literally tingling with the energies." The increased energy will rapidly change attitudes in government. All levels of human relationships will evolve to manifest the inner good in each person, resulting in sharing of the world's resources.

The peaceable KINdom comes with education and consciousness of *each* member of the human society. Corporations that succeed will be the ones who nurture the health of their customers, employees, stockholders, member/owners, and the world. Each person has unique issues and examining them is a shared road. Without raising consciousness these issues will remain a powerful driver of individual minds and lives. Unconscious people will follow the fearful into war, panic over shortages, mob mentality, and cruelty. The spiritual aspirant learns to hold the flashlight for others. Light dispels the darkness, so light one little candle, *you*!

QUANTUM PHYSICS AND THE LAW OF ATTRACTION

Quantum theory, which no one seems to really understand, attempts to explain how light and matter behave at the subatomic

230 Art Jurriaanse, *Bridges*, (Johannesburg, South Africa: Aquarian Book Centre, 1986, no copyright) (This book is dedicated to Humanity without reservation. Man's versions of the Truth should not be offered with restrictions), 214–220.

level. It is the basis of all modern electronic devices. It introduces an 'uncertainty principle,' where a particle may have an abrupt transition from one discrete energy state to another and implies, philosophically, that experiments are affected by even a noninvolved observer. Quantum theory says that before observation there is only a probability about the state of a particle and that measuring it forces the decision, determining which state will be found. It is therefore not possible to observe reality without changing it, because it is not possible to be without an opinion and truly objective. The observer then creates her own reality.

Light dispels the darkness, so light one little candle, you!

Gary Zukav writes, "We are actualizing the universe." He goes on to explain that since we are part of the universe, we too, are self-actualizing. Every person is recognized as a divine manifestation. It cannot be otherwise. Humanity relinquished this authority to scientists and now the scientists are passing the power back. "We are not sure," they tell us, "but we have accumulated evidence which indicates that the key to understanding the universe is *you*." "The new physics [quantum physics] sounds very much like old eastern mysticism."[231]

Science is discovering spiritual energy. Quantum physics demonstrates that tiny particles are conscious and that they process information. They respond to human thought and decisions without regard to location, so we are always a part of our own environment. Quantum theory, in essence supports the Law of Attraction.

It is therefore not possible to observe reality without changing it, because it is not possible to be without an opinion and truly objective.

WE EACH ARE A GROUP OF 'SELVES'

As we grow, become conscious, and evolve it becomes clear that our human personality is a composite—a collective—a 'family' of 'selves.' An adult is still the infant, child, and youth she has been,

231 Gary Zukav, *The Dancing Wu Li Master, an Overview of the New Physics*, (New York, NY: Morrow Quill Paperback, 1979), 102, 96.

as well as the adult she is, and the wiser, older woman she will be (and perhaps was before she was born). The mental adult has control of the decision and direction of the entire entity called "I," whether she chooses to grasp that concept or not. The infant subconscious merely wants to be fed, held, loved, and to feel safe; she is resilient and forgiving, but also can remain terrified long into maturity if those needs are not met. The school-child's subconscious self loves discipline and fun. She tries to see what she can get away with and will live on sugar and take risks unless guided to see the long term consequences of her behavior. She can feel lost without routine, but can take rules to an extreme and become inflexible or rebel against those same rules. The youth loves drama and is fearless, confused, and full of enthusiasm. A teen wants to embrace all her urges and, impatient with caution, is reluctant to believe her actions can cause long-term harm. The mental adult is in charge, but often refuses to admit this awesome power as she resists the nudges from her older wiser self, who sees the benefits to be reaped by paying attention to all her parts. The adult is the committee chairperson and can direct attention to each as needed, steering the 'whole' toward 'decision by consensus.'

The midlife adult determines the length of life, the relative wealth and lifestyle, the moral code that is adopted, and the legacy left behind. The wise mature crone knows that the will of her other 'selves' needs to be left intact. The younger versions of herself that still live inside need to be subtlety taught by example, gently appealing to their interests. They can be appropriately rewarded and can be reasoned with by pointing out successes which will be more fruitful than preaching and scolding. Give your infant attention, your child a dish of (raw) ice cream and your teen a new skirt for overcoming some fear. Reward yourselves.

The adult is the committee chairperson and can direct attention to each as needed, steering the 'whole' toward 'decision by consensus.

The individual adult can be likened to humanity who has memories of dark as well as thrilling happy times of the past. Humanity is approaching maturity. The human collective is on the brink of deciding to embrace all aspects of herself, heal the broken parts, heed the wisdom from wiser nonphysical helpers, clean her room (called Earth), and learn to get along peaceably with her siblings. Or she can ignore the warnings and indulge herself in sugar, perpetual war, and driving drunk off a cliff. Each human 'I-voice' gets a vote and can campaign for the outcome of her choice. The decision is up to the 'cooperative of Earth-babies.'

Give your infant attention, your child a dish of (raw) ice cream and your teen a new skirt for overcoming some fear. Reward yourselves.

EREWHON: AN EXAMPLE OF ANOTHER WAY OF THINKING

Erewhon, a 17th century novel written by Samuel Butler, portrays a traveler who stumbles upon an isolated society where the thinking is much different from the ideas of our world and presents an interesting pause for consideration. In Erewhon, for example, illness of any sort is considered highly criminal, shameful, and is severely punished, as is being poor, having bad luck, or being abused by another. It is a crime to be unfortunate. But a person who commits forgery, arson, embezzlement, even murder, is considered to be suffering from "immorality" and is put in a hospital, visited by friends, and is sent to a "straightener" (one who bends back the crooked) for painful 'treatments,' close confinement, or sometimes cruel physical tortures; yet people do not refuse the treatments. People actually pretend to be immoral (excessive alcohol use, for example) to cover up an illness. Their laws are intended to emphasize the "decrees of nature."

How much more a stretch is this than to pretend to be ill to cover a drinking problem, as done in present society? Aren't illness and fortune actually within our control as much as we believe it so for crimes? We are often deaf to the pleas of a criminal who was abused, yet believe that illness is thrust upon us from the outside.

Concerning diet, *Erewhon* tells of 'experts' who led them on several diet fads which were accepted as fact, some of which became laws. Butler writes "...that which we observe to be taken as a matter of course by those around us, we take as a matter of course ourselves." He comments, "so engrained in the human heart is the desire to believe that some people really do know what they say they know, and can thus save them from the trouble of thinking for themselves..." Butler concludes, "Indeed I can see no hope for the Erewhonians till they have got to understand that reason uncorrected by instinct is as bad as instinct uncorrected by reason."[232]

I include this story because we too are led by others who claim to know what is 'best' for us without considering the truth of the recommendation or what the 'prescriber' stands to gain from our buying into their plan. Eating and doing what others do is easy; being conscious takes more effort. Instinct and reason must be balanced. Seek your own truth.

THE NEW EARTH

Eating and doing what others do is easy; being conscious takes more effort. Instinct and reason must be balanced.

The Earth in the New Age will be the one we humans collectively *predominately* visualize. One person alone cannot bring about a new higher consciousness for the planet, but each individual holds a thread that weaves the tapestry which determines the destiny of the whole. Utilizing the assistance of the new energies we can create the world we truly want to live in—the one Jesus, Thoreau, Gandhi, and King envisioned.

Each one walks a different path, as a different aspect of 'creator energy.' 'Be still' and 'know' which path is best for you. Get out of your

232 Samuel Butler, *Erewhon,* (Mineola, NY: Dover Publications, Inc., 2002—unabridged, unaltered replication of 1901 revised and expanded edition of the work originally published in 1872), 150.

mind and drift into the profound wisdom of your SELF. How do you want the book of your life to end? Where do you fit in the process of the birth of the New Age? Ask your wiser, higher SELF "What is mine to do?"

In times to come
Human beings will have to exist
The one for the other
And not the one through the other.
Thus is reached the world's ultimate aim:
That each one is with themselves
And each would give to the other what none would demand.

—Rudolf Steiner

Appendix A

Spiritual Effects of Live Food (S.E.L.F.) – Data Collection Documents

Student name____
Address____
Phone__________________ Email____________________________
Date______________________ Intake_____ Grad_____ FU_____
Birth date__________ Age____ Sex ____Occupation (opt)___________
Please list your CURRENT diagnoses______________________________

PHYSICAL SYMPTOMS

Please show to what extent you have these physical symptoms, using the phrase "I have ____" (if applicable).

I HAVE:	NONE	LITTLE	MODERATE	LOT	OVERWHELMING
Poor general health					
Fatigue					
Tremor					
Restlessness					
Offensive body odor					
Lack of energy to do what I like to do					
Excessive body weight					
Too little body weight					
Bad complexion					
Itchy skin					
Wrinkles					
Sores on my skin					

Skin that bruises easily					
Dry skin					
Excessively dry hair					
Stiff joints					
Pain in joints					
Pain when I exercise					
Poor flexibility					
Trouble walking					
Runny nose					
Chronic cough					
Asthma/hay fever					
Shortness of breath					
Trouble getting to sleep					
Trouble staying asleep					
Excessive hunger					
Nausea					
Craving for meat					
Craving for sugar					
Craving for cooked foods					
Craving for coffee/chocolate					
Belching					
Constipation					
Diarrhea					
Stools that smell bad					
Lack of appetite					
Flatulence					
Indigestion					
Abdominal pain or pressure					
Hard stools					
Hemorrhoids					
Painful Bowel movements					
Low Blood sugar					
Rapid heart beat					
High Blood Pressure					

I HAVE:	NONE	LITTLE	MODERATE	LOT	OVERWHELMING
Swollen feet or legs					
Hot flashes					
Sexual difficulties					
Numbness					
Body aches					
Headaches					
Allergies					
Tobacco cravings					
Drug cravings					
Paralysis					
Muscle weakness					
Female: Menstrual problems					
Sore breasts					
Vaginal infections or vulvar itching					
Excessive Sleep					

Please add any comments about your physical health:

EMOTIONAL STATES

Please show how often you have these feelings, using the phrase "I feel ____".

I FEEL:	NEVER	AT TIMES	OFTEN	A LOT	ALWAYS
Resentful					
Unhealthy					
Picked on					
Useless					
Sad					
Humorless					
No interest in things					

I FEEL:	NEVER	AT TIMES	OFTEN	A LOT	ALWAYS
Helpless					
Fear about the future					
I am unattractive					
Unsupported					
Annoyed or Irritable					
Like crying					
I am unable to cry					
Guilt over something					
Ashamed of myself					
Out of control					
Stressed					
Incompetent					
Anger out of all proportion					
Confused about good food choices					
Hopeless about future					
Disconnected from other people					
Unsure of myself					
Depressed					
Panic attacks					
Fear for no reason					
Excessive worry					
Excessive shyness					
Moodiness					
Indecisiveness					

What do you see as factors that influence a person's decision to "go raw"?

Please add any comments about your emotional health:

MENTAL SYMPTOMS

Please show how often you have these symptoms:

I have:	NEVER	ATTIMES	OFTEN	A LOT	ALWAYS
Grogginess in the morning					
Trouble concentrating					
Trouble getting organized					
Mental stress					
Lots to worry about					
Trouble learning new things					
Negative thoughts					
Lack of discipline to eat what I know is really good for me					
Lack of clear goals for my life					
Few good friends					
Lost my mental sharpness					
Poor memory					
No discipline in my life					
A cluttered home					
Trouble finding things					
Trouble being on time					
Procrastination problems					
Trouble meditating					
Forgetfulness					
Bad thoughts about myself					
Lack of willpower					
Laziness					
Trouble remembering					
Problems calming my "logical" thinking					
Mental confusion					
"Foggy" thinking					
Trouble understanding what others mean					

Please add any comments about your mental health:

SPIRITUAL BELIEFS

Here are some spiritual statements. To what extent are they true for you?

SPIRITUAL BELIEFS/FEELINGS:	NEVER	AT TIMES	OFTEN	A LOT	ALWAYS
Dreams are important					
I am in control of my life and health					
I enjoy my life					
Meditation is easy for me					
I can trust my instincts					
Tolerant of others					
A connection with a nonphysical energy					
My life has bigger meaning					
I am responsible for my life condition					
I am a Divine being					
Life has purpose					
The creator is loving					
Grateful for what I have					
Love for God					
Love for myself					
I can follow through with my intentions					
I deserve good health					
There is a "higher plan" for my life					
I am more than just a body					
I can forgive myself when I make mistakes					
I can accurately tell what others are feeling					
Peace of mind					
My "inner guide" will lead me to good health					

SPIRITUAL BELIEFS/FEELINGS:	NEVER	AT TIMES	OFTEN	A LOT	ALWAYS
My life has worth to the world					
I can trust my "inner guide" in choosing food					
There are lots of people who will help me if I ask					
We have guardian angels					
I deserve to be loved					
I can trust in "Divine Order"					
God loves me					
I am using my talents					

Please add any comments about your spiritual health:

Please list all prescription drugs, nonprescription drugs and supplements you take:

RELEASE: I hereby grant permission for Janet Allen to use the above information, for any research, studies, or publication on the general subject of health and well being without using my name or personal information. I understand published written work may be sold for profit.

Name (print)____

Signature____

Appendix B

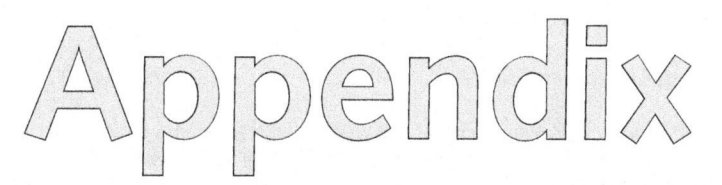

Spiritual Effects of Live Food (S.E.L.F.)—Study Results by Individual Student

Table 1, *Participant Number 1*

Student number one, M.G., is a strong, attractive, single, 35 year old Hispanic woman with no serious health problems. She became interested in natural health by reading author Kevin Trudeau. A mother of one teenaged boy, she teaches parenting to "at risk" families in a large city, and was in the process of breaking up with her boyfriend. At graduation she said "I was a wreck when I came and I learned to forgive and I learned to be grateful. "

Student # 1 M.G.	Physical		Emotional		Mental		Spiritual	
Total problems at intake	29	N/A	28	N/A	23	N/A	19	N/A
Problems resolved at graduation	20	69%	26	93%	15	65%	4	21%
Problems improved at graduation	9	31%	1	4%	5	22%	10	53%
Total either improved or resolved at graduation	29	100%	27	97%	20	87%	14	74%
Problems unchanged at graduation	0	0%	1	3%	3	13%	4	21%
Problems worse at graduation	0	0%	0	0%	0	0%	1	5%

Table 2, *Participant Number 2*

Student two, C.H., is an outgoing 72 year old single male, retired medical technician, with diabetes and obesity. At graduation he had lost 17 pounds, his blood pressure had gone from 132/70 to 104/60, his blood sugar went from 260 to 140, and his swelling of his lower legs went from 3+ to 1+. At graduation he said "my blood sugar hasn't been down to 100 in years," "the equipment is home waiting for me" [to continue eating the live food diet].

Student # 2 C.H.	Physical		Emotional		Mental		Spiritual	
Total problems at intake	21	N/A	23	N/A	17	N/A	16	N/A
Problems resolved at graduation	6	29%	21	91%	13	76%	4	25%
Problems improved at graduation	7	33%	0	0%	2	12%	7	44%
Total either improved or resolved at graduation	13	62%	21	91%	15	88%	11	69%
Problems unchanged at graduation	5	24%	2	9%	2	12%	3	19%
Problems worse at graduation	3	14%	0	0%	0	0%	2	12%

Table 3, *Participant Number 3*

Student three, M.P., was a 55 year old woman with glaucoma problems who felt changing her eating habits was "the last straw" if she wanted to get well and remains 100% raw after one year. She had dizziness during her program but felt it was a mineral imbalance and was still glad she came. Before she came she said she was determined to get rid of the glaucoma herself and to avoid surgery. At graduation she said she had been influenced by Elizabeth Baker to change her diet to raw vegetarian and since she usually never goes outside her "comfort box" she was glad her family did not come with her.

Student # 3 M.P.	Physical		Emotional		Mental		Spiritual	
Total problems at intake	14	N/A	19	N/A	22	N/A	13	N/A
Problems resolved at graduation	10	71%	19	100%	22	100%	10	77%
Problems improved at graduation	0	0%	0	0%	0	0%	0	0%
Total either improved or resolved at graduation	10	71%	19	100%	22	100%	10	77%
Problems unchanged at graduation	4	29%	0	0%	0	0%	2	15%
Problems worse at graduation	0	0%	0	0%	0	0%	1	8%

Table 4, *Participant Number 4*

Student four, C.B., is a 46 year old married woman who is an accomplished artist, with acid reflux, seborrheic dermatitis, and insomnia. She was a devoted daughter and brought her mother with her (subject number five) to CHI. At graduation she said she was committed to two months at 100% raw and indeed she stayed 90% raw for two months (until her mother became terminally ill).

Student # 4 C.B.	Physical		Emotional		Mental		Spiritual	
Total problems at intake	28	N/A	12	N/A	21	N/A	21	N/A
Problems resolved at graduation	22	79%	12	100%	18	86%	14	67%
Problems improved at graduation	2	7%	0	0%	2	10%	6	29%
Total either improved or resolved at graduation	24	86%	12	100%	20	96%	20	96%
Problems unchanged at graduation	4	14%	0	0%	1	4%	1	4%
Problems worse at graduation	0	0%	0	0%	0	0%	0	0%

Table 5, *Participant Number 5*

Student five, N.B., was an 83 year old woman from Michigan, mother of C.B., whose husband is in an adult care facility with dementia. N. B. complains of severe shortness of breath and was on many prescription medications. She said she was disappointed the surgery she had to help her breathing (heart valves replaced and fluid aspirated from around her lungs) did not help much. On intake she left many blanks on the questionnaire, but on the graduation form she just missed one (mental) page. She died in January, 2008.

Student # 5 N.B.	Physical		Emotional		Mental		Spiritual	
Total problems at intake	13	N/A	6	N/A	0	N/A	13	N/A
Problems resolved at graduation	0	0%	2	33%	0	0%	1	8%
Problems improved at graduation	3	23%	0	0%	0	0%	6	46%
Total either improved or resolved at graduation	3	23%	2	33%	0	0%	7	54%
Problems unchanged at graduation	9	69%	4	67%	0	0%	4	31%
Problems worse at graduation	1	8%	0	0%	0	0%	2	15%

Table 6, *Participant Number 6*

Student six, K.B., is a 60 year old woman from Georgia who loves to golf. She had high blood pressure and high cholesterol. She dropped ten pounds and lowered her blood pressure from 172/100 before to 130/78 after the course.

Student # 6. K.B.	Physical		Emotional		Mental		Spiritual	
Total problems at intake	21	N/A	20	N/A	24	N/A	12	N/A
Problems resolved at graduation	5	24%	14	70%	7	29%	8	67%
Problems improved at graduation	6	29%	1	5%	3	12%	2	17%
Total either improved or resolved at graduation	11	52%	15	75%	10	42%	10	83%
Problems unchanged at graduation	9	43%	5	25%	14	58%	2	17%
Problems worse at graduation	1	5%	0	0%	0	0%	0	0%

Table 7, *Participant Number 7*

Student number seven, C.J., from Virginia is the 62 year old sister of subject six and is a professional dog trainer. C. J. had high blood pressure and cholesterol and while she dropped thirteen pounds during the program, she did not see the change in blood pressure her sister did. Her follow up form shows a note stating she knows she is an "addictive" type and must do it "all or nothing" because alcohol, breads, fats, and sugar are hard for her to manage. She said, "It is not easy giving up all that comfort. "

Student # 7 C.J.	Physical		Emotional		Mental		Spiritual	
Total problems at intake	29	N/A	20	N/A	23	N/A	0	N/A
Problems resolved at graduation	9	31%	2	10%	0	0%	0	0%
Problems improved at graduation	17	59%	2	10%	2	9%	0	0%
Total either improved or resolved at graduation	26	90%	4	20%	2	9%	0	0%
Problems unchanged at graduation	3	10%	14	70%	19	83%	0	0%
Problems worse at graduation	0	0%	2	10%	2	9%	0	0%

Table 8, *Participant Number 8*

Student eight, B.N., is a 62 year old single male engineer from Chicago area still grieving the death of his mother, five months before he entered the study. He also had weight issues and shed thirteen pounds by the end of the program. His blood pressure went from 140/86 to 104/80 and he had stopped the medication he was taking for flexibility and sciatic pain.

Student # 8 B.N.	Physical		Emotional		Mental		Spiritual	
Total problems at intake	47	N/A	25	N/A	25	N/A	28	N/A
Problems resolved at graduation	39	83%	25	100%	8	32%	28	100
Problems improved at graduation	8	17%	0	0%	10	40%	0	0%
Total either improved or resolved at graduation	47	100%	25	100%	18	72%	28	100%
Problems unchanged at graduation	0	0%	0	0%	7	28%	0	0%
Problems worse at graduation	0	0%	0	0%	0	0%	0	0%

Table 9, *Participant Number 9*

Student nine, M.L., is a 48 year old woman from New Zealand with multiple issues including systemic candida, exhaustion, digestive problems, numbness in her hands, weak sex drive, and joint issues. She had severe detoxification issues during her stay and had already decided to stay three months in Michigan. She came with her husband (subject 11). At graduation she said "[the program] can put your life back on track. " She gave a tribute of gratitude to Don (founder of CHI).

Student # 9 M.L.	Physical		Emotional		Mental		Spiritual	
Total problems at intake	42	N/A	26	N/A	25	N/A	17	N/A
Problems resolved at graduation	13	31%	14	54%	8	32%	6	35%
Problems improved at graduation	19	45%	9	35%	10	40%	6	35%
Total either improved or resolved at graduation	32	76%	23	88%	18	72%	12	71%
Problems unchanged at graduation	7	17%	3	12%	7	28%	5	29%
Problems worse at graduation	3	7%	0	0%	0	0%	0	0%

Table 10, *Participant Number 10*

Student ten, P.B., is a 51 year old married massage therapist from Indiana who wanted to prevent illness in her own body and help her clients become healthier.

Student # 10 P.B.	Physical		Emotional		Mental		Spiritual	
Total problems at intake	24	N/A	1	N/A	15	N/A	1	N/A
Problems resolved at graduation	6	25%	1	100%	4	27%	0	0%
Problems improved at graduation	5	21%	0	0%	6	40%	0	0%
Total either improved or resolved at graduation	11	46%	1	100%	10	67%	1	100%
Problems unchanged at graduation	13	54%	0	0%	4	27%	0	0%
Problems worse at graduation	0	0%	0	0%	1	7%	0	0%

Table 11, *Participant Number 11*

Student eleven, R.S., husband of M.L. had prostate cancer for several years. He had done a resident intensive experiment with Gary Craig, originator of Emotional Freedom Technique and felt it was very beneficial. He is a friendly, ambitious and enthusiastic man who invited all to come and visit them in New Zealand.

Student # 11 R.S.	Physical		Emotional		Mental		Spiritual	
Total problems at intake	10	N/A	2	N/A	25	N/A	10	N/A
Problems resolved at graduation	3	30%	2	100%	7	28%	2	20%
Problems improved at graduation	0	0%	0	0%	0	0%	1	10%
Total either improved or resolved at graduation	3	30%	2	100%	7	28%	3	30%
Problems unchanged at graduation	7	70%	0	0%	18	72%	6	60%
Problems worse at graduation	0	0%	0	0%	0	0%	1	10%

Table 12, *Participant Number 12*

Student twelve, D.J., is a 67 year old male, retired psychologist from Canada. His problems were hypertension, obesity and some arthritis. His weight went from 228 pounds to 216, his blood pressure went from 164/96 to 124/90 and his pretibial edema went from 3+ to 0 at graduation. He lowered his blood pressure medication while there. He was a good sport about the spiritual questions, given that he described himself as a "secular humanist. "He said "I believe we need to be guided by moral principles but not a personalized God. "

Student # 12 D.J.	Physical		Emotional		Mental		Spiritual	
Total problems at intake	25	N/A	10	N/A	12	N/A	24	N/A
Problems resolved at graduation	14	56%	3	30%	1	8%	0	0%
Problems improved at graduation	8	32%	0	0%	1	8%	8	33%
Total either improved or resolved at graduation	22	88%	3	30%	2	16%	8	33%
Problems unchanged at graduation	3	12%	7	70%	10	83%	15	63%
Problems worse at graduation	0	0%	0	0%	0	0%	1	4%

Appendix C

Spiritual Effects of Live Food (S.E.L.F.)—Study Results by Group.

Tables 13-16 represent a summary of all 12 students' responses for each aspect. The numbers at the top represent the number each student was assigned and each column reflects one student's responses in each change-category. The number of problems in each change-category was compiled and the percent was calculated by dividing the total number in each change-category into the total number of problems in that aspect ever reported by the group (including "new at graduation"). This percentage is in the last column. Each row shows the number of problems in that change-category. The rows depict problems resolved, improved, worse, unchanged, and new at graduation.

Table 13- PHYSICAL ASPECT (61 physical questions)

(Percent of all 323 physical problems ever reported by all 12 students)

Subject Number	1	2	3	4	5	6	7	8	9	10	11	12	Tot	Percent of 323 problems reported
Problem at intake—resolved	20	6	10	22	0	5	9	39	13	6	3	14	147	45. 5%
Problem at intake—improved	9	7	0	2	3	6	17	8	19	5	0	8	84	26%
Problem at intake—unchanged	0	5	4	4	9	9	3	0	7	13	7	3	64	19. 8%
Problem at intake—worse	0	3	0	0	1	1	0	0	3	0	0	0	8	2. 4%
Problem new at graduation	0	3	0	0	0	5	3	0	0	1	8	0	20	6%
Problem never present	32	33	46	32	0	33	27	9	17	36	38	32	335	
No answer	0	4	1	1	48	2	2	5	2	0	5	4	74	

Table 14- EMOTIONAL ASPECT (31 questions)

(Percent of all 212 emotional problems ever reported by the 12 students)

Subject number	1	2	3	4	5	6	7	8	9	10	11	12	Tot	Percent of 212 problems reported
Problem at intake—resolved	26	21	19	12	2	14	2	25	14	1	2	3	141	66. 5%
Problem at intake—improved	1	0	0	0	0	1	2	0	9	0	0	0	13	6. 1%
Problem at intake—unchanged	1	2	0	0	4	5	14	0	3	0	0	7	36	16. 9%
Problem at intake—worse	0	0	0	0	0	0	2	0	0	0	0	0	2	. 94%
Problem new at graduation	0	0	0	0	7	1	6	0	0	2	0	4	20	9. 4%
Problem never present	3	8	12	19	18	10	5	6	4	28	27	17	157	
No answer	0	0	0	0	0	0	0	0	1	0	2	0	3	

Table 15- MENTAL ASPECT (27mental questions)

(Percent of all 242 physical problems ever reported by the 12 students)

Subject number	1	2	3	4	5	6	7	8	9	10	11	12	Tot	Percent of 242 problems reported
Problem at intake—resolved	15	13	22	18	0	7	0	27	8	4	7	1	122	50. 4%
Problem at intake—improved	5	2	0	2	0	3	2	0	10	6	0	1	31	12. 8%
Problem at intake—unchanged	3	2	0	1	0	14	19	0	7	4	18	10	78	32. 2%
Problem at intake—worse	0	0	0	0	0	0	2	0	0	1	0	0	3	1. 2%
Problem new at graduation	1	0	0	0	0	0	3	0	0	1	0	3	8	3. 3%
Problem never present	3	10	4	4	0	3	1	0	1	9	2	11	48	
No answer	0	0	1	2	27	0	0	0	1	2	0	1	34	

Table 16- SPIRITUAL ASPECT (31 physical questions)

(Percent of all 183 physical problems ever reported by the 12 students)

Subject number	1	2	3	4	5	6	7	8	9	10	11	12	Tot	Percent of 183 problems reported
Problem at intake—resolved	4	4	10	14	1	8	0	28	6	1	2	0	78	42. 6%
Problem at intake—improved	10	7	0	6	6	2	0	0	6	0	1	8	46	22. 9%
Problem at intake—unchanged	4	3	2	1	4	2	0	0	5	0	6	15	42	23. 4%
Problem at intake—worse	1	2	1	0	2	0	0	0	0	0	1	1	8	4. 3%
Problem new at graduation	0	1	0	1	2	0	0	0	2	3	0	0	9	4. 9%
Problem never present	12	14	18	9	11	18	0	3	12	25	21	0	143	
No answer	0	0	0	0	5	1	31	0	0	2	0	7	46	

Bibliography

Akers, Keith. *The Lost Religion of Jesus.* New York, NY: Lantern Books, 2000.

Albrecht, William A. *The Albrecht Papers.* Raytown, MO: Acres U.S.A., 1975.

Alder, Vera Stanley. *The Fifth Dimension.* York Beach, ME: Samuel Weiser, Inc., 1940.

Alder, Vera Stanley. *The Finding of the Third Eye.* York Beach, ME: Samuel Weiser, Inc., 1970.

Alexander, Joe. *Blatant Raw Foodist Propaganda!* Grass Valley, CA: Blue Dolphin Press, 1990.

Appleton, Nancy. *Rethinking Pasteur's Germ Theory.* Berkeley, CA: Frog, Ltd, 2002.

Arlin, Stephen, Dini, Fouad, and Wolfe, David. *Nature's First Law.* San Diego, CA: Maul Brothers, 2003.

Baba, Meher. *The Everything and the Nothing.* Berkeley, CA: The Beguine Library, 1963.

Bailey, Alice A. *Esoteric Healing.* New York, NY: Lucis Publishing Company, 1993.

Bailey, Alice A. *From Bethlehem to Calvary.* New York, NY: Lucis Publishing Company, 1965.

Bailey, Alice A. *A Treatise on White Magic.* New York, NY: Lucis Publishing Company, 1979.

Bailey, Alice A. *Esoteric Psychology I.* New York, NY: Lucis Publishing, 1962.

Bailey, Alice A. *Rays and the Initiations.* New York, NY: Lucis Publishing Company, 1988.

Baker, Elizabeth. *Does The Bible Teach Nutrition?* Mukilteo, WA: Winepress Publishing, 1997.

BidWell, Victoria. *The Health Seekers' Yearbook.* Mt. Vernon, WA: GetWell StayWell, America!, 1990.

Boutenko, Victoria. *12 Steps to Raw Food.* Ashland, OR: Raw Family Publishing, 2002.

Boutenko, Victoria. *Green for Life.* Ashland, OR: Raw Family Publishing, 2005.

Braden, Gregg. *Fractal Time.* Carlsbad, CA: Hay House, 2009.

Bragdon, Emma. *A Sourcebook for Helping People with Spiritual Problems.* Aptos, CA: Lightening Up Press, 1993.

Brownell, Kelly. *Food Fight.* New York, NY: McGraw-Hill, 2004.

Campbell, T. Colin. *The China Study.* Dallas, TX: BenBella Books, 2004.

Carey, Ken. *The Starseed Transmissions.* San Francisco: Harper, 1995.

Cichoke, Anthony J. *The Complete Book of Enzyme Therapy.* New York, NY: Avery, 1999.

Clement, Brian. *Living Foods for Optimal Health.* Rocklin, CA: Prima Health Publishing, 1998.

Cousens, Gabriel. *Conscious Eating.* Berkeley, CA: North Atlantic Books, 2000.

Cousens, Gabriel. *Rainbow Green Live—Food Cuisine.* Berkeley, CA: North Atlantic Books, 2003.

Cousens, Gabriel. "Simply Raw: Reversing Diabetes in 30 days," DVD, website: rawfor30days.com.

Cousens, Gabriel. *Spiritual Nutrition.* Berkeley, CA: North Atlantic Books, 2005.

Cousins, David. *A Handbook for Light Workers.* Dartmouth, UK: Barton House, 1993.

Crawford, Ina. *Guide to the Mysteries.* London: The Lucis Trust, 1990.

Davis, John. *Revelation for our Time.* Wyoming, MI: Spiritual Unity of Nations Publishing, 1998.

Day, Lorraine. "Sorting Through the MAZE of Alternative Medicine" videotape website: drday.org.

Dethlefsen, Thorwald & Dahlke, Rudiger. *The Healing Power of Illness.* Rockport, MA: Element Books, Inc, 1991.

Diamond, Harvey and Marilyn. *Fit For Life.* New York, NY: Warner Books, 1985.

Emoto, Masaru. *The Hidden Messages in Water.* Hillsboro, OR: Beyond Words Publishing, 2004.

Essene, Virginia and Nidle, Sheldon. *You are Becoming a Galactic Human.* Santa Clara, CA: S.E.E. Publishing, 1994.

Essene, Virginia. *New Cells, New Bodies, NEW LIFE!* Santa Clara, CA: S.E.E. Publishing Company, 1991.

Ferguson, Marilyn. *The Aquarian Conspiracy.* New York, NY: Jeremy P. Tarcher/ Putnam, 1980.

Gerber, Richard. *Vibrational Medicine.* Rochester, VT: Bear & Company, 2001.

Graham, Douglas N. *80/10/10.* Key Largo, FL: FoodnSport Press, 2006.

Grof, Stanislaf and Christina. *Spiritual Emergency.* New York, NY: Jeremy P. Tarcher/ Putnam, 1989.

Hay, Louise L. *Heal Your Body.* Carson, CA: Hay House, 1988.

Hay, Louise L. *You Can Heal Your Life.* Carlsbad, CA: Hay House, Inc., 1987.

Hicks, Jerry and Esther. *The Science of Deliberate Creation Journal.* San Antonio, TX: Abraham-Hicks Publications.

Holy Bible, King James Version. Cleveland, OH and New York, NY: The World Publishing Company, n.d.

Hotema, Hilton. *Man's Higher Consciousness.* Mokelumne Hill, CA: Health Research, 1962.

Howell, Edward. *Enzyme Nutrition.* Wayne, NJ: Avery Publishing, 1985.

Initiates, Three. *The Kybalion, Hermetic Philosophy.* Chicago, IL: Yogi Publication Society, 1940.

John, Da Free. *Raw Gorilla.* Clear Lake, CA: Dawn Horse Press, 1982.

Jubb, Annie Padden and David. *LifeFood Recipe Book.* Berkeley, CA: North Atlantic Books, 2003.

Jurriaanse, Aart. *Bridges.* Johannesburg, South Africa: Aquarian Book Centre 1986. No copyright: (This book is dedicated to Humanity without reservation. Man's versions of the Truth should not be offered with restrictions.)

Karagulla, Shafica. *Breakthrough to Creativity.* Marina del Rey, CA: DeVorss & Co, 1967.

Keyes, Ken Jr. *The Hundredth Monkey.* Coos Bay, OR: Vision Books, 1983.

Kulvinskas, Viktoras H. *Survival in the 21st Century.* Mt. Ida, AR: 21st Century Publishers, 2002.

Kunz-Bircher, Ruth. *The Bircher-Benner Health Guide.* Santa Barbara, CA: Woodbridge Press, 1980.

Lamsa, George M. *Holy Bible.* San Francisco: HarperSanFrancisco, 1968.

LeShan, Lawrence. *How to Meditate.* Boston: Little, Brown & Company, 1974.

Liberman, Jacob. *Light: Medicine of the Future.* Santa Fe, NM: Bear & Company, 1991.

Lipton, Bruce. *The Biology of Belief.* Carlsbad, CA: Hay House, 2009.

Long, Max Freedom. *What Jesus Taught in Secret.* Marina del Rey, CA: DeVorss & Company, 1983.

Myss, Caroline. *Anatomy of the Spirit.* New York, NY: Three Rivers Press, 1996.

Nestle, Marion. *Food Politics.* Berkeley, CA: University of California Press, 2002.

Nightingale, Florence. *Notes on Nursing.* New York, NY: Dover Publications, 1969.

Page, Christine R. *Frontiers of Health.* Essex England: C.W. Daniel Company Limited, 1992.

Parrish-Harra, Carol E. *Messengers of Hope, The Walk-In Phenomenon.* Tahlequah, OK: Sparrow Hawk, 2001.

Parrish-Harra, Carol E. *The New Dictionary of Spiritual Thought.* Tahlequah, OK: Sparrow Hawk, 2002.

Pert, Candace B. "Your Body is Your Subconscious Mind, New Insights into the Body-Mind Connection," Audiotape website: soundstrue.com, circa 1995.

Pottenger, Francis M. Jr. *Pottenger's Cats.* Lemon Grove, CA: Price-Pottenger Nutrition Foundation, 1983.

Price, Weston A. *Nutrition and Physical Degeneration.* LaMesa, CA: Price-Pottenger Nutrition Foundation, 2003.

Robbins, John. *Diet for a New America.* Tiburon, CA: H. J. Kramer, 1987.

Robbins, John. *May All Be Fed.* New York, NY: William Morrow, 1992.

Robbins, John. *The Food Revolution.* Berkeley, CA: Conari Press, 2001.

Roerich, Helena. *Letters of Helena Roerich 1929–1938, Volume I.* New York, NY: Agni Yoga Society, 1954.

Roerich, Helena. *Letters of Helena Roerich 1935–1939, Volume II.* New York, NY: Agni Yoga Society, 1967.

Rosen, Steven. *Food for the Spirit.* New York, NY: Bala Books, 1987.

Sanford, John. *Healing and Wholeness.* New York, NY: Paulist Press, 1977.

Saraydarian, Torkom. *Breakthrough to Higher Psychism.* Cave Creek, AZ: T.S.G. Publishing, 1990.

Satprem. *The Mind of the Cells.* New York, NY: Institute for Evolutionary Research, 1982.

Sheldrake, Rupert. *The Rebirth of Nature, Science and God.* Rochester, VT: Park Street Press, 1994.

Shelton, Herbert. *Superior Nutrition.* San Antonio, TX: Willow Publishing, 1994.

Smith, Huston. *The World's Religions.* New York, NY: HarperCollins, 1991.

Szekely, Edmond Bordeaux. *The Essene Gospel of Peace.* Nelson, B.C., Canada: International Biogenic Society, 1981.

Szekely, Edmond Bordeaux. *The Essene Way—Biogenic Living.* Nelson, B.C., Canada: International Biogenic Society, 1989.

Taylor, Jill Bolte. *My Stroke of Insight.* New York, NY: Viking, 2006.

Teilhard de Chardin, Pierre. *The Phenomenon of Man.* New York, NY: Perennial Library, Harper and Row, 1959).

Thomas, Lewis. *The Lives of a Cell.* New York, NY: Penguin Books, 1974.

Tilden, John. *Toxemia Explained.* No publisher listed.

Trigueirinho Netto, José. *Calling Humanity.* Tahlequah, OK: Sparrow Hawk Press, 2002.

Tuttle, Will. *The World Peace Diet.* New York, NY: Lantern Books, 2005.

Walker, N. W. *Become Younger.* Prescott, AZ: Norwalk Press, 1978.

White, Ellen. *Finding Peace Within.* Jemison, AL: Inspiration Books East, 2001.

White, John. *The Meeting of Science and Spirit, Guidelines for a New Age.* New York, NY: Paragon House, 1990.

Wigmore, Ann. *Be Your Own Doctor.* Wayne, NJ: Avery Publishing Group, 1982.

Wigmore, Ann. *Naturama Living Textbook.* Boston, MA: Hippocrates Health Institute, around 1978.

Wigmore, Ann. *Scientific Appraisal of Dr. Ann Wigmore's Living Foods Lifestyle.* Boston, MA: Ann Wigmore Press, 1993.

Wigmore, Ann. *Why Suffer?* Wayne, NJ: Avery Publishing, 1985.

Williams, Howard. *The Ethics of Diet.* Urbana and Chicago: University of Illinois Press, 2003.

Wolfe, David. *The Sunfood Diet Success System.* San Diego, CA: Maul Brothers Publishing, 2002.

Young, Robert O. with Shelley Redford Young. *Sick and Tired?* Pleasant Grove, UT: Woodland Publishing, 2001.

Zukav, Gary. *The Dancing WuLi Masters.* New York, NY: William Morrow, 1979.

Index

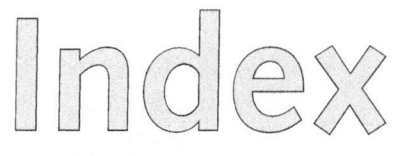

B

D

E

F

G

H

I

J

K

L

M

N

O

P

T

X

Y

Z

Contact Janet through her website drjanetallen.com

CPSIA information can be obtained at www.ICGtesting.com
Printed in the USA
BVOW09s1030020315

389264BV00002B/5/P